Mosby's

Review
Questions
for the NBCE®
EXAMINATION

PARTS I and II

Mosby's

Review
Questions
for the NBCE®
Examination

PARTS I and II

Edited by

Claire Johnson, DC, MSEd, DACBSP
Clinical Professor
Southern California University of
  Health Sciences
Whittier, California
Editor
University Publications
National University of Health Sciences
Lombard, Illinois

Bart N. Green, DC, MSEd, DACBSP
Adjunct Professor
Post Graduate and Continuing Education
Southern California University of
  Health Sciences
Whittier, California
Associate Editor
University Publications
National University of Health Sciences
Lombard, Illinois

Jill M.Davis, MA
Chair
Basic Science Department
Cleveland Chiropractic College
Kansas City, Missouri

Carl S. Cleveland III, DC
President
Cleveland Chiropractic College
Kansas City, Missouri, and
  Los Angeles, California

MOSBY

ELSEVIER

11830 Westline Industrial Drive
St. Louis, Missouri 63146

MOSBY'S REVIEW QUESTIONS FOR THE NBCE®
EXAMINATION, PARTS I AND II
Copyright © 2006 by Mosby Inc., an affiliate of Elsevier Inc.

ISBN-13: 978-0-323-03172-1
ISBN-10: 0-323-03172-2

Notice

Knowledge and best practice in this field are constantly changing. As new research and experience broaden our knowledge, changes in practice, treatment and drug therapy may become necessary or appropriate. Readers are advised to check the most current information provided (i) on procedures featured or (ii) by the manufacturer of each product to be administered, to verify the recommended dose or formula, the method and duration of administration, and contraindications. It is the responsibility of the practitioner, relying on their own experience and knowledge of the patient, to make diagnoses, to determine dosages and the best treatment for each individual patient, and to take all appropriate safety precautions. To the fullest extent of the law, neither the Publisher nor the Editors assumes any liability for any injury and/or damage to persons or property arising out or related to any use of the material contained in this book.

The Publisher

Mosby's Review Questions for the NBCE® Examination: Parts I and II is a resource for chiropractic students preparing to take the NBCE® examination, state or local boards, as well as for the chiropractor seeking state licensure. The publisher makes no claims regarding the effectiveness or relevance of the content or presentation of this material and makes no guarantee regarding any individual's performance on any of these examinations.

ISBN-13: 978-0-323-03172-1
ISBN-10: 0-323-03172-2

Publishing Director: Linda Duncan
Acquisitions Editor: Kathy Falk
Senior Developmental Editor: Christie M. Hart
Publishing Services Manager: Julie Eddy
Senior Project Manager: Joy Moore
Senior Designer: Kathi Gosche

Printed in United States of America

Last digit is the print number: 9   8   7   6   5   4   3

Contributors

Sameh A. Awad, MD
Assistant Professor
Department of Basic Sciences
Southern California University of
  Health Sciences
Whittier, California

Samir Ayad, MD
Assistant Professor
Department of Basic Sciences
Southern California University of
  Health Sciences
Whittier, California

John M. Bassano, DC, DACBR
Associate Professor
Department of Diagnosis
Los Angeles College of Chiropractic
Southern California University of
  Health Sciences
Los Angeles, California

**Robyn Beirman, MB, BS (Hons),
  MHPEd**
Lecturer and Director of
  Undergraduate Studies
Department of Health and
  Chiropractic
Macquarie University
Sydney, Australia

Antonio E. Bifero, DC, MBA
Instructor of Clinical Microbiology
  and Infectious Diseases
Department of Pathology,
  Microbiology, and Public Health
National University of Health
  Sciences
Lombard, Illinois

**Susan Boger-Wakeman, PhD,
  MS, BS, RD**
Dean
Department of Basic Science
Sherman College of Straight
  Chiropractic
Spartanburg, South Carolina

Pierre Boucher, DC, PhD
Department of Chiropractic
Université du Québec à
  Trois-Rivières
Trois-Rivières, Canada

Geracimo Bracho, PhD
Associate Professor
Department of Basic Sciences
Cleveland Chiropractic College
Kansas City, Missouri

Kay Hachtel Brashear, BS, MA
Chair, Associate Professor
Department of Physiologic and
  Pathologic Sciences
Parker College of Chiropractic
Dallas, Texas

André Bussières, BSc, DC,
   FCCS (C)
Department of Chiropractic
Université du Québec à
   Trois-Rivières
Trois-Rivières, Canada

Alan L. Campbell, PhD
Professor
Department of Physiologic and
   Pathologic Sciences
Parker College of Chiropractic
Dallas, Texas

Marni Capes, MS, DC
Assistant Professor
Department of Clinical Sciences
Life University
Marietta, Georgia

Carol Claus, BS, MA, DC, FICPA
Chair, Professor
Department of Chiropractic
   Sciences
Cleveland Chiropractic College
Los Angeles, California

Carl S. Cleveland III, DC
President
Cleveland Chiropractic College
Kansas City, Missouri, and
   Los Angeles, California

Jesse Thomas Coats, RPh, DC
Department Head, Associate
   Clinical Professor
Department of Clinical Sciences
Texas Chiropractic College
Pasadena, Texas
Chief of Staff
Friendswood Doctors of
   Chiropractic, Inc.
Friendswood, Texas

Gregory D. Cramer, DC, PhD
Professor and Dean of Research
National University of Health
   Sciences
Lombard, Illinois

Susan Darby, PhD
Professor of Anatomy
Department of Basic Sciences
National University of Health
   Sciences
Lombard, Illinois

Jill M. Davis, MA
Chair
Basic Science Department
Cleveland Chiropractic College
Kansas City, Missouri

Martin Descarreaux, DC, PhD
Department of Chiropractic
Université du Québec à
   Trois-Rivières
Trois-Rivières, Canada

Roger Engel, BSc (Hons), DC, DO
Director of Clinics
Department of Health &
   Chiropractic
Macquarie University
Sydney, Australia

Jason Flanagan, DC
Associate Professor of Clinical
   Sciences
Dean of Academic Affairs
Texas Chiropractic College
Pasadena, Texas

Martha J. Friesen, BS, MS, PhD
Professor
Microbiology
Texas Chiropractic College
Pasadena, Texas

Gene F. Giggleman, BS, DVM
Dean of Academic Affairs
Professor
Department of Anatomical Sciences
Parker College of Chiropractic
Dallas, Texas

Brian J. Gleberzon, BA, DC
Associate Professor
Department of Applied Chiropractic
   and Clinical Diagnosis
Canadian Memorial Chiropractic
   College
Toronto, Canada

Emile Goubran, MD, PhD
Professor of Anatomy
Department of Basic Sciences
Southern California University of
   Health Sciences
Whittier, California

Donald F. Gran, DC, MSEd
Dean of Academic Affairs
Palmer College of Chiropractic,
   Florida
Port Orange, Florida

Bart N. Green, DC, MSEd,
  DACBSP
Adjunct Professor
Post Graduate and Continuing
   Education
Southern California University of
   Health Sciences
Whittier, California
Associate Editor
University Publications
National University of Health
   Sciences
Lombard, Illinois

Julie-Marthe Grenier, DC,
  DACBR, FCCR(c)
Assistant Professor
Palmer College of Chiropractic,
   Florida
Port Orange, Florida

Rocco C. Guerriero, BSc, DC,
  FCCSS(C), FCCRS(C), FCCO(C)
Associate Professor
Department of Clinical Diagnosis
Canadian Memorial Chiropractic
   College
Toronto, Canada

Jerry Hochman, BA, DC
Professor
Department of Chiropractic
   Sciences
Life University
Marietta, Georgia
Diplomate
International Craniopathic Society
Sacro Occipital Research Society,
   International
Leawood, Kansas

Fiona Jarrett-Thelwell, DC
Assistant Professor
New York Chiropractic College
Seneca Falls, New York

Norman W. Kettner, DC, DACBR
Chair
Department of Radiology
Logan College of Chiropractic
Chesterfield, Missouri

Lisa Zaynab Killinger, DC
Associate Professor
Department of Research and
 Diagnosis
Palmer College of Chiropractic
Davenport, Iowa
Immediate Past Chair
American Public Health Association
 Chiropractic Health Care Section

Curt A. Krause, BS, DC
Clinician and Instructor
Clinical Sciences and Diagnostic
 Sciences
Cleveland Chiropractic College
Kansas City, Missouri

Christian G. Linard, PhD, DEPD,
 CSPQ
Professor of Biochemistry and
 Clinical Chemistry
Department of Chiropractic
Université du Québec à
 Trois-Rivières
Trois-Rivières, Canada
Clinical Chemist
Ordre des Chimistes du Québec
Québec, Canada

Johanne Martel, BSc, DC,
 FCCS(C)
Clinic Director
Department of Chiropractic
 Université du Québec à
 Trois-Rivières
Trois-Rivières, Canada

Stephan Nicholas Mayer, DC
Associate Professor
Diagnostic Sciences
Cleveland Chiropractic College
Los Angeles, California

William McGimsey, PhD
Chairman, Associate Professor of
 Anatomy
Department of Anatomy
Texas Chiropractic College
Pasadena, Texas

Michael D. Moore, AA, DC
Associate Professor
Department of Diagnosis and
 Clinical Sciences
Cleveland Chiropractic College
Kansas City, Missouri

Anita M. Mork, MS
Chair, Associate Professor
Department of Basic Sciences
Cleveland Chiropractic College
Los Angeles, California

Amanda Louisa Neill, BSc, MSc,
 MBBS, PhD, FACBS
Director of Anatomy
Department of Health and
 Chiropractic
Macquarie University
Sydney, Australia
Secretary of the College of
 Biomedical Scientists
New South Wales Institute of
 Forensic Medicine
Sydney, Australia

J. Michael Perryman, MD
Professor
Department of Physiological and
 Pathologic Sciences
Parker College of Chiropractic
Dallas, Texas

Seva Philomin, MD
Associate Professor
Department of Basic Sciences
New York Chiropractic College
Seneca Falls, New York

Jaya Prakash, MD, SM (NRM)
Chairperson
Department of Basic Sciences
National University of Health
Sciences
Lombard, Illinois

Djamel Ramla, DMV, DEA, PhD
Professor of Histology and
Pathology
Department of Chiropractic
Université du Québec à
Trois-Rivières
Trois-Rivières, Canada

**Vinnavadi C. Ravikumar,
MPharm, PhD**
Associate Professor
Palmer College of Chiropractic,
Florida
Port Orange, Florida

Richard Raymond, PhD
Texas Chiropractic College
Pasadena, Texas

**Thomas M. Redenbaugh,
DC, FICPA**
Chair
Department of Chiropractic
Philosophy and Techniques
Parker College of Chiropractic
Dallas, Texas

John H. Romfh, PhD
Associate Professor of Anatomy
Division of Basic Sciences
Life University
Marietta, Georgia

Brent da Silva Russell, DC
Assistant Professor
Division of Clinical Sciences
College of Chiropractic
Life University
Marietta, Georgia

David Seaman, DC, MS
Palmer College of Chiropractic,
Florida
Port Orange, Florida

David M. Sikorski, DC
Professor, Chair
Department of Principles and
Practice
Southern California University of
Health Sciences
Whittier, California

Virgil Stoia, BS, DC
Assistant Professor
Department of Clinical Diagnosis
National University of Health
Sciences
Lombard, Illinois

Rodger Tepe, PhD
Administrator of Research
Logan College of Chiropractic
Chesterfield, Missouri

Richard Valente, BSc, DC
Supervising Clinician
Department of Chiropractic
Université du Québec à
Trois-Rivières
Trois-Rivières, Canada

Michael R. Valentine, PhD
Assistant Professor
Department of Basic Sciences
Cleveland Chiropractic College
Los Angeles, California

Subramanyam Vemulpad, MSc, PhD
Senior Lecturer
Department of Health and Chiropractic
Macquarie University
Sydney, Australia

Vrajlal H. Vyas, MD, ASCP
Professor
Department of Pathology, Microbiology, and Public Health
National University of Health Sciences
Lombard, Illinois

Robert W. Ward, DC
Associate Professor
Department of Diagnosis
Los Angeles College of Chiropractic
Southern California University of Health Sciences
Whittier, California

Keith Wells, DC, MA
Professor
Department of Clinical Diagnosis
Southern California University of Health Sciences
Whittier, California

Lawrence H. Wyatt, DC, DACBR, FICC
Professor
Division of Clinical Sciences
Texas Chiropractic College
Pasadena, Texas

Kenneth J. Young, DC, DACBR, FCC (UK)
Senior Lecturer in Radiology
Welsh Institute of Chiropractic
University of Glamorgan
Pontypridd, United Kingdom

Isis Edward Zaki, MD, MS, PhD
Professor
Department of Histology /Anatomy
Faculty of Medicine
Cairo University
Giza, Egypt
Professor
Department of Basic Science
Cleveland Chiropractic College
Los Angeles, California

Steve Zylich, BSc, DC
Assistant Professor
Department of Clinical Diagnosis
Canadian Memorial Chiropractic College
Toronto, Canada

Preface

HOW TO USE THIS TEXT

Examinations are a means of strengthening our intellect, gymnasiums for our minds. This text is a tool to help prepare students for taking the board examinations and to point out strengths and weaknesses so they can better use their study time. For only by pointing out our weaknesses can we become stronger. This text is not meant to replace years of professional training nor give away questions so that students may pass examinations if they memorize the answers. Instead, this book and CD-ROM will help direct students to the topic areas that they may need to review and strengthen knowledge and examination-taking skills.

The chiropractic colleges do well in preparing their students for practice as well as boards. In addition, for many colleges there is a good correlation between students who do well in their chiropractic courses and those who score well on their board examinations. Therefore, to best prepare for board examinations, students should focus on doing well in their courses at their chiropractic college. It is also in the best interest of students to focus more study time for their board examinations on the areas that they have not scored as well on in their chiropractic programs. This is good news for students because most are aware of their areas of weakness and, therefore, have the opportunity to focus more resources on these areas when studying for boards.

BOARD EXAMINATIONS ARE LIKE MARATHONS

Taking most board examinations is similar to running a marathon; board examinations take both mental and physical stamina, and they should be prepared for like one is preparing to partake in a long endurance event. If one has never run a mile, he or she cannot expect to prepare adequately in only 1 week for a 26-mile race. Therefore, preparation in advance is most appropriate, and perhaps this is why there is a correlation between performance in the academic programs and the board scores.

HELPFUL HINTS FOR PREPARING TO TAKE YOUR BOARD EXAMINATIONS

1. Know your weaknesses and focus more of your resources on strengthening these areas. Look back at your grades from the courses that relate to the

examination topics. These will help point to areas that need more attention. Also, use this book as a trial run to help point to content areas that may need more review.

2. Practice makes perfect. Just re-reading old course notes may not be enough. The skill of taking an examination is more about pulling information from your brain, not stuffing more information into it. Therefore, when practicing to take board examinations, consider practicing retrieving information from your brain by taking practice examinations. You can do this in several ways: study with others by asking each other questions, test yourself with flashcards or notes that are partially covered from view, or answer questions from this text. In each case, be sure to check your answer to find out if you achieved the correct answer.

3. Practice answering examination questions in the same environment that the test will be given. In other words, most board examinations are not given in your living room with the TV or stereo blaring; therefore, do not practice in this environment. Consider practicing in an environment like the examination location using the examination questions from this text.

4. If possible, eat and sleep well during the weeks before the examination. It is difficult to compete successfully in a marathon if one is malnourished or sleep deprived. Set regular bed times and eating schedules so that your routine stays as familiar and comfortable as possible.

5. If you have a regular exercise routine, stick to it. It will help you deal with the additional stress and provide consistency in your life.

6. Block off time for practice examinations such as the examinations in this text. Try to use the same amount of time and number of questions that will be given during the actual examination. This will help prepare you for the amount of pressure in the examination environment.

7. Stay away from naysayers and people who create hype around the board examinations. Some of these people may have their own interests in mind (e.g., Are they representing a board review company? Are they the type of people who make themselves feel better by making others feel worse?). Instead, find people who are positive and demonstrate good study behaviors. Consider making a study group of people who are able to help the other members in the group stay positive.

8. If your college offers board reviews, consider taking them. These may assist you in building your confidence with the material you have already mastered and may help you focus on materials that you need to spend more time studying.

HELPFUL HINTS DURING PRACTICE EXAMINATIONS AND FOR TAKING THE ACTUAL EXAMINATION

1. It is important to note that questions that are considered "good" questions by examination standards will have incorrect choices in their answer bank that are very close to the correct answer. These wrong choices are called "distracters" for a reason; they are meant to distract the test taker.

Because of this, some test takers do better by reading the question and trying to guess the answer before looking at the answer bank. Therefore, consider trying to answer questions without looking at the answer bank.

2. Cross out answers that are obviously wrong. This will allow a better chance of picking the correct answer and reduce distraction from the wrong answers.

3. Only go back and change an answer if you are absolutely certain you were wrong with your previous choice or if a different question in the same examination provides you with the correct answer.

4. Read questions carefully. Circle, or underline, negative words in questions, such as "except," "not," and "false." If these words are missed when reading the question, it is nearly impossible to get the correct answer; marking these key words will make sure you do not miss them.

5. If you are stuck on one question, consider treating the answer bank like a series of true/false items relevant to the question. Most people consider true/false questions easier than multiple choice. At least if you can eliminate a few choices, you will have a better chance at selecting the correct answer from whatever is left.

6. Never leave blanks on the Scantron, unless the specific examination has a penalty for wrong answers. It is better to guess wrong than leave an item blank. Check with those giving the examination to find out if there are penalties for marking the wrong answer.

7. Some people do better on examinations by going through the examination and answering known questions first, then returning to the more difficult questions later. This helps to build up confidence during the examination. This also helps the test taker avoid spending too much time on a few questions and running out of time on the easy questions that may be at the end.

8. Pace yourself on the examination. Figure out ahead of time how much time each question will take to answer. Do not rush, but do not spend too much time on only one question. Sometimes it is better to move to the next question and come back to the difficult ones later because a fresh look is sometimes helpful.

9. Bring appropriate supplies to the examination, such as pencils and erasers. If you get distracted by noise, consider bringing ear plugs. It is inevitable that someone will take his or her examination next to the guy in the squeaky chair, or the one with the sniffling runny nose. Most examinations will provide you with instructions as to what you may or may not bring to the examination. Be sure to read these instructions in advance.

10. Some people find that they do better on examinations by marking all of their answers on the test packet and then, at the end, fill in their Scantron or answer sheet. If you do this, be careful to fill in the answer that corresponds with the question.

11. Make sure that once you have completed the examination all questions are appropriately filled in. Find out how many questions there are for each section before taking the examination, so that you make sure you answer the correct number of questions.

PREPARING FOR WHEN THE EXAMINATION IS OVER

It may be good to think about what you will be doing after the examination.

1. Most people are exhausted after taking board examinations. Some reasons for this exhaustion may be the amount of hours, mental focus, and the anxiety that examinations cause some people. Be aware that you may be tired, so avoid planning anything that one should not do when exhausted, such as driving across country, operating heavy machinery/power tools, or studying for final examinations. Instead, plan a day or two to recuperate before you tackle any heavier physical or mental tasks.
2. Consider a debriefing or "detoxification" meeting with your positive study partners after the examination. Talking about the examination afterwards may help reduce stress. However, remember that the feelings one has after an examination may not always match the examination score (e.g., someone who feels they did poorly may have done well or someone who feels they did well may not have.)
3. Consider planning on doing something nice for yourself. After all, you will have just completed a major examination. It is important to celebrate this milestone in your life.

We wish you the very best with taking your examinations and hope that this text provides you with an excellent training tool for your preparations.

Contents

Part I

Section Three: Physiology   109

Kay Hachtel Brashear, Vinnavadi C. Ravikumar, Richard Raymond, Robert W. Ward

Section Four: Chemistry   167

Susan Boger-Wakeman, Geracimo Bracho, Alan L. Campbell, Christian G. Linard, Richard Valente, Michael R. Valentine

Section Five: Pathology 219

Jill M. Davis, J. Michael Perryman, Seva Philomin, Djamel Ramla,
Virgil Stoia, Vrajlal H. Vyas

Section Six: Microbiology and Public Health 275

Sameh A. Awad, Samir Ayad, Jill M. Davis, Martha J. Friesen, Jaya Prakesh,
Subramanyam Vemulpad

Part II

Section Seven: General Diagnosis 323

Fiona Jarrett-Thelwell, Curt A. Krause, Stephan Nicholas Mayer,
Brent da Silva Russell, Keith Wells, Steve Zylich

Section Ten: Principles of Chiropractic   495

Carol Claus, Carl S. Cleveland III, Jason Flanagan, Thomas M. Redenbaugh, David Seaman

Section Eleven: Chiropractic Practice   549

Roger Engel, Brian J. Gleberzon, Donald F. Gran, Jerry Hochman, David M. Sikorski

Section Twelve: Associated Clinical Sciences   593

PART I

General Anatomy

Emile Goubran, William McGimsey, Anita M. Mork, John H. Romfh

Topographic Anatomy

1. Which nerve is not located in the carotid triangle?
   a. vagus nerve
   b. accessory nerve
   c. hypoglossal nerve
   d. cervical sympathetic chain

2. The sternal angle lies at the level of what intervertebral disc?
   a. T2/T3
   b. T3/T4
   c. T4/T5
   d. T5/T6

3. The skin dimples over the posterior superior iliac spines are at which spinal level?
   a. L4
   b. L5
   c. S1
   d. S2

4. Which of the following anatomical planes divide the body into anterior and posterior portions?
   a. median plane
   b. sagittal plane
   c. coronal plane
   d. horizontal plane

5. Which of the following layers of the epidermis is responsible for the constant renewal of epidermal cells?
   a. stratum germinativum
   b. stratum granulosum
   c. stratum lucidum
   d. stratum corneum

6. The transverse thoracic plane separates which two regions of the mediastinum?
    a. anterior from the middle
    b. middle from the posterior
    c. anterior from the posterior
    d. superior from the inferior

7. Which plane would indicate the origin of the inferior vena cava?
    a. transumbilical plane
    b. subcostal plane
    c. transtubercular plane
    d. transpyloric plane

8. Which plane would indicate the termination of the abdominal aorta?
    a. supracristal or intercristal plane
    b. transtubercular plane
    c. transumbilical plane
    d. subcostal plane

9. Your patient had a laceration anterior to the medial malleolus, which required stitches. He is now in your office complaining of pain along the medial border of the foot. Which nerve is most likely involved?
    a. sural nerve
    b. deep fibular
    c. tibial nerve
    d. saphenous nerve

10. When the upper limb is in anatomical position, the medial end of the scapular spine is at which vertebral level?
    a. spinous process of second thoracic vertebra
    b. spinous process of third thoracic vertebra
    c. body of the third thoracic vertebra
    d. spinous process of fourth thoracic vertebra

11. While examining a patient, you notice that the right scapula is farther from the midline than the left. You would suspect paralysis of which muscles?
    a. rhomboid major and minor
    b. latissimus dorsi
    c. supraspinatus
    d. deltoid

12. Which of the following movements occurs within the frontal plane?
    a. flexion of the leg
    b. abduction of the thigh
    c. pronation of the forearm
    d. medial rotation of the arm

13. Which anatomical plane divides the body into superior and inferior
parts?
   a. sagittal plane
   b. frontal plane
   c. transverse plane
   d. coronal plane

Answers

1. b. The accessory nerve is located in the occipital triangle, which is posterior to the sternocleidomastoid muscle. The carotid triangle is anterior to the sternocleidomastoid muscle.

2. c. The jugular notch lies at the inferior border of the body of T2. The manubrium is at the level of the T3 and T4 bodies. The sternal angle is the manubriosternal joint, which is at the level of the T4/T5 intervertebral disc.

3. d. The superior part of the iliac crests is at the L4/L5 intervertebral disc. The dimples are at the S2 level.

4. c. The coronal plane is a vertical plane passing through the body at right angle to the median plane, dividing it into anterior and posterior portions.

5. a. The stratum germinativum (basale) contains stem cells characterized by intense mitotic activity indicative of cellular division since the main function of this layer is the continual renewal of epidermal cells.

6. d. The transverse thoracic plane is a horizontal plane that cuts through the sternal angle anteriorly and the intervertebral disc between T4 and T5 posteriorly. It separates the superior mediastinum above from the inferior mediastinum below.

7. c. The inferior vena cava begins with the uniting of the common iliac veins. This occurs on the body of the fifth lumbar vertebra. The relevant surface anatomy plane is the transtubercular plane, which interconnects the iliac tubercles. This plane passes through the fifth lumbar vertebra.

8. a. The abdominal aorta terminates on the fourth lumbar vertebral body. A plane interconnecting the highest points of the iliac crest passes through the body of the fourth lumbar vertebra.

9. d. The saphenous nerve lies just anterior to the medial malleolus along side of the great saphenous vein. This nerve is most likely to be injured by the sutures.

10. b. The spinous process of the third thoracic vertebra is usually found at the level of where the spinous process meets the medial border of the scapula.

11. a. The rhomboid major and minor originate on the nuchal ligament and spinous processes of C7 through T5 and insert on the medial border of the scapula. Their main function is to retract and fix the scapula to the thoracic wall.

12. b. The frontal plane cuts the body into anterior and posterior parts. Abduction of the thigh is movement of the thigh away from the midline of the body. This movement is parallel to or within the frontal plane.

13. c. The transverse plane divides the body into superior and inferior segments. The frontal or coronal plane divides the body into anterior and posterior segments while the sagittal plane divides the body into right and left segments.

Osteology of the Appendicular Skeleton

1. The coracoid process is a feature of which bone?
   a. scapula
   b. ulna
   c. clavicle
   d. humerus

2. The linea aspera is found on the posterior surface of which bone?
   a. humerus
   b. tibia
   c. ilium
   d. femur

3. The epiphyseal disc of a developing long bone is formed from what kind of tissue?
   a. fibrocartilage
   b. hyaline cartilage
   c. elastic cartilage
   d. spongy bone

4. The medial malleolus is a component of which bone?
   a. fibula
   b. femur
   c. tibia
   d. calcaneus

5. Which is FALSE concerning the anatomical position of the hip bone?
   a. the tip of the coccyx is typically on a level with the superior half of the body of the pubis
   b. the pelvis major is situated between the two iliac fossae
   c. the anterior superior iliac spine and the anterosuperior aspect of the pubis lie in the horizontal plane
   d. ischial spine and superior end of the pubic symphysis are approximately in the same horizontal plane

6. Which group attaches to the first cuneiform bone in the foot?
    a. fibularis (peroneus) longus and adductor hallucis muscles
    b. tibialis anterior and posterior and fibularis (peroneus) longus muscles
    c. tibialis anterior and quadratus plantae muscles
    d. quadratus plantae and abductor hallucis

7. At what approximate age does the secondary center of ossification of the medial end of the clavicle completely fuse together?
    a. between 18th and 20th years
    b. between 14th and 16th years
    c. between 16th and 20th years
    d. between 25th and 31st years

8. Which muscle does NOT attach to the medial border of the scapula?
    a. subscapularis
    b. serratus anterior
    c. rhomboid major
    d. levator scapulae

9. Which carpal bone is most commonly fractured?
    a. lunate
    b. hamate
    c. scaphoid
    d. capitate

10. Which of the following bone cells are located within bone matrix?
    a. osteocytes
    b. osteoblasts
    c. osteoclasts
    d. osteoprogenitor cells

11. Which of the following is the lateral continuation of the spine of the scapula?
    a. coracoid process
    b. acromion
    c. glenoid cavity
    d. head of scapula

12. What is the broad rough line on the posterior aspect of the shaft of the femur called?
    a. medial supracondylar line
    b. lateral supracondylar line
    c. spiral line
    d. linea aspera

13. After limb bones develop through intracartilaginous (endochondral) ossification, further increase in length is carried out through the activity of what structure?
    a. periosteum
    b. endosteum
    c. articular cartilage
    d. epiphyseal cartilage

14. Which of the following bone cells causes bone resorption (breakdown)?
    a. osteoblasts
    b. osteoclasts
    c. osteocytes
    d. osteoprogenitor cells

15. What is the name of the medial fossa of the distal anterior surface of the humerus?
    a. olecranon fossa
    b. coronoid fossa
    c. radial fossa
    d. radial notch

16. Which carpal bone is known for its wedge shape?
    a. scaphoid
    b. trapezoid
    c. triquetrum
    d. trapezium

17. Which ridge of bone is most closely associated with the lesser trochanter?
    a. pectineal line
    b. medial supracondylar line
    c. linea aspera
    d. gluteal tuberosity

18. The cuboid bone is located just posterior to what structure?
    a. base of the first metatarsal
    b. head of the first metatarsal
    c. medial cuneiform bone
    d. tuberosity of the fifth metatarsal

19. At puberty, the Y-shaped triradiate cartilage is still present in which bone?
    a. scapula
    b. innominate bone
    c. femur
    d. sacrum

1. a. The coracoid process projects anteriorly from the scapula. It serves as an attachment for muscles and ligaments of the upper limb. It should not be confused with the conoid tubercle of the clavicle or the coronoid process of the ulna.

2. d. The linea aspera is a rough line running down the posterior surface of the femur. It serves as an important attachment for several muscles that originate on the innominate bone and move the thigh.

3. b. The epiphyseal disc is composed of hyaline cartilage. It represents the remainder of the original hyaline cartilage model developed in the fetal period of growth. Elastic cartilage and fibrocartilage are not involved in the process of bone formation.

4. c. The medial malleolus is the tibia's contribution to the medial side of the ankle joint. It forms the bony knob on the medial side of the joint. The lateral malleolus is a component of the fibula.

5. c. The anterior superior iliac spine and the anterosuperior aspect of the pubic tubercle lie in the same vertical plane.

6. b. All of these muscles have an attachment to the first cuneiform bone. The fibularis (peroneus) muscles plantarflex and evert the foot, whereas the tibialis anterior and posterior invert the foot.

7. d. The secondary center of ossification on the medial end of the clavicle completely ossifies between the 25th and 31st years.

8. a. The subscapularis muscle attaches to and fills the subscapular fossa. It also has a small attachment to the inferior lateral border of the scapula. The serratus anterior attaches to the ventral surface of the medial border, while the rhomboids major and minor attach to more dorsal aspects of the medial border.

9. c. The scaphoid is the most commonly fractured carpal bone. It usually results from falling and landing on the palm of the hand.

10. a. Osteocytes are found within bone matrix inside spaces between bone lamellae called lacunae. All other types of bone cells are found in relation to bone surfaces in the cellular layer of the periosteum and in the endosteum.

11. b. The acromion is a flat expansion of the lateral end of the spine of the scapula, which articulates with the lateral (acromial) end of the clavicle.

12. d. The linea aspera is a broad vertical ridge prominent on the posterior aspect of the middle third of the shaft of the femur. It is continuous inferiorly with the medial and lateral supracondylar lines and superiorly with the spiral line and gluteal tuberosity.

13. d. The epiphyseal cartilage plate (one at each end of the shaft) connects the two epiphyses to the diaphysis and is responsible for the growth in length of the limb bones. When the epiphyseal plates disappear, at around 20 years of age, long bones cease to grow.

14. b. The osteoclasts secrete enzymes, including collagenase enzyme, which bring about the breakdown of collagen and organic bone matrix as well as the dissolution of calcium salt crystals, leading to bone resorption.

15. b. The coronoid fossa is the depression that receives the coronoid process of the ulna during full flexion of the elbow. It is superior to the trochlea.

16. b. The scaphoid is boat shaped, the triquetrum is a three-cornered pyramid, the trapezium is four sided and has a tubercle, and the trapezoid is wedged between the trapezium and the capitate.

17. a. The linea aspera is located on the central posterior femur. The lateral lip of the linea aspera is continuous superiorly with the gluteal tuberosity. The medial lip is continuous with a line called the spiral line, which blends anteriorly with the intertrochanteric line. The pectineal line is an intermediate ridge from the linea aspera to the lesser trochanter.

18. d. The tuberosity of the fifth metatarsal is at the base of the metatarsal. The base of the metatarsal is proximal and the head is distal. The medial cuneiform is on the high medial side of the transverse arch of the foot. The cuboid bone is on the lower lateral side of the foot.

19. b. The immature innominate bone has three parts, the ilium, ischium, and pubis, which are joined by cartilage. As a person grows, the cartilage is replaced by bone. At puberty, the innominate bone/hipbone is ossified except in the acetabulum, where the Y-shaped triradiate cartilage separates the three areas of bone.

CHAPTER 3

Arthrology and Syndesmology of the Appendicular Skeleton

1. A joint that moves in one plane only is called what type of joint?
   a. plane
   b. hinge
   c. saddle
   d. condyloid

2. The acromioclavicular joint is classified as what type of joint?
   a. plane
   b. hinge
   c. pivot
   d. condyloid

3. The hip joint is classified as what type of joint?
   a. plane
   b. hinge
   c. pivot
   d. ball and socket

4. The metacarpophalangeal joints are classified as what type of joint?
   a. plane
   b. hinge
   c. condyloid
   d. saddle

5. The interosseous membrane located between the radius and ulna is classified as what type of fibrous joint?
   a. syndesmosis
   b. gomphosis
   c. suture
   d. synchondrosis

6. The proximal radioulnar joint is classified as what type of synovial joint?
   a. pivot joint
   b. condyloid joint
   c. gliding joint
   d. hinge joint

7. Which of the following does the deltoid ligament reinforce?
   a. lateral side of the shoulder joint
   b. medial side of the ankle joint
   c. lateral side of the knee joint
   d. medial side of the elbow joint

8. The wrist joint is classified as what type of joint?
   a. synovial hinge joint
   b. syndesmosis
   c. synovial condyloid joint
   d. symphysis

9. The middle joint between the radius and the ulna is classified as what type of joint?
   a. symphysis
   b. synovial joint
   c. syndesmosis
   d. pivot joint

10. Which joint of the hand is a condyloid type of synovial joint?
    a. carpometacarpal joint of the thumb
    b. metacarpophalangeal joint of the fourth digit
    c. carpometacarpal joint of the second digit
    d. third distal interphalangeal joint

11. The tendon of the popliteus passes between the lateral meniscus and which ligament of the knee?
    a. oblique popliteal ligament
    b. tibial collateral ligament
    c. arcuate popliteal ligament
    d. fibular collateral ligament

12. What does the superior articular surface of the talus fit into?
    a. capitulum
    b. meniscus
    c. trochlea
    d. mortise

Answers

1. b. Hinge joints move in one plane around one axis only and permit flexion and extension only. The elbow joint is a hinge joint.

2. a. The acromioclavicular joint is classified as a plane joint. Plane joints have flat opposing surfaces and are mostly small. They allow gliding or sliding movements.

3. d. The hip joint is classified as a ball and socket joint. The ball is the head of the femur and the socket is the acetabulum. These joints are multiaxial and therefore are highly movable joints.

4. c. Metacarpophalangeal joints are condyloid joints. These are biaxial joints allowing flexion/extension around one axis and abduction/adduction around another axis.

5. a. A syndesmosis is defined as a type of fibrous joint that unites bones with a sheet of fibrous tissue, either a ligament or a fibrous membrane.

6. a. The proximal radioulnar joint is classified as a synovial pivot joint. The head of the radius pivots or turns within the ring formed by the radial notch of the ulna and the annular ligament. It allows for pronation and supination movements of the forearm.

7. b. The deltoid ligament is a triangular-shaped ligament that reinforces the medial side of the ankle joint. It is frequently injured with an eversion sprain.

8. c. The wrist joint is classified as a synovial condyloid joint between the carpal surface of the radius and the scaphoid and lunate bones. It has motion in two body planes, allowing flexion and extension as well as abduction and adduction.

9. c. The proximal and distal radioulnar joints are pivot-type synovial joints. A symphysis is a joint where the two bones are united by fibrocartilage. The fibrous connective tissue of the interosseous membrane joins the radius and the ulna together in a fibrous joint or syndesmosis.

10. b. The carpometacarpal joint of the thumb is a saddle joint. The medial four carpometacarpal joints are planar synovial joints. All of the metacarpophalangeal joints are condyloid joints. All of the interphalangeal joints are hinge joints.

11. d. The oblique popliteal ligament is an expansion of the tendon of the semimembranosus into the posterior capsule of the knee. The arcuate popliteal ligament passes over the tendon of the popliteus posteriorly and blends into the fibrous capsule posteriorly. The tibial collateral ligament is attached to the medial meniscus. The cordlike fibular collateral ligament is separated from the lateral meniscus by the tendon of the popliteus.

12. d. The medial and lateral malleoli form a mortise or deep socket into which fits the rounded trochlea of the talus.

Myology of the Appendicular Skeleton

1. Plantarflexion and eversion of the foot are functions of which muscle?
   a. gastrocnemius
   b. peroneus longus
   c. peroneus tertius
   d. soleus

2. The head of the fibula is the insertion of which muscle?
   a. peroneus longus
   b. semimembranosus
   c. biceps femoris
   d. adductor magnus

3. Which muscle of the rotator cuff group allows medial rotation of the glenohumeral joint?
   a. supraspinatus
   b. infraspinatus
   c. teres minor
   d. subscapularis

4. Which nerve innervates the muscles of the anterior arm?
   a. musculocutaneous nerve
   b. median nerve
   c. ulnar nerve
   d. radial nerve

5. Which muscle does NOT rotate the humerus?
   a. infraspinatus
   b. supraspinatus
   c. teres minor
   d. subscapularis

6. The obturator nerve innervates which lateral rotator of the thigh?
   a. obturator internus
   b. piriformis
   c. quadratus femoris
   d. obturator externus

7. Besides the anterolateral abdominal muscles, which muscle assists in forced expiration, coughing, sneezing, vomiting, urinating, defecating, and fixation of the trunk during strong movements of the upper limb?
   a. piriformis
   b. pelvic diaphragm
   c. trapezius
   d. gluteus maximus

8. Which nerve is NOT in direct physical contact with the humerus?
   a. radial nerve
   b. median nerve
   c. musculocutaneous nerve
   d. ulnar nerve

9. The flexor carpi ulnaris muscle has proximal origins from the medial epicondyle and what other site?
   a. posterior border of the ulna
   b. anterior base of the fifth metacarpal
   c. interosseous membrane
   d. ulnar tuberosity

10. Which muscle would move the abducted (90°) arm anteriorly?
    a. sternocostal head of the pectoralis major
    b. clavicular head of the pectoralis major
    c. inferior fibers of the serratus anterior
    d. pectoralis minor

11. Which of the following is an intrinsic muscle of the hand and a muscle of the thenar eminence and does NOT attach to a phalange?
    a. adductor pollicis
    b. opponens pollicis
    c. abductor pollicis brevis
    d. flexor pollicis longus

12. Identify the flexor of the elbow, which arises from the lateral supracondylar crest and is innervated by a branch of the posterior cord.
    a. brachioradialis
    b. brachialis
    c. long head of the biceps brachii
    d. medial head of the triceps brachii

13. Which muscle does NOT flex the knee and extend the hip?
    a. semitendinosus
    b. hamstring portion of the adductor magnus
    c. long head of the biceps femoris
    d. semimembranosus

14. Which muscle provides the powerful "push-off" used during walking?
    a. tibialis posterior
    b. flexor hallucis longus
    c. peroneus longus
    d. quadratus plantae

15. Which of the following muscles does the inferior gluteal nerve supply?
    a. obturator internus
    b. gluteus maximus
    c. gluteus medius
    d. gluteus minimus

16. Which of the following nerves provides motor supply to the deltoid muscle?
    a. spinal accessory
    b. axillary
    c. musculocutaneous
    d. radial

17. Which of the following represents the action of the soleus muscle?
    a. flexion of the leg at the knee joint
    b. flexion of the leg at the knee and dorsiflexion of the foot at the ankle joint
    c. plantarflexion of the foot at the ankle joint
    d. dorsiflexion of the foot at the ankle joint

18. Which of the following is the embryonic primordial cell of skeletal muscle fibers?
    a. osteoblast
    b. fibroblast
    c. hemocytoblast
    d. myoblast

19. Which of the following is a characteristic histological feature of skeletal muscle?
    a. nuclei are peripheral in position
    b. there are transverse striations
    c. individual fibers are covered by endomysium
    d. cytoplasm contains myofibrils

20. While performing a surgical biopsy of the lymph nodes in the mid to lower portions of the axilla, which nerves would be in danger of being severed?
    a. thoracodorsal and long thoracic
    b. median and radial
    c. suprascapular and axillary
    d. ulnar and musculocutaneous

Answers

1. b. The tendon of the peroneus longus runs posterior to the lateral malleolus of the fibula and then crosses the plantar surface of the foot to insert on the medial side of the foot. It thus has the ability to plantarflex and evert the foot in addition to helping to maintain the transverse arch of the foot.

2. c. The head of the fibula is the insertion for the tendon of the biceps femoris. The biceps femoris muscle runs along the posterolateral side of the thigh and thus inserts into the head of the fibula (lateral bone of the leg). The semimembranosus and adductor magnus muscles are located on the medial side of the posterior thigh.

3. d. The subscapularis muscle is the only muscle of the rotator cuff group that rotates the arm medially. This is because it is the only muscle in the group that crosses the shoulder joint anteriorly and thus pulls the arm internally during rotation. The supraspinatus abducts the arm while the other two muscles are lateral rotators of the arm.

4. a. The musculocutaneous nerve innervates the three muscles of the anterior compartment of the arm. The median and ulnar nerves pass through the anterior arm but have no function until they reach the anterior forearm and hand. The radial nerve supplies all of the muscles and skin on the posterior side of the upper limb.

5. b. Supraspinatus, although one of the rotator cuff muscles, is the only abductor of the group.

6. d. The obturator nerve innervates the obturator externus muscle, which laterally rotates the thigh. The obturator internus, piriformis, and quadratus femoris are all innervated by branches of the sacral plexus.

7. b. The pelvic diaphragm is composed of the levator ani and coccygeus muscles. This pelvic diaphragm assists in forced expiration, coughing, sneezing, vomiting, urinating, defecating, and fixation of the trunk during strong movements of the upper limb.

8. c. The musculocutaneous nerve enters the coracobrachialis muscle and then lies between the biceps brachii and the brachialis before it ultimately enters the forearm.

9. a. The flexor carpi ulnaris has two heads. The humeral head attaches to the medial epicondyle. The other head, as the name implies, attaches to the ulna. The muscle covers much of the medial portion of the forearm.

10. b. These actions can be easily demonstrated and palpated. Resisting anterior movement of the arm abducted to 60° tests the sternocostal head of the pectoralis major; the clavicular head is tested after the arm is abducted to 90°.

11. b. All four muscles are muscles of the thumb. The flexor pollicis longus is an extrinsic muscle of the hand; the other three are intrinsic muscles of the hand. The adductor pollicis is a short muscle of the thumb but is not part of the thenar eminence. The opponens pollicis originates from carpal bones and inserts on the first metacarpal. The other three muscles insert on phalanges of the thumb.

12. a. The brachioradialis is an elbow flexor innervated by the radial nerve, which is a terminal branch of the posterior cord. The triceps brachii is an extensor. A branch of the lateral cord innervates the brachialis and biceps brachii.

13. b. All four muscles are hamstring muscles of the posterior thigh. All four muscles extend the hip. Only the hamstring portion of adductor magnus does not cross the knee. It inserts on the adductor tubercle of the femur. The other three muscles cross the knee posteriorly and therefore flex the knee.

14. b. The flexor hallucis longus inserts on the plantar surface of the distal phalange of the big toe where it is in position to provide the "push-off."

15. b. The gluteus maximus receives motor supply from the inferior gluteal nerve. The gluteus medius and minimus receive their motor supply through the superior gluteal nerve, and the obturator internus muscle is supplied by the nerve to obturator internus.

16. b. The axillary nerve provides motor supply to the deltoid muscle and is a branch of the posterior cord of the brachial plexus.

17. c. The soleus muscle acts on the ankle joint in conjunction with the gastrocnemius and plantaris muscle to plantarflex the foot.

18. d. The myoblast is an embryonic cell that differentiates from the mesenchymal cells of the mesoderm in the myotome regions of the somites. The prefix *myo* means "muscle," and the suffix *blast* means "precursor cell."

19.   a.   The peripheral location of the nuclei in skeletal muscle is characteristic and helps to differentiate skeletal muscle from cardiac and smooth muscles, whose nuclei are central in position.

20.   a.   The only pair that could be damaged in this location would be the thoracodorsal and long thoracic nerves. The thoracodorsal courses inferiorly along the posterior wall of the axilla and enters the anterior surface of the latissimus dorsi muscle. The long thoracic nerve courses along the medial wall superficial to the serratus anterior muscle.

Cardiovascular and Lymphatic Systems

1. Which of the following valves of the heart is made up of two cusps?
   a. right atrioventricular valve
   b. left atrioventricular valve
   c. pulmonary valve
   d. aortic valve

2. The abdominal aorta divides into two common iliac arteries at the level of the lower border of which vertebra?
   a. L2
   b. L3
   c. L4
   d. L5

3. The left testicular vein drains its blood into what vein?
   a. left renal vein
   b. left common iliac vein
   c. inferior vena cava
   d. splenic vein

4. Which of the following is a characteristic histological feature of the thymus?
   a. presence of a capsule of connective tissue
   b. presence of lymphatic nodules in the cortex
   c. presence of Hassall's corpuscles in the medulla
   d. presence of blood vessels in the capsule

5. Which two nerves are in danger during axillary lymph node dissection and excision?
   a. thoracodorsal and long thoracic nerves
   b. median and ulnar nerves
   c. radial and axillary nerves
   d. musculocutaneous and suprascapular nerves

6. What is the origin of the suprascapular artery?
   a. thoracoacrominal artery
   b. axillary artery
   c. thyrocervical trunk (artery)
   d. circumflex scapular artery

7. Which is branch of the internal iliac artery supplies the spinal meninges and the dorsal and ventral rootlets?
   a. inferior vesicular artery
   b. vaginal artery
   c. internal pudendal artery
   d. lateral sacral artery

8. What is located in the posterior wall of the omental foramen of Winslow?
   a. inferior vena cava
   b. portal triad
   c. first part of duodenum
   d. caudate lobe of liver

9. The sinoatrial node is located in what chamber of the heart?
   a. left atrium
   b. right atrium
   c. left ventricle
   d. right ventricle

10. Which of the following is the thickest layer in the wall of an artery?
    a. tunica intima
    b. tunica media
    c. tunica adventitia
    d. tunica externa

11. Which is the valve that is located between the right atrium and the right ventricle?
    a. aortic valve
    b. pulmonary valve
    c. mitral valve
    d. tricuspid valve

12. Which of the following allows blood to bypass the lung during fetal development?
    a. ductus venosus
    b. ligamentum teres
    c. ductus arteriosus
    d. umbilical artery

13. Which named peripheral nerve is responsible for pain sensation from the pericardium, mediastinal pleura, diaphragmatic pleura, and diaphragmatic peritoneum?
   a. vagus nerve
   b. phrenic nerve
   c. greater thoracic splanchnic nerve
   d. tenth intercostal nerve

14. Which statement is TRUE of the coronary arteries?
   a. coronary arteries have substantial anastomoses
   b. coronary arteries have no anastomoses
   c. coronary arteries are functionally end arteries
   d. coronary arteries have no anastomoses with extracardiac vessels

15. Which veins are located in the falciform ligament?
   a. esophageal veins
   b. paraumbilical veins
   c. superficial epigastric veins
   d. retroperitoneal veins

16. The lymphatic vessels, which accompany the great saphenous vein, drain into which lymph nodes?
   a. superficial inguinal lymph nodes
   b. deep inguinal lymph nodes
   c. popliteal lymph nodes
   d. external iliac lymph nodes

17. The diaphragmatic surface of the heart is formed mainly by what area of the heart?
   a. right atria
   b. right ventricle
   c. left atria
   d. left ventricle

18. The portal vein results from the union of which two veins?
   a. superior mesenteric and renal
   b. superior mesenteric and inferior mesenteric
   c. splenic and superior mesenteric
   d. splenic and inferior mesenteric

Answers

1.   b.   The left atrioventricular (mitral) valve is made up of only two cusps. It is often referred to as the bicuspid valve. The other three heart valves have three cusps.

2.   c.   The abdominal aorta divides into two common iliac arteries at the lower level of the fourth lumbar vertebra just to the left of the midline.

3.   a.   The left testicular vein originates from the left pampiniform plexus and drains its blood into the left renal vein. The right testicular vein, however, drains into the inferior vena cava.

4.   c.   Hassall's corpuscles are characteristic to the thymus. They are composed of concentric lamellate bodies found in the medulla of the thymus and is made up of degenerating epithelial reticular cells found only in the thymus.

5.   a.   Because the thoracodorsal and long thoracic nerves are found coursing unprotected through the axilla, they may be traumatized during axillary lymph node dissection and biopsy.

6.   c.   The thyrocervical trunk (artery), a branch of the subclavian artery, has several branches. One of them, the suprascapular artery, travels laterally close to the inferior belly of the omohyoid muscle and the suprascapular nerve to the scapula. The other branches of the thyrocervical trunk mainly supply neck structures.

7.   d.   The lateral sacral artery, a branch of the internal iliac artery, enters the ventral sacral foramina to supply some of the spinal nerve roots of cauda equina.

8.   a.   The omental foramen of Winslow is posterior to the lesser omentum. The posterior wall of the foramen is formed by parietal peritoneum covering the inferior vena cava and the right crus of the diaphragm.

9.   b.   The sinoatrial node is located in the right atrium of the heart. It serves as the pacemaker for the heart. Impulses generated there are passed on from right to left and inferiorly to the atrioventricular node in the lower end of the interatrial septum.

10. b. The thickest layer in the wall of an artery is the tunica media. This layer contains elastic tissue and/or smooth muscle. The muscle is important in helping to keep the blood flowing away from the heart to the tissues. The internal and external tunics are thin layers of epithelium and connective tissue, respectively.

11. d. The valve between the right atrium and the right ventricle of the heart is the tricuspid valve. The mitral or bicuspid valve serves the same purpose but on the left side of the heart. The pulmonary and aortic valves guard the exit points of the heart into the pulmonary and systemic circulations.

12. c. The ductus arteriosus is the fetal bypass of the lungs. It connects the pulmonary artery to the arch of the aorta so that blood is diverted into the aorta. It becomes the ligamentum arteriosum after birth, when a baby breathes on its own and blood enters the lungs through the pulmonary arteries. The ductus venosus is associated with the liver, the ligamentum teres with the umbilical vein, and the umbilical artery with oxygenated blood from the placenta.

13. b. The phrenic nerve arises from ventral rami of C3, C4, and C5 spinal nerves. The sensory neurons of the dorsal root ganglia of C3, C4, and C5 supply axons for somatic pain from the named area of parietal serous membranes. C3, C4, and C5 also supply the shoulder with the cutaneous innervation by the supraclavicular nerves. This is why pericardial or diaphragmatic pain will refer to the shoulder.

14. c. The branches of the coronary arteries have small anastomoses between each other and subepicardial and extracardiac thoracic vessels, but these collateral routes are of little use in the case of a sudden occlusion of a coronary artery. These arteries are functionally end arteries.

15. b. The esophageal veins and the paraumbilical veins are tributaries of the hepatic portal venous system. The epigastric veins and the retroperitoneal veins are tributaries of the caval venous system. Portal-caval anastomoses may become sites of varicose veins following portal hypertension. An example is the caput medusae on the anterior abdominal wall, that is due to the anastomoses between the paraumbilical and superficial epigastric veins.

16. a. The great saphenous vein is a cutaneous vein. The lymphatic vessels, which accompany it, drain into the superficial inguinal lymph nodes, which in turn drain mostly into the external iliac lymph nodes. The deep inguinal lymph nodes are deep to the fascia lata and accompany the femoral veins.

17.   d.   The large left ventricle forms most of the surface area of the heart. The right ventricle forms most of the anterior surface. The left ventricle forms most of the diaphragmatic surface.

18.   c.   The portal vein is a short but wide vein that results from the union of the splenic and superior mesenteric veins. It then divides into right and left branches, which enter the corresponding lobe of the liver.

CHAPTER 6

Digestive System

CONTENT AREAS

- Oral cavity and pharynx
- Digestive viscera
- Development
- Histology

1. A brush border is found on the epithelial cells of which organ?
   a. stomach
   b. colon
   c. esophagus
   d. duodenum

2. Which of the following structures is a derivative of the embryonic midgut?
   a. liver
   b. jejunum
   c. pancreas
   d. stomach

3. The columns of Morgagni are located in the walls of what part of the digestive system?
   a. anal canal
   b. stomach
   c. duodenum
   d. rectum

4. Which abdominal organs does the thoracic cage protect?
   a. spleen, liver, adrenal gland, and upper portion of kidneys and stomach
   b. pancreas, liver, and vermiform appendix
   c. gallbladder, urinary bladder, liver, and uterus
   d. spleen, pancreas, adrenal gland, and ovaries

5. What is located in the anterior wall of the omental foramen of Winslow?
   a. gastroduodenal artery
   b. right crus of diaphragm
   c. inferior vena cava
   d. portal triad

6. Which forms from the embryonic ventral mesentery of the foregut?
   a. transverse mesocolon
   b. greater omentum
   c. lesser omentum
   d. gastrosplenic ligament

7. The superior mesenteric artery passes over the anterior surface of what part of the duodenum?
   a. first
   b. second
   c. third
   d. fourth

8. Which is NOT a characteristic of the ileum?
   a. long vasa recta
   b. many short loops of the vascular arcades
   c. few and low plicae circulares
   d. many Peyer's patches

9. The main pancreatic duct joins with what structure?
   a. common bile duct
   b. common hepatic duct
   c. major duodenal papilla
   d. second part of the duodenum

10. Which of the following palatine muscles is innervated by mandibular nerve fibers?
    a. tensor veli palatini
    b. levator veli palatini
    c. palatoglossus
    d. palatopharyngeus

11. Which of the following muscles of the pharynx is supplied by the glossopharyngeal nerve (CN IX)?
    a. palatopharyngeus
    b. stylopharyngeus
    c. superior constrictor
    d. middle constrictor

12. In abdominal examination, the spleen lies in which of the following quadrants?
    a. upper left quadrant
    b. upper right quadrant
    c. lower left quadrant
    d. lower right quadrant

13. Which of the following cells of the gastric gland secrete the intrinsic factor?
    a. mucous neck cells
    b. peptic (chief) cells
    c. parietal (oxyntic) cells
    d. stem cells

1.   d.   A brush border of microvilli is a characteristic feature of the small intestine of which the duodenum is the first section. The brush border increases the surface area of the mucosa to maximize absorption of nutrients into the blood. There is no absorption in the esophagus, and minimal absorption in the stomach and colon, so no brush border is present or necessary.

2.   b.   The jejunum is a derivative of the embryonic midgut. The midgut includes part of the duodenum through a portion of the transverse colon. The liver and biliary duct system along with the pancreas and its duct system are outgrowths of the original foregut. The stomach is a foregut derivative also, because it forms proximal to the duodenum.

3.   a.   The columns of Morgagni are located in the mucosal lining of the anal canal. These folds allow for expansion of the canal as the feces pass out of the body. The stomach has similar folds called rugae, and the duodenum has folds called the plicae circulare. The rectum is void of folds in the mucosa.

4.   a.   The abdominal cavity extends superiorly into the thoracic cage. Subsequently, the ribs protect several abdominal organs. These are the spleen, liver, adrenal gland, and upper portions of the kidneys and stomach.

5.   d.   The omental foramen of Winslow is the communication between the greater peritoneal cavity and lesser peritoneal cavity or omental bursa. The foramen is situated posterior to the free edge of the lesser omentum. The portal triad is situated in the free edge of the lesser omentum and thus part of the anterior wall of the omental foramen of Winslow.

6.   c.   The foregut, but not the midgut or hindgut, had a ventral mesentery during development. After the development of the liver and rotation of the gut, the ventral mesogastrum becomes the lesser omentum. The other three structures named are from dorsal mesenteries.

7.   c.   The superior mesenteric artery and vein and the root of the mesentery of the jejunum and ileum all pass over the third part of the duodenum as it lays across the L3 vertebrae. The inferior vena cava and the aorta are also posterior to the third part of the duodenum.

8. a. The ileum has more levels of the vascular arcades and shorter vasa recta than the jejunum. The ileum also has more fat in the mesentery surrounding the vasa recta, occluding the little windows seen between the vasa recta of the jejunum.

9. a. Right and left hepatic ducts join together to form the common hepatic duct, which joins with the cystic duct to form the (common) bile duct. The bile duct passes posterior to the first part of the duodenum and joins with the main pancreatic duct to form the hepatopancreatic ampulla (of Vater), which forms the major duodenal papilla as it opens into the second part of the duodenum.

10. a. All of the palatine muscles are supplied by the vagus nerve (CN X) except the tensor veli palatini muscle, which is supplied by fibers from the mandibular (CN V.1) nerve via the branch to medial pterygoid muscle.

11. b. All the pharyngeal muscles are supplied by the vagus nerve (CN X) except the stylopharyngeus muscle, which is supplied by the glossopharyngeal nerve (CN IX).

12. a. The spleen lies in the upper left quadrant or left hypochondrium of the abdomen under the diaphragm, adjacent to the 9th, 10th and 11th ribs.

13. c. Parietal (oxyntic) cells secrete hydrochloric acid and the intrinsic factor, which helps with the absorption of vitamin B12. A deficiency of intrinsic factor causes a type of anemia called pernicious anemia.

Respiratory System

1. The horizontal fissure parallels which rib?
   a. right fourth rib
   b. right sixth rib
   c. left fourth rib
   d. left sixth rib

2. The parasympathetic motor axons of the vagus nerve cause what action?
   a. decreased secretion from type II alveolar gland cells
   b. vasoconstriction of pulmonary arteries
   c. bronchodilation
   d. bronchoconstriction

3. Which statement is TRUE regarding the vasculature of the lungs?
   a. bronchial arteries and pulmonary arteries contain deoxygenated blood
   b. branches of the bronchial arteries anastomose with branches of pulmonary arteries in the walls of the bronchioles
   c. pulmonary veins and bronchi are paired and have the same branching pattern
   d. pulmonary arteries follow an intersegmental path in the connective tissues between the lung segments

4. The parasympathetic fibers to the pulmonary plexuses are provided by which nerve?
   a. facial
   b. glossopharyngeal
   c. vagus
   d. accessory

5. Which of the following laryngeal muscles abduct the vocal folds?
   a. thyroarytenoid
   b. transverse arytenoid
   c. lateral cricoarytenoid
   d. posterior cricoarytenoid

6. Which of the following cells in the lung secrete pulmonary surfactant?
    a. alveolar type I cells
    b. alveolar type II cells
    c. alveolar phagocytes
    d. alveolar capillary endothelia

7. The vocal cords are attached posteriorly to which laryngeal cartilages?
    a. arytenoid cartilages
    b. cricoid cartilages
    c. thyroid cartilages
    d. cuneiform cartilages

8. The alveoli of the lungs are lined with what type of epithelium?
    a. pseudostratified columnar
    b. simple columnar
    c. stratified squamous
    d. simple squamous

Answers

1. a. Both lungs have an oblique fissure. The left lung has two lobes, the right has three lobes. The right lung has the horizontal fissure, which follows the fourth rib.

2. d. The first three answers are actions of sympathetic motor axons. The parasympathetic motor axons cause contraction of the smooth muscle of the bronchi.

3. b. Bronchial arteries supply oxygenated blood to the lung stroma and the visceral pleura. The most distal branches of the bronchial arteries do have anastomoses with branches of the pulmonary arteries. The pulmonary arteries and the bronchi are the paired vessels. It is the pulmonary veins that follow a separate path between the segments.

4. c. The anterior and posterior pulmonary plexuses contain parasympathetic fibers from the vagus nerve. These fibers are motor to the bronchial muscles causing bronchoconstriction and are also secretomotor to bronchial glands.

5. d. The posterior cricoarytenoid muscles pull the muscular process of each arytenoid cartilage posteriorly resulting in lateral rotation of the vocal process, thus opening the rima glottides.

6. b. Alveolar type II cells secrete the pulmonary surfactant. The surfactant is spread over the surface of the alveolar cells and helps to reduce the surface tension, and therefore prevents the alveoli from collapsing during expiration.

7. a. The vocal cords cross the larynx from the thyroid cartilage anteriorly to the arytenoid cartilages posteriorly. The cords have no attachment to the cricoid cartilage at the lower end of the larynx, nor to the cuneiform cartilages.

8. d. The alveoli of the lung are lined with simple squamous epithelium. The alveoli are the sites of external respiration (between the air and the blood). Diffusion of gases can occur very rapidly due to the one-layer-thick epithelium. A stratified epithelium would hinder the process. Simple columnar epithelium functions in absorption and secretion.

Urogenital System

1. What epithelium lines the urinary tract of the body?
   a. transitional epithelium
   b. pseudostratified columnar epithelium
   c. simple columnar epithelium
   d. stratified squamous epithelium

2. Which part of the male urethra passes through the urogenital diaphragm?
   a. spongy urethra
   b. prostatic urethra
   c. membranous urethra
   d. penile urethra

3. What is the origin of the cavernous nerves?
   a. dorsal nerve of penis
   b. perineal nerve
   c. prostate nerve plexus
   d. superior hypogastric nerve

4. Inhibition of the internal urethral sphincter allows the body to:
   a. micturate
   b. defecate
   c. hold the urine until later
   d. ejaculate

5. Which is NOT found in the spermatic cord?
   a. ilioinguinal nerve
   b. pampiniform plexus of veins
   c. sympathetic and parasympathetic nerves
   d. genital branch of the genitofemoral nerve

6. Which nerves supply motor and sensory innervation to the perineum?
   a. pelvic splanchnic nerves
   b. sacral parasympathetic nerves
   c. sacral splanchnic nerves
   d. pudendal nerves

7. Which of the following describes the pelvic diaphragm?
    a. it is composed of striated muscle of somatic origin
    b. it is composed of striated muscle of visceral origin
    c. it is composed of smooth muscle
    d. it is part of the perineum

8. An accumulation of blood in the tunica vaginalis is the definition of what term?
    a. spermatocele
    b. varicocele
    c. hydrocele
    d. hematocele

9. Which of the following renal structures contains the macula densa?
    a. afferent glomerular arteriole
    b. efferent glomerular arteriole
    c. proximal convoluted tubule
    d. distal convoluted tubule

10. The trigone is located on what internal surface of the bladder?
    a. superior surface
    b. inferolateral surface
    c. apex
    d. base

11. Which of the following spermatogenic cells perform the first meiotic division?
    a. spermatogonia
    b. primary spermatocytes
    c. secondary spermatocytes
    d. tertiary spermatocytes

Answers

1. a. The urinary tract is lined by transitional epithelium. This is the only epithelium that has the ability to change its appearance if it is in a stretched versus a collapsed state. This property is necessary for the urinary system due to its capacity to store urine in the urinary bladder. Simple squamous epithelium functions in diffusion, while a stratified and pseudostratified epithelium serves a protective role in the body. None of these tissues require the ability to stretch.

2. c. The male urethra is divided into three parts: prostatic, membranous, and penile. The prostatic urethra runs through the prostate gland that lies superior to the urogenital diaphragm. The membranous urethra runs through the urogenital diaphragm and is surrounded by the internal urethral sphincter. The spongy or penile urethra lies within the corpus spongiosum of the penis.

3. c. The prostate nerve plexus is composed of parasympathetic nerve fibers. These are thought to arise from the pelvic splanchnic nerves. From the prostatic nerve plexus, the cavernous nerve arises and then courses through the connective capsule of the prostate and the deep transverse perineal muscle to innervate the deep artery of the penis. With stimulation of these nerves, the penis becomes erect.

4. a. Parasympathetic fibers inhibit the smooth muscles of the internal urethral sphincter, which allows urine to flow into the urethra.

5. a. The ilioinguinal nerve exits the abdominal wall through the superficial inguinal ring. It is not a constituent of the spermatic cord.

6. d. The pelvic splanchnic nerves are parasympathetic nerves from S2, S3, and S4. The cavernous nerves are a subset of the parasympathetic nerves that supply motor innervation to the helicine arteries of the erectile tissues. The pudendal nerves are also from S2, S3, and S4 but follow a different path than the parasympathetic nerves. The pudendal nerves are motor to the somatic muscles of the perineum and sensory to the skin of the perineum.

7. a. The pelvic diaphragm is striated muscle of somatic origin, which forms the muscular floor of the pelvis. It is innervated by general somatic efferent axons from S3 and S4. The muscles of the face and jaws are composed of striated muscle formed from the upper portion of the gastrointestinal tract, the pharyngeal arches.

8. d. These are all swellings in the scrotum. The varicocele is a dilated, varicose, pampiniform plexus (testicular veins). The hydrocele is excess serous fluid in the tunica vaginalis. The spermatocele is a collection of excess fluid in the epididymis.

9. d. The macula densa is a modified segment of the distal convoluted tubule in which the cells appear tall columnar with their nuclei densely packed. These macula densa cells are sensitive to the ionic content and water volume in the tubular lumen.

10. d. The smooth triangular area between the openings of the ureters and urethra is called the trigone and is found on the internal surface of the base of the urinary bladder.

11. b. Primary spermatocytes arise from spermatogonia through mitotic division and differentiation, and then they perform the first meiotic division to give rise to secondary spermatocytes. These perform the second meiotic division to give rise to spermatids, which do not divide but undergo metamorphosis to become spermatozoa.

Endocrine System

1. Which of the following zones of the suprarenal gland secrete mineralocorticoids?
   a. zona glomerulosa
   b. zona fasciculata
   c. zona reticularis
   d. zona medullaris

2. Rathke's pouch is a diverticulum of the embryonic stomodeum that gives rise to what structure?
   a. thyroid gland
   b. parathyroid gland
   c. adenohypophysis
   d. neurohypophysis

3. Which of the following hormones is secreted by the acidophil cells of the pituitary gland?
   a. somatotropin
   b. thyrotropin
   c. corticotropin
   d. gonadotropins

4. The thyroid gland is derived from the epithelia of what structure?
   a. clefts of the first pharyngeal arch
   b. dorsum of the tongue
   c. pouches of the third pharyngeal arch
   d. roof of the mouth

5. The right adrenal gland is in contact with what structure?
   a. spleen
   b. inferior vena cava
   c. pancreas
   d. stomach

6. Pancreatic endocrine secretions pass through what structure(s)?
   a. pancreaticoduodenal veins
   b. bile duct
   c. pancreatic duct
   d. hepatopancreatic ampulla

7. Releasing hormones that regulate the anterior lobe of the pituitary gland are synthesized in what brain region?
   a. hypothalamus
   b. cerebral cortex
   c. thalamus
   d. basal ganglia

8. The interstitial cells of Leydig secrete which of the following hormones?
   a. estrogen
   b. somatotropin
   c. testosterone
   d. prolactin

Answers

1. a. The mineralocorticoids represent a group of hormones secreted by the zona glomerulosa of the suprarenal cortex. The primary hormone of this group is aldosterone, which controls and maintains water and electrolyte balance.

2. c. Rathke's pouch, also known as hypophyseal diverticulum, develops in the middle of the fourth week from the stomodeum (future mouth) and then becomes detached from the oral epithelium in the sixth week. This part of the pituitary gland, which develops from the ectoderm of the stomodeum, gives rise to the adenohypophysis.

3. a. Somatotropin (growth hormone) is secreted by the acidophil cells of the pars distalis of the pituitary gland. Thyrotropin (thyroid-stimulating hormone [TSH]), corticotropin (adrenocorticotrophic hormone [ACTH]), and gonadotropins (follicle-stimulating hormone [FSH] and luteinizing hormone [LH]) are all secreted by the basophil cells of the pituitary gland.

4. b. The thyroid gland is derived from the surface epithelia of the tongue; a site marked by the opening of the thyroglossal duct, the foramen cecum. The parathyroid glands are derived from the pouches of the third and fourth arches. No endocrine glands form from the pharyngeal clefts.

5. b. The right adrenal gland is in contact with the inferior vena cava anteromedially. It is separated from the pancreas by the duodenum. The left adrenal is in contact with the posterior wall and the stomach and the body-tail of the pancreas.

6. a. Endocrine glands are ductless glands. Endocrine hormones are absorbed and distributed by the circulatory system. Exocrine glands have ducts.

7. a. The anterior lobe of the pituitary gland is regulated by releasing hormones produced by the hypothalamus. These hormones are sent to the anterior lobe via the hypophyseal-portal vascular system. The other three components of the central nervous system do not affect or connect to the anterior lobe.

8. c. The interstitial cells of Leydig of the testes secrete the hormone testosterone.

Section One Recommended Reading

Agur A, Dalley A: *Grant's atlas of anatomy*, ed 11, Philadelphia, 2004, Lippincott Williams & Wilkins.

Drake RL, Vogl, MA: *Gray's anatomy for students,* Oxford, 2005, Churchill Livingstone.

Junqueira L, Carneiro J: *Basic histology*, ed 11, Stamford, Conn, 2005, Appleton & Lange.

Moore K, Dalley A: *Clinically oriented anatomy*, ed 5, Philadelphia, 2005, Lippincott Williams & Wilkins.

Moore K, Persaud T: *The developing human: clinically oriented embryology*, ed 7, Philadelphia, 2003, WB Saunders.

Standring S, ed: *Gray's anatomy: the anatomical basis of clinical practice,* ed 39, New York, 2004, Churchill Livingstone.

Spinal Anatomy

*Pierre Boucher, Gregory D. Cramer, Susan Darby,
Gene F. Giggleman, Amanda Louisa Neill, Isis Edward Zaki*

Osteology of the Axial Skeleton

1. Which of the following forms the posterior border of a typical intervertebral foramen?
   a. pedicle
   b. zygapophyseal joint
   c. uncinate process
   d. lamina

2. The vertebral foramina and sacral canal are circular (as viewed from above) and are the smallest in which of the following regions?
   a. cervical
   b. thoracic
   c. lumbar
   d. sacral

3. The atlas (C1) has which of the following features?
   a. superior articular processes that are concave inferiorly
   b. an articulation with the occiput that is categorized as a planar joint
   c. inferior articular processes that are oval
   d. prominent anterior and posterior tubercles on the transverse processes

4. Each typical thoracic vertebra (T2 to T9) has which of the following features?
   a. a prominent superior vertebral notch
   b. rectangular vertebral bodies (when viewed from above)
   c. superior articular processes that face posteriorly and medially and lie within a vertical plane
   d. a transverse costal facet on the transverse process that articulates with the rib with the same number

5.   Which is TRUE regarding the sacrum and the coccyx?
      a.   There are typically five pairs of pelvic sacral foramina
      b.   The anteriormost aspect of the body of S1 is known as the ala
      c.   The transverse processes of the coccyx line up with (are in register with) the sacral cornua
      d.   The superior aspect of the coccyx is known as its base

6.   Which structure of a typical vertebra does NOT arise from the pediculolaminar junction?
      a.   spinous process
      b.   transverse process
      c.   superior articular process
      d.   inferior articular process

7.   Which structure does NOT participate in the formation of the boundaries of the intervertebral foramen (IVF)?
      a.   the pedicle of the vertebra above
      b.   the vertebral body of the vertebra above
      c.   the transverse process of the vertebra above
      d.   the pedicle of the vertebra below

8.   In a typical cervical vertebra, which structures arise as elevations of the lateral and posterior rim on the top surface of the vertebral body?
      a.   uncinate processes
      b.   intertubercular lamellae
      c.   pedicles
      d.   anterior tubercles

9.   Which thoracic vertebra contains only a single facet on each side for articulation with the ribs?
      a.   4
      b.   6
      c.   8
      d.   10

10.   What is the normal minimum dimension of the anteroposterior canal in an adult lumbar vertebra?
      a.   5 mm
      b.   9 mm
      c.   11 mm
      d.   15 mm

11.   Which of the following is NOT a feature of the atlas vertebra?
      a.   anterior tubercle
      b.   bifid spinous process
      c.   posterior arch
      d.   fovea dentalis

12. Uncinate processes are characteristic of what area of the vertebral column?
    a. cervical vertebrae
    b. thoracic vertebrae
    c. lumbar vertebrae
    d. sacrum

13. Which of the following foramina is NOT located in the middle cranial fossa?
    a. foramen ovale
    b. foramen rotundum
    c. foramen spinosum
    d. foramen cecum

14. Which of the following is NOT transmitted through foramen magnum?
    a. spinal cord
    b. internal carotid artery
    c. vertebral artery
    d. spinal part of accessory nerve

15. Which of the following is NOT a part of the ethmoid bone?
    a. crista galli
    b. cribriform plate
    c. superior nasal concha
    d. inferior nasal concha

16. Select the FALSE statement concerning the atlantoaxial joint.
    a. it is a synovial joint
    b. it has two plane joints between the superior and inferior articular facets of the atlas and axis
    c. it has one pivot joint between the dens of the axis and the anterior arch of the atlas
    d. it permits flexion and extension of the head

17. Which bone is NOT part of the cranial vault?
    a. frontal
    b. parietal
    c. ethmoid
    d. maxilla

18. The os coxae is composed of what structures?
    a. fused vertebra of the coccyx
    b. fused vertebra of the sacrum
    c. ilium, ischium, and pubic bones
    d. facial bones of the skull

19. Which of the following is a feature of the sphenoid bone?
    a. sella turcica
    b. mastoid process
    c. cribriform plate
    d. external occipital protuberance

20. What type of ribs are the first seven ribs?
    a. real ribs
    b. true ribs
    c. floating ribs
    d. false ribs

21. Choose the INCORRECT statement.
    a. the anterior fontanel closes at 18 to 24 months of age and becomes the bregma
    b. the posterolateral fontanel is located at the intersection of the squamous and lambdoidal sutures
    c. the posterior fontanel closes by 2 months of age and becomes the lambda
    d. the metopic suture is usually obliterated by age 6 and connects the glabella to the pterion

22. Which two bones form the structure called the clivus?
    a. occipital bone, temporal bone
    b. temporal bone, zygomatic bone
    c. vomer bone, occipital bone
    d. sphenoid bone, occipital bone

23. The inferior articular facets of T12 face in which direction?
    a. anterolateral
    b. anteromedial
    c. posterolateral
    d. posteromedial

24. Which one of the following structures does NOT pass through the foramen magnum of the occipital bone?
    a. spinal cord
    b. meninges
    c. cranial nerve XII
    d. vertebral artery

25. In the growing infant, which fontanel typically closes first?
    a. anterior
    b. posterior
    c. anterolateral
    d. posterolateral

26. Which of the following is the list of ATYPICAL vertebrae?
    a. C1, T1, L1, S1
    b. C1, C2, T10, T12, L5
    c. C2, C7, T2, T8, L2, S5
    d. C1, C2, C7, T1, T12, L3
    e. C1, C7, T8, T9, T10, L2, L5, S3

27. Choose the INCORRECT statement concerning vertebral ossification centers.
    a. a typical vertebra has five ossification centers that develop during puberty
    b. typical vertebrae have three initial ossification centers
    c. the three ossification centers of a typical vertebra are the two transverse processes and the centrum
    d. fusion of the vertebral arch is complete by age 6 in the lumbar vertebrae
    e. secondary ossification centers unite with the vertebrae by age 25

28. The anterior curve present in the normal adult cervical spine would be classified as what type of curve?
    a. primary
    b. secondary
    c. tertiary
    d. quaternary

29. The first intervertebral foramen is located between which two bones?
    a. occiput, atlas
    b. atlas, axis
    c. axis, third cervical vertebra
    d. third cervical vertebra, fourth cervical vertebra

30. The neural canal is smallest and circular in shape in the _____ region of the vertebral canal.
    a. cervical
    b. thoracic
    c. lumbar
    d. sacral

Answers

1. b. The borders of a typical intervertebral foramen are as follows: superior, pedicle of the vertebra above; anterior (from superior to inferior), vertebral body of the vertebra above; intervertebral disc, vertebral body of the vertebra below; inferior, pedicle of the vertebra below; posterior, zygapophyseal (facet) joint (formed by the superior articular facet of the vertebra below, the inferior articular facet of the vertebra above, and lined by the ligamentum flavum anteriorly).

2. b. The vertebral foramina in the cervical region are the largest of the spine and are trefoil in shape. The thoracic vertebral foramina are the smallest of the spine (the spinal cord is also smaller in this region) and are rounded in shape. The vertebral foramina in the lumbar region are of intermediate size between the cervical, which are larger, and the thoracic, which are smaller. The lumbar vertebral foramina are trefoil in shape. The sacral canal, which is also trefoil in shape, is slightly smaller than the lumbar vertebral canal.

3. c. The right and left superior articular processes of the atlas are very irregular in shape and are concave superiorly in order to accommodate the convex occipital condyle of the corresponding side. The joint between the occiput and the atlas is categorized as a condyloid (ellipsoid), synovial (diarthrodial) joint. The left and right transverse processes are each large and possess a single lateral process (not an anterior and posterior tubercle as is the case with typical cervical vertebrae).

4. d. The typical thoracic vertebrae include T2 through T9. The 1st, 10th, 11th, and 12th thoracic vertebrae can best be described as unique rather than the term "atypical," which is best used to describe C1 and C2. The vertebral bodies of the thoracic spine are larger than those of the cervical region. The bodies are more or less heart-shaped as seen from above (concave posteriorly). The pedicles of the thoracic spine are quite stout. They attach very high up on their respective vertebral bodies and, as a result, there is no superior vertebral notch associated with typical thoracic vertebrae. The transverse processes of typical thoracic vertebrae have a facet for articulation with the articular tubercle of the corresponding rib (e.g., the transverse process of T6 articulates with the sixth rib. This facet is appropriately named the transverse costal facet or costal facet of the transverse process. The superior articulating facets of the thoracic spine are oriented in a plane that lies approximately 30 degrees to a vertical plane. They face posteriorly, superiorly, and laterally.

5. d. The sacrum is made of five fused segments. It is triangular in shape, and therefore the superior surface of the sacrum is known as the base (same with the coccyx), and the inferior surface is known as the apex. The most anterior portion of the sacral base is known as the sacral promontory. The anterior portions of the sacral base located on both the left and right sides (lateral to) the body of the first sacral segment are known as the sacral ala. The ventral surface of the sacrum displays four pair of ventral (pelvic, anterior) sacral foramina. The coccyx is formed by three to five fused segments. It, too, is triangular in shape with the superior surface being the base and the inferior surface forming the apex. The transverse process projects laterally from the first coccygeal segment. The coccygeal cornua are found on the posterior (dorsal) surface of the first coccygeal segment and are in register with the sacral cornua.

6. a. The spinous processes arise from the laminae only.

7. c. The boundaries of the IVF include the following: (1) pedicle of the vertebra above, (2) vertebral body of the vertebra above, (3) the intervertebral disc, (4) the vertebral body of the vertebra below, (5) the pedicle of the vertebra below, and (6) the Z joints form the posterior wall of the IVF.

8. a. The intertubercular lamella and the anterior tubercle are part of the transverse process. Pedicles attach to the posterior and lateral aspects of the vertebral bodies.

9. d. Thoracic vertebrae 4, 6, and 8 are typical thoracic vertebrae that contain two facets on each side.

10. d. Values regarding the vertebral canal dimensions are important because of their clinical significance (i.e., canal stenosis). An adult anteroposterior canal measurement of less than 15 mm indicates stenosis.

11. b. Bifid spinous processes are features of C2-C6 cervical vertebrae. The atlas has no spinous process; instead it has a posterior tubercle. All the other structures listed are features of the atlas.

12. a. Uncinate processes are unique features of the C3-C7 cervical vertebrae. They form uncovertebral joints of Luschka that are found only in the cervical region of the vertebral column.

13. d. The foramen cecum is located in the anterior cranial fossa, between the crista galli and frontal crest. It transmits emissary veins between the superior sagittal sinus and nasal veins. All other foramina are located on the greater wing of the sphenoid bone that forms part of the floor of the middle cranial fossa.

14. b. The internal carotid artery enters the cranial cavity through the carotid canal, which is located in the petrous part of temporal bone in the base of the skull.

15. d. The inferior nasal concha is a separate skull bone. The superior and middle nasal conchae are parts of the ethmoid bone. All other structures listed are parts of the ethmoid bone.

16. d. The principal motion seen in the atlantoaxial joint is rotation. The dens blocks flexion and extension at this joint.

17. d. The cranial vault is made of bones that form the cavity for the brain. This includes the frontal, parietal, ethmoid, sphenoid, temporal, and occipital bones. The maxillary bone is considered a facial bone.

18. c. The os coxa, or hip bone, is composed of three bones before puberty. These are the ilium, ischium, and pubis. They fuse at the acetabulum following puberty, and fusion is complete by the early 20s.

19. a. The sella turcica is the bony structure that houses the pituitary gland, and it is part of the sphenoid bone. The mastoid process is part of the temporal bone, the cribriform plate is part of the ethmoid bone, and the external occipital protuberance is part of the occipital bone.

20. b. Ribs 1 through 7 are true or vertebrosternal ribs because they articulate with both the vertebrae and to the sternum by their own costal cartilage. False ribs are the 8th to 12th ribs, of which the 11th and 12th are considered floating ribs.

21. d. The metopic suture is typically "closed" by age 6, but it connects the bregma to the glabella and not to the pterion, which is the adult equivalent of the anterolateral or sphenoidal fontanel.

22. d. The clivus is the area of the skull located in the posterior fossa that slopes from the foramen magnum to the dorsum sellae. It is formed by part of the basilar portion of the occipital bone and part of the body of the sphenoid bone.

23. a. The inferior articular facets located on the articular process of the thoracic vertebrae face in an anterior direction, but those on T12 have turned slightly lateral to articulate with the superior articular facets of L1.

24. c. The structures that pass through the foramen magnum include the spinal cord, the meninges, the spinal components of cranial nerve XI, and the vertebral arteries. Cranial nerve XII exits the skull through the hypoglossal canals.

25. b. The fontanels "close" in a predictable pattern. The first to close or ossify is the posterior or occipital fontanel. This fontanel closes by 2 months of age and becomes the anatomic structure called the lambda.

26. b. Vertebrae are listed as typical or atypical. The atypical vertebrae are those that do not look like or possess the same attributes as other vertebrae in its group. The atypical vertebrae in the cervical region are C1, C2, and C7; thoracic region, T1, T9, T10, T11, and T12; and lumbar region, L5.

27. c. The primary ossification centers of a typical vertebra are the centrum and the two halves of the neural arch.

28. b. The spinal column has basically a "C-shape" at birth and begins to take on more of a sigmoid shape as the child begins to stand erect. Those spinal curves that are present at birth (posterior) and that remain into adult life are considered primary curves. Those spinal curves that change and become anterior are considered secondary curves.

29. c. The first intervertebral foramen is the exit for C1 spinal nerve and is located between the occiput and C1. Intervertebral discs, however, are present, starting between the vertebral bodies of C2 and C3 vertebrae and ending between the vertebral bodies of L5 and S1.

30. b. The neural canal (vertebral canal) is largest and most triangular in the cervical region and smallest and most circular in the thoracic region.

Myology of the Axial Skeleton

1. Which of the following muscles does NOT attach to the mastoid process of the temporal bone?
   a. digastric muscle
   b. longissimus capitis muscle
   c. splenius capitis muscle
   d. semispinalis capitis muscle

2. Choose the INCORRECT statement.
   a. the iliocostalis lumborum muscle attaches to the ilium and the inferior six ribs
   b. the longissimus muscles form the middle column of the erector spinae group and extends from the ilium to the skull
   c. the erector spinae muscles will extend the spine, laterally flex the spine, and rotate the spine
   d. the iliocostalis thoracis muscle attaches from the transverse processes of T12-L4 and to ribs 8 through 12

3. Which of the following muscles does NOT attach to the atlas?
   a. levator scapulae
   b. rectus capitis posterior minor
   c. rectus capitis posterior major
   d. obliquus capitis superior

4. Choose the INCORRECT statement.
   a. the multifidus muscles attach from the transverse process of one vertebra to the spinous processes of the 2 to 4 superior vertebrae
   b. the short rotator muscles in the lumbar region attach to the transverse muscle of one vertebra and insert on the spinous process of the vertebra directly superior to its origin
   c. the interspinalis muscles attach from spinous process to spinous process
   d. the long rotator muscles in the cervical region attach from the transverse muscle of one vertebra and insert on the spinous process of the vertebra directly above it up to the level of C2

5. Which of the following is TRUE of the latissimus dorsi muscle?
    a. it originates from the vertebra of the thoracic spine, thoracolumbar fascia, and ilium
    b. it inserts into the intertubercular sulcus of the humerus
    c. it adducts and medially rotates the arm
    d. all of the above

6. Which of the following is the most lateral portion of the erector spinae muscle group?
    a. multifidus
    b. spinalis
    c. semispinalis
    d. iliocostalis

7. Where does the semispinalis capitis muscle have its superior attachment?
    a. between the superior and inferior nuchal lines of the occiput
    b. mastoid process of the temporal bone
    c. spinous processes of the first three cervical vertebrae
    d. transverse processes of the first three cervical vertebrae

8. Which muscle of the transversospinalis group crosses only one vertebral joint?
    a. spinalis
    b. semispinalis
    c. rotatores
    d. multifidus

9. Which of the following back muscles is innervated by dorsal primary rami of spinal nerves?
    a. latissmus dorsi
    b. rhomboid major
    c. serratus posterior superior
    d. splenius capitis

10. Which of the following muscles does NOT attach to transverse processes of vertebrae?
    a. semispinalis
    b. multifidus
    c. spinalis
    d. intertransversarii

11.   Which of the following muscles is attached to mamillary processes of lumbar vertebrae?
    a.   longissimus thoracis
    b.   multifidus
    c.   rotatores
    d.   spinalis

12.   The trapezius muscle is innervated by which nerve?
    a.   spinal accessory nerve
    b.   thoracodorsal nerve
    c.   dorsal scapular nerve
    d.   dorsal primary rami of spinal nerves

13.   Contraction of which muscle produces extension of the head?
    a.   spinalis cervicis
    b.   longus capitis
    c.   longus colli
    d.   sternocleidomastoid

14.   In the lumbar spine, the multifudus lumborum muscle originates from which structure?
    a.   spinous processes of the lumbar vertebrae
    b.   sacrotuberous ligament
    c.   posteromedial iliac crest
    d.   mamillary processes of the lumbar vertebrae

15.   Which muscles constitute the deepest muscle fasciculi located in the groove between the spinous and transverse processes?
    a.   multifudus
    b.   semispinalis
    c.   rotatores
    d.   longissimus

16.   Which muscle originates on the spinous process of the axis and inserts onto the transverse process of the atlas?
    a.   rectus capitis posterior major
    b.   obliquus capitis inferior
    c.   rectus capitis posterior minor
    d.   obliquus capitis superior

17.   Which of the following portions of the multifidus muscle group is the most highly developed in humans?
    a.   lumborum
    b.   thoracis
    c.   cervicis
    d.   capitis

18. Which of the following muscles is innervated by a posterior primary division (dorsal ramus)?
    a. trapezius
    b. rhomboid major
    c. serratus posterior superior
    d. obliquus capitis superior

19. Which of the following muscles is located most laterally?
    a. longissimus thoracis
    b. iliocostalis thoracis
    c. semispinalis thoracis
    d. spinalis thoracis

20. Which of the following muscles is considered to be an accessory muscle of respiration?
    a. latissimus dorsi
    b. rhomboid major
    c. serratus posterior superior
    d. iliocostalis thoracis

Answers

1. d. The mastoid process of the temporal bone serves as an attachment for several muscles, including the sternocleidomastoid, the longissimus capitis, the digastricus, and the splenius capitis muscles. The semispinalis capitis muscle attaches to the transverse processes of C4-T6 vertebrae and to the superior nuchal line of occipital bone but not to the mastoid process of the temporal bone.

2. d. The iliocostalis thoracic muscle attaches from the inferior six ribs to the superior six ribs, the rest of the statements are correct.

3. c. The rectus capitis posterior major muscles attache from the spinous process of the axis to the inferior nuchal line of the occipital bone and has no attachments to the atlas. The other muscles listed do attach to the atlas (C1 vertebra). The levator scapulae muscle attaches to the transverse process of the atlas, the rectus capitis posterior minor attaches to the posterior tubercle of the atlas, and the obliquus capitis superior attaches to the transverse process of the atlas.

4. d. The long rotator muscles attach from the transverse process of one vertebra to the spinous process of the second vertebra superior to its origin as opposed to short rotator muscles, which attach from the transverse process of one vertebra and insert on the spinous process of the vertebra above its origin.

5. d. This superficial muscle covers the inferior portion of the back. The origin of the latissimus dorsi is the spinous processes of T6-T12, the thoracolumbar fascia, iliac crest, and ribs 10 through 12. This muscle inserts in the floor of the intertubercular groove of the humerus. The actions of this muscle include extension, adduction, and medial rotation of the shoulder joint.

6. d. The three muscles of the erector spinae are the iliocostalis, longissimus, and spinalis in order from lateral to medial. The semispinalis, multifidus, and rotatores are parts of the deeper transversospinalis group.

7. a. The semispinalis muscle extends has three parts: the semispinalis thoracis, cervicis, and capitis, each named according to their superior attachment.

8. c. The rotators are short muscles that arise from the transverse process of one vertebra and insert into the spinous process of the vertebra above.

9. d. The splenius capitis is a deep back muscle. All deep back muscles are innervated by dorsal primary rami of spinal nerves. The latissmus dorsi is innervated by the thoracodorsal nerve, the rhomboid major by the dorsal scapular nerve, and the serratus posterior superior by the ventral rami of upper thoracic nerves.

10. c. Spinalis muscles originate from spinous processes and insert into spinous processes. The semispinalis and multifidus are two muscles of the fifth layer of back muscles that are also known as the transversospinalis muscles. They originate from transverse processes and insert into spinous processes. The intertransversarii muscles are located between transverse processes of successive vertebrae.

11. b. Multifidus muscles originate partially from mamillary processes of lumbar vertebrae. Longissimus thoracis originate partially from accessory processes of lumbar vertebrae.

12. a. The spinal part of the accessory nerve innervates the trapezius and sternocleidomastoid muscles. The thoracodorsal nerve innervates the latissmus dorsi muscle. The dorsal scapular nerve innervates the levator scapulae and the rhomboid major and minor muscles (second layer of back muscles). The dorsal primary rami of spinal nerves innervate deep back muscles.

13. a. The longus capitis, longus colli, and sternocleidomastoid muscles are all associated with the anterior aspect of the cervical vertebrae and thus produce flexion of the head.

14. d. The multifudus lumborum inserts on the spinous processes of vertebrae located two to four segments above; the sacrotuberous ligament and the posteromedial iliac crest represent the location of some of the insertions of the iliocostalis lumborum.

15. c. The longissimus muscle is part of the fifth layer of the back muscles. All others are part of the sixth layer, but the rotators are the deepest.

16. b. The rectus capitis posterior major begins at the spinous process of C2 and terminates at the occiput. The rectus capitis posterior minor begins at the posterior tubercle of the atlas and terminates at the occiput. The obliquus capitis superior arises from the transverse process of the atlas and inserts on the occiput.

17. a.   The multifidus lumborum is much more substantial than any of the
          other regions of this muscle (thoracic and cervicis regions). The
          other contributors to the transversospinalis muscle group (sixth
          layer of back muscles) also are most highly developed in a specific
          region of the spine. More specifically, the semispinalis capitis and
          rotatores thoracis muscles are the most highly developed portions
          of the other transversospinalis muscles.

18. d.   The first three layers of back muscles are either innervated by
          anterior primary divisions (ventral rami) or in the case of the
          trapezius muscles by cranial nerve IX (spinal accessory nerve).
          The deep back muscles (layers 4 through 6, i.e., splenius capitis
          and cervicis muscles, erector spinae muscle group, and the
          transversospinalis muscle group), suboccipital muscles,
          intertransversarii muscles, and interspinales muscles are all
          innervated by posterior primary divisions (dorsal rami). The
          obliquus capitis superior muscle is one of the suboccipital muscles
          and is therefore innervated by a posterior primary division
          (specifically the suboccipital nerve, which is the posterior primary
          division of the first cervical spinal cord segment).

19. b.   From lateral to medial, the erector spinae muscles are composed
          of the iliocostalis, longissimus, and spinalis muscles. The
          transversospinalis muscle group (semispinalis, multifidus, and
          rotatores muscles) is located medial to the iliocostalis and
          longissimus muscles.

20. c.   The third layer of back muscles, which are composed of the
          serratus posterior superior and serratus posterior inferior muscles,
          are considered to be accessory muscle of respiration. They are
          thought to help with forced inspiration and expiration, respectively.
          The latissimus dorsi muscle functions to adduct, internally rotate,
          and extend the upper extremity by acting on the humerus; the
          rhomboid major (muscle) retracts the scapula; and the iliocostalis
          thoracic muscle laterally flexes the thoracic region to the
          same side.

CHAPTER 12

Arthrology and Syndesmology of the Axial Skeleton

1. What kind of cartilage covers the articulating surfaces of each superior and inferior articular process of the vertebrae?
   a. annular
   b. reticular
   c. elastic
   d. hyaline

2. Which component has been found to be the primary load-bearing structure of the intervertebral disc?
   a. annulus fibrosus
   b. nucleus pulposus
   c. vertebral end-plate
   d. Sharpey's fibers

3. The nucleus pulposus is thickest in which region of the spine?
   a. lumbar spine
   b. inferior half of the thoracic spine
   c. superior half of the thoracic spine
   d. cervical spine

4. Which statement is FALSE concerning the intervertebral foramen (IVF)?
   a. a pair (left and right) of IVFs are located between all of the adjacent vertebrae from C2 to the sacrum
   b. the pedicles of adjacent vertebrae form the roof and the floor of the IVF
   c. IVFs become smaller in spinal flexion and larger in spinal extension
   d. the IVFs are smaller in the cervical region

5. Which is TRUE of the zygapophysial joints (also known as Z joints, or facet joints)?
   a. they are classified as condylar joints
   b. they are surrounded by a fibrous joint capsule along both their anterior and posterior surfaces
   c. they are oriented in approximately the same plane of articulation throughout the spine
   d. they are innervated by posterior primary divisions (dorsal rami) of spinal nerves

6. Which is TRUE of the transverse ligament of the atlas (transverse portion of the cruciform ligament)?
   a. it is the weakest part of the cruciform ligament
   b. it prevents the atlas from rotating upon the axis
   c. it forms a synovial joint with the odontoid process
   d. it has broad attachments to the medial aspect of the left and right occipital condyles

7. The tectorial membrane lies most directly between the cruciform ligament and which of the following?
   a. ligamentum flavum
   b. dura mater
   c. anterior atlanto-occipital membrane
   d. posterior atlanto-occipital membrane

8. Which of the following ligaments courses from the crest of the head of a rib to the intervertebral disc, dividing the costovertebral (costocorporeal) synovial articulation into two halves?
   a. articular capsule
   b. intra-articular ligament
   c. radiate ligament
   d. superior costocorporeal ligament

9. Which of the following joints is a syndesmosis?
   a. axial-occipital
   b. lateral atlantoaxial
   c. sacroiliac
   d. costotransverse

10. Which of the following ligaments limits hyperextension of the vertebral column?
    a. interspinous
    b. intertransverse
    c. ligamentum flavum
    d. anterior longitudinal

11. Whiplash injury from a rear-end collision would tear which of the following ligaments?
    a. posterior longitudinal ligament (PLL)
    b. anterior longitudinal ligament (ALL)
    c. ligamentum nuchae
    d. ligamentum flavum

12. Which of the following is a symphysis type of joint?
    a. facet joints
    b. atlanto-occipital joints
    c. intervertebral discs
    d. sternoclavicular joints

13. Which of the following ligaments is anterior to the spinal cord?
    a. ligamentum flavum
    b. interspinous ligament
    c. supraspinous ligament
    d. posterior longitudinal ligament (PLL)

14. What is the main motion at the atlantoaxial joints?
    a. rotation
    b. flexion
    c. extension
    d. lateral flexion

15. What type of joint are synchondroses?
    a. fibrous joint
    b. synovial joint
    c. cartilaginous joint
    d. suture

16. Which bony structure does NOT border the intervertebral foramen?
    a. intervertebral disc
    b. superior facet
    c. lamina
    d. inferior facet

17. Which of the following is NOT part of the axial skeleton?
    a. coccyx
    b. sternum
    c. rib
    d. ilium

18. What is a secondary curve of the vertebral column?
    a. scoliosis
    b. curve that developed during the fetal period
    c. kyphosis
    d. curve that develops after birth

19. The tectorial membrane is the superior continuation of what structure?
    a. ligamentum nuchae
    b. anterior longitudinal ligament
    c. ligamentum flavum
    d. posterior longitudinal ligament

20. The ligamentum nuchae extends from what structure to what structure?
    a. atlas to T12
    b. inion and median nuchal crest to the spinous process of C7
    c. lateral masses of the axis to the transverse processes of T1
    d. external occipital protuberance and occipital crest to the spinous process of T12

21. Which ligament attaches the transverse ligament of the atlas to the anterior margin of the foramen magnum?
    a. cranial crus of the cruciate ligament
    b. anterior atlanto-occipital membrane
    c. alar ligament
    d. apical ligament

22. Which of the following classifications does NOT describe the zygapophyseal joints?
    a. syndesmosis
    b. gliding
    c. plane
    d. diarthrodial

23. Which ligament is found within the confines of the neural canal?
    a. anterior longitudinal ligament
    b. posterior longitudinal ligament
    c. interspinous ligament
    d. supraspinous ligament

24. What type of cartilage directly covers the articular surfaces of the bodies of adjacent vertebrae?
    a. fibrous
    b. hyaline
    c. elastic
    d. they are not covered with cartilage

25. Which of the following structures attaches from the tip of the odontoid process to the anterior margin of the foramen magnum?
    a. transverse ligament of the atlas
    b. alar ligament
    c. apical ligament
    d. tectorial membrane

26. Choose the INCORRECT statement regarding the intervertebral discs.
    a. there are 23 of them in the adult
    b. they account for approximately 25% of the height of the vertebral column
    c. they form part of the anterior wall of the IVF
    d. in regions of the anterior spinal curves, the disc is thicker on its posterior margin

Answers

1. d. Hyaline cartilage is flexible and somewhat elastic. Elastic or reticular cartilages do not cover the articular processes. The annular cartilage is located in the trachea.

2. a. The annulus fibrosus can maintain its function (e.g., load bearing) even when the nucleus has been removed.

3. a. The nucleus pulposus is thickest in the lumbar spine, followed by the cervical region; it is thinnest in the thoracic spine.

4. c. Flexion of the spine creates a separation of the zygapophyseal joints, creating an augmentation of the size of the IVF.

5. d. The junction between a superior articular facet and inferior articular facet of two adjacent vertebrae is known as a zygapophyseal joint (Z joint). These joints are also known as facet joints, apophyseal joints, and interlaminar joints. The Z joints are classified as diarthrodial, planar joints. Each Z joint is surrounded by a capsule, which in turn is internally lined by a synovial membrane. Anteriorly, the ligamentum flavum takes the place of the joint capsule. The Z joint side of the ligamentum flavum is also lined by a synovial membrane. Each Z joint of a typical vertebra receives innervation from posterior primary divisions, or dorsal rami (more specifically, the medial branches of these nerves). The shape and plane of articulation of each of these joints are very important in determining the direction of movement and the range of motion that can occur between adjacent vertebrae. These variables (shape and plane of articulation) change in each region of the vertebral column (cervical, thoracic, and lumbar regions).

6. c. The transverse ligament of the atlas (transverse portion of the cruciform ligament) courses from one lateral mass (medial aspect) of the atlas to the other and is very strong. It passes posterior to the odontoid process and forms a diarthrodial (synovial) trochoid joint with that structure. This ligament allows the atlas to pivot on the axis and also holds the atlas in its proper position. This latter function protects the spinal cord. It also prevents the atlas from gliding anteriorly during forward flexion.

7. b. The tectorial membrane is the superior extension of the posterior longitudinal ligament. It begins by attaching to the posterior aspect of the vertebral body of C2, crosses over the odontoid process, and inserts onto the anterior rim of the foramen magnum (clivus). This ligament limits both flexion and extension of the atlas and occiput. It is located between the cruciform ligament, which is anterior, and the anterior aspect of the spinal dura mater, which is posterior.

8. b. There are three types of ligaments associated with the costocorporeal (costovertebral) articulation: (1) the joint capsules (for both the superior and inferior parts of these joint), (2) the intra-articular ligaments (which course from the crest of the head of the rib directly to the adjacent and medially located intervertebral disc), and (3) the radiate ligaments (which cover the other two ligaments and course from the head of a rib to the two vertebral bodies and the intervertebral disc in between). Note: There is no superior costocorporeal ligament. The superior costotransverse ligament is associated with the costotransverse joint and passes from a transverse process to the neck of the rib below.

9. a. A syndesmosis is a joint consisting of two bones connected by one or more ligaments. The spine is unique in that it has several examples of such joints. The unique syndesmoses include (listed from posterosuperior to anteroinferior): (1) axial-occipital syndesmosis (located between the axis and the occiput, ligaments includes the tectorial membrane, cruciform, apical-odontoid, and alar ligaments); (2) ligamentum nuchae (syndesmosis between occiput and C1-C7); (3) supraspinous syndesmosis (supraspinous ligament); (4) interspinous syndesmosis (interspinous ligament); (5) laminar syndesmosis (ligamentum flavum); and (6) intertransverse syndesmosis (intertransverse ligament).

10. d. The anterior longitudinal ligament is quite wide and covers the anterior aspect of the vertebral bodies from the level of C1 to the sacrum. Generally speaking, this ligament has rather strong attachments to the vertebral bodies but rather weak attachments to the intervertebral discs. However, the precise attachments are somewhat more complex than this. The anterior longitudinal ligament functions to limit extension of the spine. The interspinous ligament, supraspinous ligament, and ligamentum flavum all function to limit hyperflexion of the vertebral column.

11. b. Whiplash injury includes hyperextension of cervical vertebrae that may tear the anterior longitudinal ligament that limits extension of cervical spine. All of the other ligaments limit flexion of the cervical spine; accordingly, they may be torn in hyperflexion injuries.

12. c. IVDs are fibrocartilaginous joints (symphysis = secondary cartilaginous joints). Facet joints are plane synovial joints. The atlanto-occipital joint is a condylar synovial joint, and the sternoclavicular joint is a saddle type of synovial joint.

13. d. The posterior longitudinal ligament connects the back of vertebral bodies and forms an anterior boundary to the vertebral canal; accordingly, it is anterior to the spinal cord. All other ligaments are posterior to the spinal cord.

14. a. There are three atlantoaxial joints. The median atlantoaxial joint is a pivot (trochoid) type of synovial joint where the main motion is rotation. The two lateral atlantoaxial joints are plane (gliding) types of synovial joints where the main motion is also rotation.

15. c. A synchondrosis is a cartilaginous joint such as the epiphyseal plates between the diaphysis and epiphyses of long bones, and costosternal joints. Fibrous joints include syndesmoses and sutures. Synovial joints are enclosed by a joint capsule and contain synovial fluid.

16. c. The pedicle of the vertebra above forms the roof of the IVF, the two vertebral bodies and the disc between them forms the anterior border of the IVF, the pedicle of the vertebra below forms the floor of the IVF, and the zygapophyseal joint forms the posterior border of the IVF. The lamina is posterior to the IVF and does not border it.

17. d. The axial skeleton includes the skull, hyoid bone, vertebral column, and the thoracic cage. The ilium is part of the appendicular skeleton.

18. d. At birth, the spine is "C" shaped with a posterior apex. This is the primary curve. As the infant lifts the head and later begins to stand and walk, the cervical and lumbar curves reverse, forming secondary curves. Even though secondary curves are kyphotic, a "kyphosis" refers to a pathologic curve. A scoliosis is an abnormal lateral curve of the spine.

19. d. The superior continuation of the posterior longitudinal ligament is called the membranatectoria, occipitoaxial ligament, or tectorial membrane. It attaches to the occipital bone medial to the hypoglossal canal and is closely adherent to the cranial dura once inside the cranial vault.

20. b. The ligamentum nuchae is the superior continuation of the supraspinous ligament and attaches to the external occipital protuberance (inion), the median nuchal line, the posterior tubercle of the atlas, and the spinous processes of the cervical vertebrae down to C7.

21. a. The transverse ligament of the atlas attaches on the two lateral masses of the atlas and serves to hold the odontoid process of the axis tight against the anterior arch of the atlas. The transverse ligament of the atlas is stabilized by two fibrous cords, one superior and one inferior. These are known as the cranial and caudal crus, respectively, and the entire complex is called the cruciate ligament. Other names include the superior longitudinal band and inferior longitudinal band, respectively.

22. a. The zygapophyseal joint, or the Z joint, facet joints, interlaminar joints, or apophyseal joints are synovial, diarthrodial, plane (shape of the articular surfaces), gliding (surfaces glide on each other), uniaxial joints formed by the prezygapophysis (superior articular facets) and the postzygapophysis (inferior articular facets) of two adjacent vertebrae. A syndesmosis is a type of fibrous joint involving an interosseous ligament.

23. b. The posterior longitudinal ligament lies within the neural canal posterior to the vertebral bodies.

24. b. The intervertebral joint is classified as a secondary cartilaginous joint. The surfaces of the vertebral bodies are covered with a thin plate of hyaline cartilage.

25. c. The apical ligament (suspensory ligament) is a single ligament that attaches from the tip of dens (odontoid process) of the axis to the anterior margin of foramen magnum. It may be the remains of the embryonic notochord as there is no disc there.

26. d. In regions of the spinal column where the spinal curve is anterior (lordosis), the intervertebral discs are thicker on their anterior margin, thus forcing the anterior curvature to the spinal column.

CHAPTER 13

Anatomy of the Central Nervous System and Related Structures

CONTENT AREAS

- Cerebrum
- Brainstem and cerebellum
- Spinal cord and meninges
- Blood vascular relationships
- Ventricles and cerebrospinal fluid
- Development
- Histology

1. When cerebrospinal fluid is withdrawn by lumbar puncture, which structure will NOT be penetrated by the needle?
   a. dura mater
   b. subdural space
   c. pia mater
   d. subarachnoid space

2. Which structure acts as a relay station in the central nervous system?
   a. occipital lobe
   b. temporalis
   c. pituitary gland
   d. thalamus

3. Which structure is immediately external to the myelin sheath of a nerve?
   a. endoneurium
   b. Schwann cytoplasm
   c. basement membrane
   d. axolemma

4. The sacral elements of the spinal cord may be crushed by a fracture of which vertebrae?
   a. L1
   b. L3
   c. L5
   d. S1 and S2

5. The cerebellum is an outgrowth of which embryonic brain vesicle?
   a. diencephalon
   b. mesencephalon
   c. prosencephalon
   d. metencephalon

6. Which of the following is a cerebral commissure?
   a. corpus callosum
   b. crus cerebri
   c. internal capsule
   d. external capsule

7. Which of the following areas does the middle cerebral artery NOT supply?
   a. motor area
   b. primary visual area
   c. premotor area
   d. auditory projection area

8. Broca's area is located in which of the following areas?
   a. superior temporal gyrus
   b. superior frontal gyrus
   c. inferior frontal gyrus
   d. precentral gyrus

9. The cerebral aqueduct is located within which brain region?
   a. mesencephalon
   b. telencephalon
   c. metencephalon
   d. diencephalons

10. The basal ganglia do NOT include which of the following structures?
    a. putamen
    b. caudate nucleus
    c. globus pallidus
    d. red nucleus

11. Which of the following is a function of the hippocampus?
    a. smell
    b. taste
    c. memory
    d. vision

12. Which of the following is NOT an ascending tract in the spinal cord?
    a. ventral spinothalamic
    b. corticospinal
    c. spinotectal
    d. spino-olivary

13. Which lamina of the dorsal horn of the spinal cord is known as the substantia gelatinosa of Rolando?
    a. I
    b. II
    c. IV
    d. VI

14. The fasciculus cuneatus conveys information from the:
    a. ipsilateral upper extremity
    b. contralateral upper extremity
    c. ipsilateral lower extremity
    d. contralateral lower extremity

15. The paleospinothalamic tract conveys:
    a. light touch
    b. proprioception
    c. vibration
    d. pain and temperature

16. At the caudal level of the medulla, what percentage of the fibers of the corticospinal tract cross at the pyramidal decussation?
    a. 90% to 100%
    b. 80% to 90%
    c. 70% to 80%
    d. 60% to 70%

17. This descending tract originates in the superior colliculus and is involved with the orientation toward a stimulus in the environment by reflex turning of the head.
    a. rubrospinal
    b. reticulospinal
    c. tectospinal
    d. vestibulospinal

18. The lateral division fibers of the dorsal root utilize the dorsolateral tract of _____ to enter the spinal cord.
    a. Lisfranc
    b. Lister
    c. Lissauer
    d. Lichten

19. Which of the following structures separates the primary motor cortex from the primary sensory cortex?
    a. central sulcus
    b. longitudinal fissure
    c. cingulate sulcus
    d. lateral fissure

20. Which of the following innervates the meninges located within the supratentorial region of the cranial cavity?
    a. C1-C3 spinal nerves
    b. vagus nerve
    c. suboccipital nerve
    d. trigeminal nerve

21. Cerebrospinal fluid courses between which layers of the meninges?
    a. dura mater and pia mater
    b. arachnoid mater and pia mater
    c. dura mater and arachnoid mater
    d. pia mater and the cortex

22. Which of the following is the group of crossing fibers that convey information to perform voluntary, purposeful movements?
    a. internal arcuate fibers
    b. ventral white commissural fibers
    c. dorsal tegmental decussation fibers
    d. pyramidal decussation fibers

23. An occlusion of the posterior cerebral artery would result in a deficit of which of the following?
    a. motor speech
    b. general sensation from the knee, leg, and foot
    c. vision
    d. voluntary, purposeful movements of muscles located in the region of the head to the hip

24. The cell bodies of the oculomotor nerve are located within what part of the central nervous system?
    a. midbrain
    b. frontal lobe
    c. rostral pons
    d. floor of the fourth ventricle

25. The spinal cord ends at what vertebral level?
    a. T10
    b. L1
    c. L6
    d. S1

26. What are cells that produce myelin in the peripheral nervous system called?
    a. microglia
    b. oligodendrocytes
    c. astrocytes
    d. neurolemmocytes (Schwann) cells

27. Ascending tracts in the white matter of the spinal cord carry what kind of information?
    a. sensory
    b. motor
    c. both sensory and motor
    d. autonomic

28. At what vertebral level would the spinal segment that gives rise to the L5 spinal nerve be located?
    a. between L4 and L5 vertebrae
    b. between L5 and S1 vertebrae
    c. between T5 and T6 vertebrae
    d. between T11 and T12 vertebrae

29. What kind of information is found in the ventral root of a spinal nerve?
    a. GSE, GVE
    b. GSA, GVA
    c. GVE, GVA
    d. GSE, GSA

30. The thalamus and hypothalamus are part of what brain region?
    a. prosencephalon
    b. diencephalon
    c. mesencephalon
    d. telencephalon

1. c. The pia mater is adherent to the spinal cord, which ends at the L2 spinal level in the adult. Inferior to the termination of the spinal cord (conus medularis), the pia mater continues as the filum terminale. Because lumbar punctures are administered below the L2 spine, it is unlikely to puncture pia mater.

2. d. The thalamus is composed of several nuclei, many of which serve as important relay centers for the sensory pathways.

3. b. The myelin sheath is composed of the membrane of Schwann cells that is wrapped around axons for insulation. Most of the cytoplasm is excluded from this part of the membrane and therefore it is external to the sheath itself.

4. a. The inferior end of the spinal cord is at the L2 spinal level, which corresponds to the sacral cord. Inferior to L2 is the location of the cauda equina. Therefore, a fracture of L1 would potentially crush the spinal cord.

5. d. The telencephalon forms the cerebral hemispheres, the diencephalon forms the thalamus and hypothalamus, the mesencephalon forms the midbrain, the metencephalon forms the pons and cerebellum, and the myelencephalon forms the medulla oblongata.

6. a. Commissures are white matter tracts that communicate between hemispheres of the brain, and thus cross the midline. They include the corpus callosum, anterior commissure, and posterior commissure. The crus cerebri, internal capsule, and external capsule carry information ipsilaterally.

7. b. The middle cerebral artery supplies the motor and premotor areas and the auditory projection areas. The posterior cerebral artery supplies the primary visual area.

8. c. Broca's area occupies the opercular and triangular parts of the inferior frontal gyrus. This area is involved with speech. Damage to this area results in motor or expressive aphasia. The patients are unable to express themselves using language; however, they are capable of understanding language. The control of muscles used in speech is not affected.

9. a. The mesencephalon or midbrain contains a narrow cavity called the cerebral aqueduct of Sylvius. It transmits the cerebrospinal fluid from the third to the fourth ventricle.

10. d. The basal ganglia are groups of neurons related to the diencephalon but separated from it by the internal capsule. They include caudate nucleus, putamen, globus pallidus, subthalamic nuclei, and substantia nigra (in the midbrain). They help to control movement. The red nucleus is located in the midbrain.

11. c. The hippocampus, which is part of the limbic system, is important in the processing, but not storage of, declarative (cognitive) memory. It is formed by the gray and white matter of two gyri rolled together and is located in the medial temporal lobe.

12. b. The major ascending tracts of the spinal cord include the ventral and dorsal spinothalamic tracts, the spinotectal tract, the ventral and dorsal spinocerebellar tracts, and the spinoreticular tract. Other ascending tracts are spino-olivary and spinovestibular tracts. The corticospinal tract is a descending motor tract.

13. b. Lamina I is known as the marginal zone of Waldeyer; laminae III and IV are known as the nucleus proprius; and laminae VI to X are not named.

14. a. The fasciculus cuneatus conveys information from the ipsilateral upper extremity. The fasciculus gracilis conveys information from the ipsilateral lower extremity.

15. d. Light touch, proprioception, and vibration are carried mainly by the dorsal columns. The ventral spinothalamic tract conveys some light touch and pressure. The paleospinothalamic tract is the subdivision of the lateral spinothalamic tract that carries slow (C-type) pain fibers.

16. b. Most anatomists agree that 80% to 90% of the fibers of the corticospinal tract cross over.

17. c. The rubrospinal tract originates in the red nucleus; the reticulospinal tract originates in the medullary and pontine reticular formation; and the vestibulospinal tract originates in the lateral vestibular nucleus.

18. c. The tract of Lissauer receives small dorsal root fibers and axons originating from dorsal horn neurons (primary afferent nociceptive axons, pain-carrying fibers).

19. a. The central sulcus separates the precentral gyrus, which is the primary motor cortex, from the postcentral gyrus, which is the primary sensory cortex. The longitudinal fissure separates the two hemispheres. The cingulate sulcus is seen on a medial view and separates the superior frontal gyrus from the cingulate gyrus. The lateral fissure separates the frontal lobe from the temporal lobe.

20. d. Branches of the trigeminal nerve innervate the meninges superior to the tentorium cerebelli (supratentorial cranial cavity). Branches of C1-C3 spinal nerves innervate the meninges in the infratentorial cranial cavity.

21. b. Cerebrospinal fluid flows in the subarachnoid space, which is between the arachnoid mater and pia mater.

22. d. Information concerning voluntary, purposeful movements is conveyed in the corticospinal or pyramidal tract. These fibers cross in the pyramidal decussation at the junction of the cord and medulla. The dorsal columns, conveying information concerning proprioception, vibration, and touch, cross as internal arcuate fibers in the caudal medulla. The spinothalamic tracts conveying pain and temperature information cross in the ventral white commissure of the spinal cord. The tectospinal tract fibers cross in the midbrain as the dorsal tegmental decussation.

23. c. The posterior cerebral artery supplies the occipital lobe as well as the inferior aspect of the temporal lobe. The primary visual cortex is located in the occipital lobe; therefore, part of the visual field would be affected if this artery were occluded. The middle cerebral artery supplies the lateral aspect of the frontal, temporal, and parietal lobes, and an occlusion would therefore affect motor speech and voluntary purposeful movements from the head to the hip, as well as other functions in these areas. The anterior cerebral artery supplies the medial aspect of the frontal and parietal lobes, and an occlusion would therefore affect general sensation from the knee, leg, and foot.

24. a. The cell bodies of the oculomotor nuclear complex are located in the midbrain of the brainstem. The oculomotor nerve emerges from the ventral side of the midbrain.

25. b. In the human, the spinal cord terminates in the neural canal of L1 (sometimes L2) vertebra as the conus medullaris.

26. d. Neurolemmocytes, sometimes called Schwann cells, produce the myelin sheath in the peripheral nervous system.

27. a. The white matter of the spinal cord carries ascending (sensory) tracts and descending (motor) tracts.

28. d. A spinal segment is the cross-sectional area of the spinal cord that gives rise to a pair of spinal nerves. There are 31 pairs of spinal nerves and therefore 31 spinal segments. The spinal segment that gives rise to spinal nerves L5 is located toward the inferior aspect of the spinal cord in the region of T11-T12 vertebrae.

29. a. Spinal nerves carry both sensory and motor information. Bell-Magendie's law says that the dorsal root of the spinal nerve carries sensory information and the ventral root carries motor information. Information carried in the neuron is classified as to GVE (motor), GSE (motor), GSA (sensory), and GVA (sensory). There are other functional components of neurons, but none of these are carried in spinal nerves (i.e., SVA, SSA, SVE).

30. b. The caudal portion of the prosencephalon is called the diencephalons and consists of the thalamus and hypothalamus.

CHAPTER 14

Anatomy of the Peripheral and Autonomic Nervous Systems

1. Which of the following structures does NOT transmit any visceral efferent information?
   a. parabrachial nucleus
   b. central gray matter
   c. thalamus
   d. amygdala

2. From which cranial nuclei do parasympathetic efferent signals emerge?
   a. II, III, and X
   b. III, V, IX, and X
   c. V, VII, and X
   d. III, VII, IX, and X

3. Which nerve roots unite to form the ansa cervicalis of the cervical plexus?
   a. C1 and C5
   b. C2 and C3
   c. C3 and C4
   d. C4 and C5

4. This nerve provides articular branches to the elbow and wrist joints and motor innervation to the majority of the muscles of the anterior forearm.
   a. ulnar
   b. radial
   c. median
   d. axillary

5. These nerves innervate the structures located on the anterior aspect of the vertebral canal.
    a. lateral branches of the posterior primary divisions
    b. recurrent meningeal nerves
    c. anterior primary divisions
    d. medial branches of the posterior primary divisions

6. Which of the following contains the cell bodies of preganglionic neurons of the parasympathetic nervous system?
    a. cranial nerve nuclei and sacral spinal cord
    b. cervical and thoracic spinal cord
    c. cranial nerve nuclei and cervical spinal cord
    d. thoracic and lumbar spinal cord

7. Following radical resection of a primary tongue tumor, a patient has lost general sensation on the anterior two thirds of the tongue. This is probably due to injuries of which of the following nerves?
    a. trigeminal nerve
    b. facial nerve
    c. glossopharyngeal nerve
    d. vagus nerve

8. Which of the following statements concerning the phrenic nerve is TRUE?
    a. contains only efferent fibers
    b. injury could cause difficulty in expiration
    c. supplies the pericardium, mediastinal pleura, and diaphragm
    d. enters the thorax by passing in front of the subclavian vein

9. Bilateral severance of which of the following nerves would be most life threatening?
    a. trigeminal nerve
    b. facial nerve
    c. vagus nerve
    d. spinal accessory nerve

10. Which of the following conditions result from severance of the abducens nerve proximal to its entrance into the orbit?
    a. ptosis of the upper eyelid
    b. loss of the pupil's ability to dilate
    c. external strabismus (lateral deviation)
    d. internal strabismus (medial deviation)

11.   Which of the following is NOT a branch originating from a spinal nerve?
a.   ventral primary rami
b.   dorsal primary rami
c.   white rami communicans
d.   gray rami communicans

12.   Preganglionic neurons of the sympathetic nervous system originate from which area?
a.   dorsal horns of the gray matter of the spinal cord
b.   lateral horns of the gray matter of the spinal cord
c.   ventral horns of the gray matter of the spinal cord
d.   dorsal root ganglia

13.   Which of the following cranial nerves does NOT contain parasympathetic fibers?
a.   oculomotor
b.   facial
c.   trigeminal
d.   vagus

14.   Which of the following does NOT give rise to secretomotor fibers?
a.   submandibular ganglion
b.   otic ganglion
c.   pterygopalatine ganglion
d.   trigeminal ganglion

15.   Which of the following cranial nerves contains preganglionic parasympathetic fibers to the parotid gland?
a.   oculomotor
b.   facial
c.   glossopharyngeal
d.   vagus

16.   A 28-year-old woman sustains an injury to the left arm during a fall off of her bicycle. Radiographs done at your clinic show an oblique fracture through the mid-shaft of the humerus. Which nerve is most likely to be injured by the mid-shaft fracture of the humerus?
a.   radial nerve
b.   median nerve
c.   musculocutaneous nerve
d.   ulnar nerve

17.   A 24-year-old man is thrown from a pick-up truck during an accident and sustains an injury to the left neck, shoulder, and upper limb. Examination in the emergency department does not reveal any cuts, fractures, or dislocations, and he is sent home. The following day, he is experiencing several maladies and seeks help from you at your clinic. You perform your examination and find that the patient has sustained a lateral traction injury to the superior roots of the brachial plexus. Which of the following signs would you NOT expect to find in this patient?
a.   dropped left shoulder
b.   left scapula that falls laterally
c.   inability to rotate the humerus medially
d.   paresis of muscles of the anterior aspect of left arm

18.   A 29-year-old man sustains a severe nerve compression injury to his left upper leg as a result of a fall from a motorcycle. Examination of this patient at your office reveals a contusion surrounding the head and neck of the fibula. Which nerve is susceptible to direct injury by a severe compression force applied to the lateral aspect of the head and neck of the fibula?
a.   common peroneal nerve
b.   tibial nerve
c.   obturator nerve
d.   saphenous nerve

19.   Gray rami communicans leave the paravertebral ganglia and carry postganglionic GVE neurons to what nerves?
a.   T1 through L2 spinal nerves
b.   C1 through T12 spinal nerves
c.   all spinal nerves
d.   only those spinal nerves below the diaphragm

20.   Choose the incorrect statement with regard to the brachial plexus.
a.   the anterior division of brachial plexus trunks innervates muscles that are flexors
b.   the cords of the brachial plexus are named according to their relationship to the axillary artery
c.   the brachial plexus is derived from dorsal rami of C5, C6, C7, C8, and T1
d.   the posterior cord is formed by the posterior divisions of all three trunks

21.   For the nervous system to detect stimuli, what must be present?
a.   neurotransmitters
b.   receptors
c.   myofibrils
d.   neurofibrils

22. Which of the following structures directly contributes to the formation of the spinal nerve?
    a. ventral rami, dorsal rami
    b. ventral root, dorsal root
    c. recurrent meningeal, dorsal rami
    d. dorsal root, dorsal rami

23. Spinal nerve C7 exits the intervertebral foramen located between which two of the following vertebrae?
    a. C4, C5
    b. C5, C6
    c. C6, C7
    d. C7, C8

24. Which branch of the spinal nerve carries GSE information to the muscles of the anterior and lateral trunk and all of the muscles of the limbs?
    a. recurrent meningeal nerve
    b. ventral ramus
    c. dorsal ramus
    d. rami communicans

25. How would axons that release, and receptors that respond to norepinephrine and/or epinephrine, be classified?
    a. adrenergic
    b. cholinergic
    c. muscarinic
    d. nicotinic

26. Preganglionic sympathetic fibers that will influence effector tissues in the orbit will synapse in which of the following structures?
    a. stellate ganglion
    b. celiac ganglion
    c. superior cervical ganglion
    d. middle cervical ganglion

27. Through what structure will preganglionic sympathetic fibers leave the spinal nerve in order to enter the sympathetic chain?
    a. ventral ramus
    b. dorsal ramus
    c. gray ramus communicans
    d. white ramus communicans

28. To say that most organs served by the autonomic nervous system (ANS) have "dual innervation" means what?
   a. it takes two postganglionic neurons to achieve the desired response
   b. the organs are innervated by both sympathetic and parasympathetic neurons
   c. both a preganglionic and a postganglionic neuron go to the organ
   d. it must receive innervation from at least two of the splanchnic nerves

29. General visceral afferent (GVA) fibers conveying pain information from viscera that converge in the dorsal horn with general somatic afferent (GSA) fibers and manifest as referred pain provide an example of which of the following?
   a. viscerosomatic pain
   b. somatovisceral pain
   c. viscerovisceral pain
   d. somatosomatic pain

30. Ventral rami contain which of the following fibers?
   a. only sensory
   b. only motor
   c. both sensory and motor
   d. both sympathetic and parasympathetic

Answers

1. c. The thalamus receives information from the periphery and transmits it to the cerebral cortex. It does not send information back to the periphery. Other structures listed in the question do.

2. d. There are no II and V cranial parasympathetic nuclei.

3. b. C1 forms the superior root of the ansa cervicalis; parts of C3, C4, and C5 nerve roots form the phrenic nerve.

4. c. The ulnar nerve provides motor innervation to the majority of the intrinsic muscles of the palm and the radial nerve to the posterior arm and forearm. The axillary nerve goes to the teres minor and deltoid muscles.

5. b. The anterior primary divisions form the lumbar plexus; the medial branches of the posterior primary divisions innervate those fibers that supply the spinous process; and the lateral branches of the posterior primary divisions supply motor innervation to the erector spinae muscles.

6. a. The cell bodies of the preganglionic parasympathetic nervous system are located in the nuclei associated with cranial nerves III, VII, IX and X and the sacral cord. The sympathetic preganglionic neuron cell bodies are located in the spinal cord segments T1-L2.

7. a. Although the facial nerve innervates the anterior two thirds of the tongue, its innervation is for taste sensation rather than general sensation. The trigeminal nerve is associated with general sensation of the anterior two thirds of the tongue.

8. c. The phrenic nerve arises from the ventral rami of C3 through C5 nerves and is the sole source of motor innervation to the diaphragm. The phrenic nerve also supplies sensory innervation to the diaphragm, pericardium, and mediastinal pleura.

9. c. Because the vagus nerve is responsible for about 75% of parasympathetic activity of the body, which regulates thoracic and abdominal visceral function, death is more likely to ensue following bilateral vagotomy. Bilateral section of the other nerves would have serious, but not life-threatening, consequences.

10. d. The abducens nerve innervates the lateral rectus muscle of the eye. Paralysis of this muscle causes medial deviation of the eye.

11. d. Gray rami communicans (31 pairs) are branches from sympathetic trunk ganglia to spinal nerves. They carry postganglionic sympathetic fibers. All of the other listed branches, as well as the recurrent meningeal nerve (sinovertebral nerve), are branches of spinal nerves.

12. b. Preganglionic neurons of the sympathetic nervous system originate in the lateral horns of TI-L2 spinal cord segments (thoracolumbar). They innervate smooth muscle, cardiac muscles, sweat glands, and adrenal medulla (GVE). Dorsal horns contain sensory neurons. Ventral horns contain motor neurons (GSE), and dorsal root ganglia contain sensory neurons (GSA).

13. c. The four cranial nerves that contain parasympathetic fibers are oculomotor, facial, glossopharyngeal, and vagus nerves.

14. d. Trigeminal ganglion is the sensory ganglion of cranial nerve V and is involved with all sensory functions of the trigeminal nerve. All of the other ganglia listed are involved with the autonomic secretomotor innervation of glands.

15. c. The parotid gland is stimulated to secrete saliva by the glossopharyngeal nerve. The preganglionic parasympathetic fibers from this nerve travel through the lesser petrosal nerve to the otic ganglion. The postganglionic parasympathetic fibers are carried through the auriculotemporal nerve to the parotid gland.

16. a. The radial nerve travels in the radial groove of the humerus and is subject to injury during midshaft fractures.

17. c. Lateral traction injuries resulting from excessive displacement of the head to the opposite side and depression of the shoulder on the same side produce signs and symptoms associated with damage to C5 and C6 nerve roots. This condition is also known as Erb-Duchenne palsy. The clinical picture involves the dorsal scapular nerve—dropped shoulder and scapula falls laterally; the suprascapular nerve—loss of lateral rotators, the axillary nerve—humerus rotates medially due to loss of lateral rotators and unopposed pectoralis major muscle, and the musculocutaneous nerve—paresis of muscles of the anterior arm and the muscles that pronate the forearm due to loss of biceps brachii muscle producing a sign called "waiter's tip." There is no loss of medial rotation of the humerus.

18. a. The common peroneal nerve travels around the proximal head of the fibula and is susceptible to injury. Damage to the common peroneal at the head of the fibula could result in a loss of innervation of the muscles that dorsiflex the foot and evert the foot.

19. c. White rami communicans carry the preganglionic axon from the spinal nerve to the paravertebral ganglia from spinal segments T1 to L2. Gray rami carry the ganglionic axon from the paravertebral chain back to the spinal nerve and connect to all spinal nerves.

20. c. All of the peripheral nerve plexi are derived from the ventral rami of the spinal nerves, not the dorsal rami.

21. b. The nervous system is a stimulus response system; for stimuli to be detected, there must be a receptor designed to detect that stimulus.

22. b. The spinal nerve is formed by the union of the dorsal (posterior) root and the ventral (anterior) root as they come together at the intervertebral foramen.

23. c. Spinal nerves exit the vertebral column through the intervertebral foramen located between two adjacent vertebrae. In the cervical region, the nerve is numbered according to the vertebra it exits above. So C7 spinal nerve would exit superior to C7, or between C6 and C7 vertebrae.

24. b. The ventral ramus (anterior primary ramus) supplies all motor, sensory, and sympathetic fibers to the anterior and lateral muscles and skin of the neck and trunk and all of the muscles and skin of the limbs, including the superficial back muscles. GSE is general somatic efferent information supplying motor input to skeletal muscles in these regions.

25. a. Adrenergic refers to those axons that release and those receptors that are activated by epinephrine or related substances (norepinephrine). The term particularly refers to the sympathetic nerve fibers that release norepinephrine.

26. c. The cell bodies of preganglionic sympathetic fibers, which will influence effector tissues in the orbit, are in the intermediolateral cell column (lateral horn) of the upper thoracic cord segments. After coursing superiorly through the sympathetic chain, the fibers will synapse in the superior cervical ganglion. Postganglionic fibers then course along the internal carotid artery to the effector tissues in the orbit.

27. d. The myelinated white rami communicans carry preganglionic sympathetic fibers. Gray rami contain postganglionic sympathetic fibers.

28. b. Most organs receive both sympathetic and parasympathetic innervations that operate in conjunction with each other. A balance in the firing of the two helps to maintain an internal stable environment in the face of changing external conditions.

29. a. The convergence of visceral afferent information with somatic afferent information in the dorsal horn of the cord can be interpreted by higher centers as being of somatic origin rather than visceral. As a result, pain from viscera can be referred to somatic structures.

30. c. Ventral rami are branches of spinal nerves and therefore contain both sensory and motor fibers. Dorsal roots contain only sensory fibers and ventral roots contain only motor fibers. The spinal nerve and nerves distal to it contain both sensory and motor fibers.

Organs of Special Senses

1. Which of the following is NOT part of the auditory pathway?
    a. spiral ganglion
    b. medial longitudinal fasciculus
    c. lateral lemniscus
    d. medial geniculate body

2. The axons that form the optic nerve arise from which neurons of the retina?
    a. bipolar cells
    b. rods and cones
    c. amacrine cells
    d. ganglion cells

3. Hair cells in the cochlea are stimulated by the shearing motion between the organ of Corti and what structure?
    a. tegmental membrane
    b. tentorial membrane
    c. basilar membrane
    d. tectorial membrane

4. These taste papillae predominate in the anterior part of the tongue.
    a. circumvallate
    b. foliate
    c. fungiform
    d. fusiform

5. If a patient's pupil remains small when room lighting is subdued, this may indicate damage to which structure?
    a. trochlear nerve
    b. superior cervical ganglion
    c. oculomotor nerve
    d. ophthalmic nerve

6. What is the name of the structure where axons of the ganglion cells leave the retina to form the optic nerve?
    a. fovea centralis
    b. opaque column
    c. fovea capitis
    d. optic disc

7. Which cranial nerve carries SSA information?
    a. CN II
    b. CN III
    c. CN VI
    d. CN V

8. The dendrites of which cranial nerve occupy the holes of the cribriform plate?
    a. CN I
    b. CN II
    c. CN V
    d. CN VIII

9. Where is the location of a lesion that results in the visual deficit known as a bitemporal hemianopia?
    a. right optic tract
    b. left optic tract
    c. occipital lobe
    d. optic chiasm

10. What part of the inner ear's vestibular system would be stimulated as one ascends in an elevator that stops at every floor?
    a. utricle
    b. semicircular ducts
    c. saccule
    d. cochlear duct

Answers

1. b. The medial longitudinal fasciculus consists of fibers that extend to the midbrain and are involved in vestibular functions and eye movements. All of the other structures listed are part of the peripheral and central connections of the auditory pathway.

2. d. The ganglion cell layer contains the cell bodies of neurons whose axons leave the eyeball as the optic nerve at the area of the optic disc (blind spot of the eye).

3. d. Hair cells are located inside the organ of Corti, which lies upon the basilar membrane. Hair bundles are in close contact with the tectorial membrane, which is located just above.

4. c. Circumvallate and foliate taste papillae predominate in the posterior part of the tongue. There is no fusiform taste papillae.

5. b. Sympathetic innervation to the intrinsic eye muscles comes from the superior cervical ganglion. Damage to this structure would prevent normal papillary dilation, and therefore the pupil would stay constricted. Damage to the oculomotor nerve (parasympathetic) would lead to ptosis, lateral strabismus, pupillary dilation, loss of accommodation, and diplopia.

6. d. The optic disc (blind spot) is the structural point of exit for the optic nerve.

7. a. Functional classifications of information carried in spinal and cranial nerves is denoted by the letters GSA, GVE, SSA, etc. SSA information is special somatic afferent information. This type of information deals with special sensory information carrying sight, sound, and equilibrium that is carried in cranial nerves II and VIII.

8. a. The cribriform plate in located in the ethmoid bone, and the dendrites of cranial nerve I occupy these holes as they innervate the nasal mucosa.

9. d. Bitemporal hemianopia is a loss of vision in the temporal or lateral aspect of each eye's visual field. Axons conveying information from the temporal visual field of each eye cross in the optic chiasm. Therefore, a lesion there would cause a deficit in the temporal visual fields bilaterally.

10.   c.   The saccule is part of the static membranous labyrinth of the vestibule of the inner ear. Fluid in the saccule of the inner ear moves in response to vertical linear acceleration or deceleration and causes the macula to shift and stimulate the hair cells. The utricle is similar but is involved with horizontal linear acceleration or deceleration. The semicircular ducts are sensitive to rotatory movements. The cochlear duct is involved with audition.

Section Two Recommended Reading

Aminoff M, Simon R, Greenburg D: *Clinical neurology*, ed 6, New York, 2005, McGraw-Hill.

Cramer G, Darby S: *Basic and clinical anatomy of the spine, spinal cord, and ANS*, ed 2, St Louis, 2005, Mosby.

Junqueira L, Carneiro J: *Basic histology*, ed 11, Stamford, Conn, 2005, Appleton & Lange.

Kiernan JA: *Barr's the human nervous system: an anatomical viewpoint*, ed 8, Philadelphia, 2004, Lippincott Williams & Wilkins.

Moore K, Persaud T: *The developing human: clinically oriented embryology*, ed 7, Philadelphia, 2003, WB Saunders.

Nolte J: *The human brain: an introduction to its functional anatomy*, ed 5, St Louis, 2002, Mosby.

Panjabi M, White A: *Biomechanics in the musculoskeletal system*, New York, 2001, Churchill Livingstone.

Snell R: *Clinical neuroanatomy for medical students*, ed 5, Philadelphia, 2001, Lippincott Williams & Wilkins.

Standring S, ed: *Gray's anatomy: the anatomical basis of clinical practice*, ed 39, New York, 2004, Churchill Livingstone.

Waxman S: *Correlative neuroanatomy*, ed 24, New York, 1999, McGraw-Hill.

Physiology

Kay Hachtel Brashear, Vinnavadi C. Ravikumar, Richard Raymond, Robert W. Ward

Neurophysiology

1. Which type of receptor does the parasympathetic nervous system activate at an effector organ?
   a. alpha-1
   b. nicotinic
   c. beta
   d. muscarinic

2. Which of the following must be activated sequentially for action potential propagation?
   a. peripheral membrane proteins
   b. ligand-gated channels
   c. voltage-gated ion channels
   d. leak channels

3. What response would result from a subthreshold stimulus to a nerve cell?
   a. action potential
   b. graded response
   c. no response
   d. resting membrane potential

4. What is generated if a graded potential should reach threshold?
   a. receptor potential
   b. pacemaker potential
   c. IPSP
   d. action potential

5. What is the origin of a receptor potential?
   a. sensory neurons
   b. neurons of the ANS
   c. hypothalamic neurons
   d. motor cortex neurons

6. Which of the following describes why an action potential is propagated without degradation?
    a. it is replaced by graded potentials at specific points on the membrane
    b. it is generated at a very high voltage, which overcomes the cable properties of the cell
    c. it is constantly regenerated all along the membrane
    d. it is reinforced by injection of a new ion species of similar charge every few millimeters of movement

7. Which organ receives preganglionic sympathetic fibers?
    a. pancreas
    b. medulla of the adrenal gland
    c. uterus
    d. testis

8. You are sleeping peacefully when your alarm clock awakens you. What part of your brain is associated with arousal?
    a. peritricial plexus
    b. sympathetic system
    c. parasympathetic system
    d. reticular formation

9. A number of significant clinical conditions involve abnormalities of neurotransmitter release or reception at the myoneural junction. The neurotransmitter associated with the motor endplate is:
    a. norepinephrine
    b. dopamine
    c. acetylcholine
    d. myasthenia gravis

10. Often, neurologic deficits can affect specific anatomical regions and not the rest of the body. Such deficits can result from damage to peripheral nerves, nerve roots, spinal tracts, or brain centers. Which is the tract responsible for carrying vibration sense to the upper extremity?
    a. rubrospinal tract
    b. fasciculus cuneatus
    c. fasciculus gracilus
    d. anterior spinothalamic tract

11. Changes in the membrane potential of excitable cells occur as rates of ion movement across the cell membrane change. Increased permeability to chloride causes an influx of chloride into cell, which results in which of the following responses?
    a. repolarization
    b. hyperpolarization
    c. depolarization
    d. plateau

12. There are a number of differences between nerve fibers that can have an influence on the time required for the neural action potential in the peripheral nervous system to travel from its site of origin to the next synapse. Which of these factors has no influence on the time between the initial and secondary synapse?
    a. the nerve fiber is in an afferent pathway rather than an efferent pathway
    b. differences in axon diameter
    c. myelinated versus nonmyelinated
    d. overall fiber length (anatomical length of nerve)

13. Which of the following autonomic responses requires sympathetic stimulation?
    a. peristalsis
    b. erection
    c. mydriasis
    d. salivation

14. The rapid influx of sodium ions into a cell that is physiologically excitable is best described as which of the following?
    a. depolarization
    b. hyperpolarization
    c. the refractory period
    d. the action potential

15. As the action potential travels along the axon or dendrite, temporary changes in membrane potential result in significant flux of various ions. The transmembrane ionic flux during the action potential that results in release of neurotransmitter vesicles from the terminal bouton of the axon is which of the following?
    a. sodium influx
    b. calcium influx
    c. potassium efflux
    d. calcium efflux

16. Which describes a cell at the resting membrane potential?
     a. hyperpolarized
     b. depolarized
     c. polarized
     d. at zero volts (resting = no electrical activity)

17. Which is the neurotransmitter responsible for the conversion of chemical energy into bioelectrical energy at the motor end plate of skeletal muscle?
     a. acetylcholine
     b. norepinephrine
     c. GABA
     d. histamine

18. What affects action potential amplitude of myelinated nerve fibers?
     a. thickness of myelination
     b. nerve fiber diameter
     c. calcium concentration of the extracellular fluid
     d. none of the above

19. The repolarization phase of an action potential is due mainly to the influence of what channel?
     a. Na^+-K^+ ATPase pump
     b. Na^+ leak channels
     c. K^+ channels
     d. Na^+-Ca^{2+} antiport

20. Which is an inhibitory neurotransmitter in the central nervous system?
     a. GABA
     b. epinephrine
     c. glutamate
     d. norepinephrine

21. A drug completely blocks voltage-gated Na^+ channels in nerves. Which of the following effects on the action potential would be expected?
     a. increase the Na^+ equilibrium potential
     b. abolish the hyperpolarizing afterpotential
     c. block the occurrence of action potentials
     d. increase the rate of rise of the upstroke of the action potential

22. Which is true of the Nernst potential of sodium in nerves?
     a. it is negative
     b. it is dependent on the threshold potential for the neuron
     c. it is positive
     d. it is unrelated to the concentrations of sodium inside and outside the cell

23. The absolute refractory period of a nerve cell is due to what mechanism?
    a. activation of potassium channels
    b. inactivation of sodium channels
    c. hyperpolarization
    d. changing the equilibrium potential to more closely approach the potassium equilibrium potential

24. Which of the following is a correct statement?
    a. microglial cells are one of the "housekeeping" cells of the CNS
    b. spatial summation occurs when a postsynaptic cell is stimulated by one synapse firing in rapid succession
    c. if a neuron resting membrane potential is changed from −70 mV to −88 mV, the cell would be "facilitated"
    d. myelinated neurons have a slower conduction velocity because the myelin sheath inhibits ion movement

25. In a nerve, the magnitude of the action potential overshoot is normally a function of which of the following?
    a. magnitude of the stimulus
    b. extracellular sodium concentration
    c. intracellular potassium concentration
    d. diameter of the axon

26. An excitable membrane will become depolarized upon influx of which of the following ions?
    a. sodium
    b. potassium
    c. chloride
    d. bicarbonate

27. During chemical neurotransmission, exocytosis of neurotransmitters is dependent upon influx of which of the following ions?
    a. sodium
    b. potassium
    c. magnesium
    d. calcium

28. Visual action potentials are generated by which of the following cells in the retina?
    a. photoreceptor
    b. bipolar
    c. horizontal
    d. ganglion

29. The parasympathetic nervous system does not regulate secretory activity in which of the following exocrine glands?
    a. salivary
    b. sweat
    c. lacrimal
    d. sebaceous glands

30. Parasympathetic innervation stimulates contractions in all except which of the following structures?
    a. intestinal smooth muscle
    b. ciliary muscle
    c. dilator pupillae muscle
    d. urinary bladder

31. Conduction velocity is slowest in which of the following nerve fibers?
    a. postganglionic sympathetic fibers
    b. somatomotor nerve fibers
    c. preganglionic autonomic nerves
    d. A-alpha proprioceptive fibers

Answers

1. d. Acetylcholine is the most common neurotransmitter released from parasympathetic postganglionic fibers. The parasympathetic receptors on effectors are muscarinic. Nicotinic receptors are found at the synapse between preganglionic and postganglionic neurons of the sympathetic and parasympathetic nervous systems as well as at neuromuscular junctions. Acetylcholine can have either an excitatory or inhibitory effect depending on the type of receptor activated.

2. c. An action potential is a rapid but transient change in membrane potential. Action potentials require specific sodium and potassium voltage-gated ion channels that occur at regions of the cell membrane that are electrically excitable. Threshold is the point at which the voltage-gated channels will open.

3. b. A graded response is a local subthreshold response. Receptor (generator) potentials, pacemaker potentials, postsynaptic membrane potentials, and end-plate potentials are some examples of graded potentials.

4. d. Graded potentials have variable changes in the magnitude of the potential. Graded potentials decrease in magnitude as they move along the cell membrane but can function as signals over a very short distance. If a graded potential reaches threshold, an action potential is generated.

5. a. Sensory receptors respond to stimuli from mechanoreceptors, thermoreceptors, nociceptors (pain), chemoreceptors, and electromagnetic (vision) receptors. A graded potential caused by a stimulus is called a receptor potential. If the graded potential reaches threshold, then an action potential is generated and sensory input is transmitted to the spinal cord and brain.

6. c. An action potential is a local event. Conduction with decrement means the signal will die out in 5 mm. Action potentials are propagated without decrement because an action potential at one location acts as a stimulus for the production of an action potential at an adjacent region of the membrane. "New" action potentials are produced along the length of the membrane.

7. b. The chromaffin cells of the medulla of the adrenal gland develop from neural crest cells, which are associated with the sympathetic portion of the autonomic nervous system. These cells function like sympathetic postganglionic neurons except that they secrete catecholamines, mainly epinephrine and norepinephrine, into the bloodstream. Thus, they receive preganglionic sympathetic fibers.

8. d. The reticular formation is a diffuse network of fibers running through the midbrain that is responsible for regulating periods of consciousness and unconsciousness. The peritricial plexus is the collection of nerve endings around a hair follicle that allows for the sensation of touch when a hair is touched.

9. c. Norepinephrine can be a motor neurotransmitter at myoneural junctions of postganglionic sympathetic neurons, but the term "motor endplate" is reserved for only skeletal muscles. Dopamine is a neurotransmitter in the basal ganglia, which is part of the motor system but nowhere near the myoneural junction. Myasthenia gravis is a condition of impaired neurotransmitter reception at the motor endplate, which is not what the question asked about.

10. b. The rubrospinal tract is a motor tract from the cerebellum. The fasciculus cuneatus carries vibration, proprioception, and complex touch from the upper extremity and the fasciculus gracilus provides the same functions for the lower extremity. The anterior spinothalamic tract carries pain and temperature.

11. b. The influx of chloride as described is typical of the IPSP (inhibitory postsynaptic potential).

12. a. While fiber length is not a factor in the velocity of nerve transmission, it is a factor in the total time required for the signal to get from its starting point to its finishing point. Transmission velocity increases (and therefore overall time therefore decreases) with increased fiber diameter and myelination.

13. c. Mydriasis is pupil dilation. The other choices here are parasympathetic functions.

14. a. While the action potential is associated with rapid sodium influx, so is the EPSP (excitatory postsynaptic potential). Both are types of depolarization, but the action potential occurs only if threshold is achieved. Thus, while "action potential" is a correct response, "depolarization" is a better response. Hyperpolarization is associated with the influx of chloride or efflux of potassium, and the refractory period is characterized by reduced sodium permeability.

15.   b.   Sodium influx causes depolarization, and potassium efflux causes repolarization and hyperpolarization.

16.   c.   The resting electrical potential of cell membranes is negative. Cells demonstrating a persistent voltage of zero are either dead or have been structurally disrupted such that cell death is in progress.

17.   a.   Norepinephrine functions as a neurotransmitter in the autonomic nervous system. GABA and histamine can serve as neurotransmitters in the central nervous system.

18.   d.   The term "amplitude" refers to the peak voltage of an action potential. Myelination and fiber diameter increase the speed of propagation but not the amplitude. Amplitude is governed by the concentration of intracellular and extracellular ions. Calcium has negligible contribution to the potential and is too well regulated by the body to allow for significant changes in its concentration.

19.   c.   As potassium leaves the cell, a net loss of positive charge occurs inside the cell membrane, causing repolarization. The electrochemical events of the action potential happen too quickly for active transport to play a meaningful role.

20.   a.   Generally, GABA (gamma-aminobutyric acid) is an inhibitory neurotransmitter in the CNS, whereas epinephrine, glutamate, and norepinephrine are excitatory.

21.   c.   The opening of sodium-gated Na^+ channels is necessary for depolarization. A drug that blocks its action would not allow an action potential to occur.

22.   c.   The Nernst potential is also known as the equilibrium potential for in individual ion. In nerves, the concentration of sodium outside the cell is greater than inside the cell; therefore, a net positive charge inside the cell relative to outside the cell would be necessary to maintain the chemical gradient. Keep in mind that the resting membrane potential is negative due to the greater influence of potassium ions. The Nernst potential for potassium is negative.

23.   b.   By preventing sodium entry during this phase, no additional action potentials will occur. Therefore, the cells are refractory to any additional stimuli.

24. a. Microglia are supportive cells of the CNS that may function as macrophages when neural tissue is damaged. Temporal summation is due to the effects of a single synapse firing in rapid succession. A neuron whose resting membrane potential is more negative would be inhibited, or hyperpolarized. Myelinated neurons have a greater conduction velocity.

25. b. The amount of sodium entry into the cell during the action potential will determine how high the action potential will go. Therefore, the concentration of extracellular sodium determines how much sodium enters the cell and affects the overshoot. The magnitude of the stimulus would only affect the frequency of action potentials.

26. a. At rest, an excitable membrane is polarized with the inside surface negative relative to the outside. Depolarization involves the inside becoming more positive. Influx of sodium ions, which are the predominant extracellular fluid cations (positively charged), will cause the membrane to depolarize. Potassium ions are predominant intracellular cations that efflux to initiate repolarization. Chloride ion influx from the ECF will cause membrane hyperpolarization, whereas bicarbonate ions are involved in ECF buffering action and not in membrane potential changes.

27. d. Sodium and potassium ions are involved in membrane depolarization and repolarization phenomena. Magnesium ions are primarily intracellular, are important for utilization of ATP, and diminish chemical neurotransmission. Neurotransmitter exocytosis is a calcium ion–dependent process.

28. d. Photoreceptors, bipolar cells, and horizontal cells of the retina develop graded potentials. Only the cells in the ganglion cell layer of the retina develop action potentials that ascend in the visual pathway to the visual cortex.

29. b. All of the glands listed are exocrine glands whose activity is stimulated by acetylcholine. The only neuroeffector junction that is part of the sympathetic nervous system and is cholinergic is the innervation of the sweat glands (sympathetic cholinergic control).

30. c. Parasympathetic stimulation causes contractions of intestinal smooth muscles to increase peristaltic activity, ciliary muscles of the eye to relax the suspensory ligaments and increase refractive power of the lens to see near objects, and the smooth muscles of the urinary bladder to initiate micturition. Contractions of the dilator pupillae of the iris to cause mydriasis is a function of sympathetic stimulation.

31.   a.   Conduction velocity is directly proportional to the diameter of the nerve fiber and degree of myelination. Postganglionic sympathetic nerve fibers have the smallest diameter, are unmyelinated, and therefore have the slowest conduction velocity.

Muscle Physiology

1. The "attenuation reflex" is a protective reflex involving contraction of which of the following muscles?
   a. dilator pupillae
   b. constrictor pupillae
   c. stapedius
   d. ciliary

2. Slow, oxidative skeletal muscles appear red due to the presence of which of the following substances?
   a. melanin
   b. myoglobin
   c. hemoglobin
   d. bilirubin

3. The speed of muscle contraction is a function of which of the following factors?
   a. resting length of the muscle fiber
   b. cross-sectional diameter of the muscle
   c. creatine phosphate of the muscle
   d. glycolytic capacity of the muscle

4. Denervation supersensitivity in skeletal muscles is the result of which of the following events?
   a. increase in density of nicotinic ACh receptors at the muscle endplate
   b. antibody-mediated destruction of endplate ACh receptors
   c. spontaneous calcium ion release from the sarcoplasmic reticulum
   d. compensatory spreading of ACh receptors over the entire sarcolemma

5. Causing muscles to fatigue by stimulating all the muscle fibers in one muscle (i.e., lifting an extremely heavy weight) is explained by what mechanism?
    a. increased muscle H^+ ion
    b. increased muscle K^+ ion
    c. depletion of muscle ATP
    d. increasing the frequency of action potentials (motor endplate potentials)

6. Which of the following is CORRECT regarding the muscle spindle?
    a. detects tension when muscle is contracted
    b. contains a lot of thin extrafusal muscle fibers
    c. annulospiral endings cause efferent motor contractions of the muscle
    d. nuclear bag fibers are the primary sensor for muscle length

7. Excitation of the Golgi tendon organ normally induces:
    a. contraction of a muscle's extrafusal fibers
    b. relaxation of a muscle's extrafusal fibers
    c. contraction of a muscle's intrafusal fibers
    d. relaxation of a muscle's intrafusal fibers

8. Alpha motor neurons innervate which of the following?
    a. nuclear chain fibers
    b. nuclear bag fibers
    c. extrafusal fibers
    d. intrafusal fibers

9. When comparing smooth muscle and striated muscle, there are many important similarities and many important distinctions. Which of the following characteristics are similar for smooth muscle and skeletal muscle?
    a. length of actin filaments
    b. contracts in response to action potentials, which begin following stimulation by motor neurons
    c. calcium ions are crucial to contraction
    d. strength of contraction per cross-sectional area of muscle

10. Neural impulses race from the brain to the muscles in the form of action potentials. These action potentials leap across the chasm of the motor endplate synapse, causing an action potential on the muscle cell surface. In response to this, calcium is released, and the muscle contracts. Examples include your eye movements to read this question and use of the pencil to mark this test. Which of the following intramuscular structures is responsible for the release of calcium to trigger contraction?

    a. actin/myosin complex
    b. troponin
    c. T-tubules
    d. sarcoplasmic reticulum

11. Where in the tissues does nutrient exchange take place?
    a. capillaries
    b. interstitial spaces
    c. arterioles
    d. venules

12. Smooth muscle and skeletal muscle both have contractility and employ similar mechanisms of contraction. However, they also have numerous physiologic differences, which account for their different functional characteristics. Which is a characteristic common to both smooth and skeletal muscle?
    a. calmodulin
    b. troponin
    c. actin
    d. spindle organs

13. Surface electromyography (SEMG) and needle electromyography (EMG) are commonly used tools in the clinical monitoring of muscular function. What is the physiologic event is measured by the electromyogram?
    a. muscle action potential
    b. muscle endplate synapse
    c. alpha motor neuron depolarization
    d. gamma motor neuron depolarization

14. Which of the following factors has no influence on the amount of contractile force created during contraction of skeletal muscle?
    a. change in the number of motor units that are facilitated
    b. change in the frequency of action potentials along each alpha motor neuron
    c. change in the amplitude of action potentials in both the alpha motor neuron and the muscle cells
    d. change in muscle size (over time, through exercise)

15. Contractile shortening of myofibrils requires that free calcium be made available on the surface of the actin/myosin complex. What protein binds to calcium leading to smooth muscle contraction?
    a. sarcolemma
    b. troponin
    c. tropomyosin
    d. calmodulin

16. While myocytes and neurons both display the trait of excitability, there are subtle differences in the characteristics of action potentials in different tissues. What physiologic phenomenon accounts for the plateau in the action potential of heart muscle?
    a. the presence of calmodulin
    b. slow passive influx of sodium into the heart cells at rest
    c. relatively slow rate of potassium efflux, resulting in longer lasting action potentials
    d. countertransport of intracellular calcium for extracellular sodium after the voltage-controlled sodium gates have closed

17. At which phase during a skeletal muscle contraction does the load begin to lift?
    a. isometric contraction phase
    b. isometric relaxation phase
    c. isotonic contraction phase
    d. isotonic relaxation phase

18. Which of the following terms describes the addition of more motor units in order to lift a load?
    a. motor addition
    b. power curve enhancement
    c. nervous enhancement
    d. recruitment

19. During the excitation-contraction coupling cycle in skeletal muscle, what must occur in order for the actin fiber to be released immediately after flexure of the myosin head?
    a. release ADP and Pi
    b. relax back to its original position
    c. bind ATP
    d. bind GMP

20. What type of muscle contraction occurs when there is tension development but there is no change in the fiber length?
    a. isotonic
    b. isometric
    c. isokinetic
    d. isoregulatory

Answers

1. c. Dilator and constrictor pupillae are smooth muscles of the iris that control pupil diameter. Sudden loud sounds cause reflex contraction of the stapedius muscle and prevent the stapes from continuing to transfer pressure to the cochlear fluid through the oval window of the middle ear. Contraction of the ciliary muscle in the eye is involved in the process of accommodation.

2. b. Melanin is the pigment in skin, hair, and iris. Hemoglobin is the oxygen transport molecule in red blood cells that has a crimson red color when oxygenated. Bilirubin is the product of hemoglobin catabolism that colors the sclera yellow (jaundice). Myoglobin stores oxygen in slow twitch muscle fibers, which helps them resist fatigue.

3. a. The speed of contraction is directly related to the resting length of the muscle fiber, whereas the force of contraction depends upon the cross-sectional diameter. Creatine phosphate content ensures availability of ATP for the contraction-relaxation cycles, and glycolytic capacity is important for endurance.

4. d. Denervation of a skeletal muscle causes loss of basal stimulus at the end plate region. Consequently, the muscle develops ACh receptors over the entire sarcolemma and responds with involuntary twitches when innervation gradually reestablishes.

5. b. Lifting an extremely heavy weight will rapidly fatigue muscles, unlike the fatigue seen with constant exercise for a long period of time. The latter will fatigue muscles by ATP depletion.

6. d. Within the muscle spindle, the nuclear bag fibers are the primary sensors of muscle length, whereas the flower spray endings are the secondary sensors.

7. b. The Golgi tendon apparatus is a tension detector. If stimulated, it will cause relaxation of the muscle.

8. c. Alpha motor neurons are termed the final common pathway and innervate the normal muscle fibers, whereas the gamma motor neurons innervate the muscle spindle and are generally used for posture and tone.

9. c. Smooth muscle has longer actin filaments. It may also contract in response to hormones, without neural stimulation and without action potentials. It also can develop more contractile force per cross-sectional area than skeletal muscle.

10. d. Actin and myosin develop the contractile force after calcium is released. Troponin keeps actin and myosin from interacting until calcium is released. T-tubules transmit the action potential from the muscle cell membrane (sarcolemma) to the sarcoplasmic reticulum within the cell.

11. b. The vessels of various sizes provide transmission conduits for body fluids, but the exchange described takes place between cell surfaces and the interstitial fluid.

12. c. Calmodulin is found only in smooth muscle. Troponin is found in skeletal and cardiac muscle. Spindle organs are found only in skeletal muscle.

13. a. Synapses do not produce electrical fields. Neural action potentials are monitored in nerve conduction studies.

14. c. The amplitude of action potentials is not variable, and all have the same amplitude. Contractile force increases with increased number of motor units, increased frequency of action potentials, and increase in muscle size with use over time.

15. d. Calcium enters the smooth muscle mainly through the sarcolemma (muscle cell membrane) and triggers contraction by binding to the protein calmodulin, which then activates myosin kinase. The phosphorylation of myosin then leads to crossbridge formation and subsequent contraction.

16. d. Countertransport of intracellular calcium for extracellular sodium after the voltage-controlled sodium gates have closed accounts for the plateau in the action potential of heart muscle. Calmodulin is not a correct answer because it is found in smooth muscle. The slow passive influx of sodium into the heart cells accounts for the heart's ability to maintain a (slow) rhythm without external stimulus. Although the relatively slow rate of potassium efflux is reasonable, it is not the mechanism used.

17. c. The initial portion of muscle contraction is isometric. When the force development by the muscle equals the load being lifted, the muscle can shorten and the muscle contraction becomes isotonic.

18. d. An alpha motor neuron plus all of the skeletal muscle fibers it innervates is called a motor unit. As skeletal muscle begins to contract, it activates more and more motor units until the entire load is lifted, or maximum tension development occurs. This graded response is called motor unit recruitment, or motor unit summation.

19. c. ATP binds with the myosin head, causing a conformational change, which releases actin. Myosin head ATPase splits ATP to ADP + P_i, returning the myosin head to its original position. The excitation-coupling cycle can again be repeated.

20. b. During isometric muscle contraction, the contractile element (CE) and the parallel elastic element (PEE) contract. The series elastic element (SEE) stretches in an amount equal to the CE and PEE contraction. The result is that the whole muscle does not change length.

Cardiovascular Physiology

1. What occurs during the rapid ejection phase of the cardiac cycle?
   a. semilunar valves are closed, and there is a rapid decrease in ventricular volume
   b. there is a rapid increase in ventricular volume, and semilunar valves are open
   c. the semilunar valves are closed, and there is a rapid increase in ventricular volume
   d. there is a rapid decrease in ventricular volume, and the semilunar valves are open

2. When does the second heart sound occur?
   a. during closure of the mitral valve
   b. during closure of the tricuspid valve
   c. during closure of the pulmonic valve
   d. during the opening of the aortic valve

3. During which phase of the cardiac cycle is ventricular volume the lowest?
   a. atrial systole
   b. isovolumetric ventricular contraction
   c. at the onset of rapid ventricular ejection
   d. isovolumetric ventricular relaxation

4. Which of the following would cause a decrease in hematocrit?
   a. decreased plasma colloid oncotic pressure (decreased albumin)
   b. increase viscosity
   c. low arterial blood pressure
   d. increase in P_c

5. According to Poiseuille's law, if the radius of a blood vessel were to double in size, how much would blood flow increase, all other factors being equal?
    a. it would double
    b. increase 4 times
    c. increase 8 times
    d. increase 16 times

6. Disorders of the heart valves can lead to hypertrophy of heart chambers, secondary to chronically increased mechanical loads. For example, stenosis of the mitral valve can result in hypertrophy of what chamber of the heart due to increased mechanical resistance during contraction?
    a. left atrium
    b. right atrium
    c. left ventricle
    d. right ventricle

7. During isovolumetric relaxation, which of the following occurs?
    a. AV valves are open, and the aortic and pulmonic valves are closed
    b. AV valves are open
    c. AV valves are closed
    d. AV valves are closed, and the aortic and pulmonic valves are open

8. The heart contains a variety of different types of muscle fibers, each with a different frequency of spontaneous contraction. Which of the following has the shortest period (highest frequency) of spontaneous contraction?
    a. Purkinje fibers
    b. SA node
    c. AV node
    d. myocardium

9. The heart contains a variety of different types of muscle fibers, each of which conducts action potentials at a different velocity. Which of the following has the most rapid conduction of action potentials?
    a. Purkinje fibers
    b. SA node
    c. AV node
    d. myocardium

10. What would happen to the cardiac rhythm if you slowed conduction through the AV node?
    a. longer PR interval
    b. shorter RT interval
    c. shorter PR interval
    d. longer RT interval

11. Return of fluids from the lower extremities is impeded in the upright posture by the ceaseless forces of gravity. Lymphatic drainage from the lower extremities is increased by what mechanism?
    a. venous stasis
    b. increased muscle contraction
    c. increased capillary colloidal osmotic pressure
    d. decreased diastolic arterial pressure

12. As blood flows through the circulatory system, the pressure decreases as the blood moves from the heart, through the systemic arterial tree, and back through venous return. Which is the part of the circulatory system where the greatest drop in pressure occurs?
    a. arteries
    b. arterioles
    c. capillaries
    d. veins

13. What wave is associated with ventricular physiologic and mechanical activity?
    a. T and P
    b. QRS and T
    c. P and QRS
    d. QRS only

14. What event causes the first heart sound (S1)?
    a. closure of the AV valves
    b. opening of the AV valves
    c. closure of the aortic and pulmonic valves
    d. opening of the aortic and pulmonic valves

15. The Frank-Starling law describes the relationship between cardiac preload and cardiac output. Consistent with the Frank-Starling law, the factor that is most important in determining cardiac output is:
    a. venous return
    b. heart rate
    c. stroke volume
    d. the inotropic state (functional contractility) of the ventricular myocardium

16. Oxygen binding affinity is greatest for which of the following molecules?
    a. iron-protoporphyrin IX
    b. myoglobin
    c. fetal hemoglobin
    d. adult hemoglobin

17. Sickle cell anemia is a genetic condition that results in replacement of a glutamate residue with valine in the structure of which of the following molecules?
    a. iron-protoporphyrin IX
    b. myoglobin
    c. hemoglobin alpha chain
    d. hemoglobin beta chain

18. Systemic blood pressure is primarily a function of which of the following factors?
    a. cardiac inotropicity
    b. cardiac chronotropicity
    c. diameter of conductance vasculature
    d. total peripheral vascular resistance

19. Inhibiting the myocardial sodium pump results in which of the following events?
    a. greater sodium influx during phase 0
    b. decrease in potassium ion influx
    c. increase in $[Ca^{2+}]_i$
    d. decrease in cardiac output

20. Stimulation of CN X will cause which of the following effects?
    a. atrial fibrillation
    b. sinus bradycardia
    c. cardiac rigor
    d. ventricular fibrillation

21. Which of the following determines preload in the cardiac muscle?
    a. volume of blood in the ventricle at the end of diastole
    b. systolic arterial blood pressure
    c. calcium availability
    d. end-systolic volume

22. What is the ability to increase cardiac output as a result of an increase in metabolism called?
    a. cardiac output
    b. cardiac index
    c. cardiac reserve
    d. ventilation-perfusion ratio

23. Which mechanism is the most important in regulating blood flow through the coronary circulation?
    a. via alpha receptors on the vascular smooth muscle
    b. metabolic control of blood flow
    c. development of collateral circulation
    d. concentration of epinephrine

24. Which of the following is most important in long-term regulation of cardiac output?
    a. sum of peripheral blood flow
    b. stroke volume
    c. level of sympathetic stimulation
    d. contractility

25. Which of the following is released from juxtaglomerular cells in the macula densa as a result of hypotension or a decrease in renal filtration pressure?
    a. aldosterone
    b. antidiuretic hormone
    c. angiotensin II
    d. renin

1. d. During this phase, the ventricles are contracting; therefore, the semilunar valves are open, allowing ejection of volume during this phase. Because the pressures in the ventricles are greater than in the atria, the AV valves are closed and ventricular volume is decreasing.

2. c. The first heart sound (S1) occurs when the atrioventricular (mitral and bicuspid) valves close. The second sound (S2) occurs when the semilunar valves (pulmonic and aortic) close. Normal valves typically do not make sounds during opening.

3. d. During this phase, all of the ventricular volume has been ejected. The semilunar and AV valves are closed and no volume is changing in the ventricles. This phase has the lowest volume.

4. c. Capillary hydrostatic pressure is a determinant of net fluid filtration. With a decrease in arterial blood pressure, less fluid is filtered out of the vascular compartment, whereas the same volume is reabsorbed. This causes dilution of the blood and results in a decrease in hematocrit.

5. d. The radius is the major determinant of blood flow because it is radius to the 4th power. If the radius doubles, then the blood flow would increase by 2nd to the 4th power, or a 16-fold increase.

6. a. Stenosis can create only additional load during contraction as a heart chamber tries to push blood through it. Thus, mitral stenosis can load the left atrium, tricuspid stenosis can load the right atrium, aortic stenosis can load the left ventricle, and pulmonic stenosis can load the right ventricle.

7. c. During the brief interlude of isovolumetric relaxation, all of the valves are closed. To use the left side of the heart for illustration, pressure is higher in the aorta than the left ventricle, so the aortic valve is closed. Pressure is still higher in the left ventricle than in the left atrium, so the mitral valve is still closed. Analogous conditions occur on the right side.

8. b. The SA node has a frequency of 70 to 80 depolarizations per minute; the AV node frequency is 40 to 60; and the Purkinje cell frequency is 15 to 40; the myocardium is even slower. This question refers to how often these fibers will have action potentials, not how fast they travel.

9. a. The velocity of action potentials in Purkinje fibers is 1.5 to 4 m/sec, and the velocity in the myocardium is 0.3 to 0.5; the SA node is probably similar. The AV node is 0.02 to 0.05. This question refers to how fast action potentials will travel in these tissues, not how often they occur.

10. a. The P wave represents atrial depolarization, and the QRS represents ventricular depolarization. Slowed conduction through the AV node increases the time interval between these two events, as seen by a longer PR interval.

11. b. Venous stasis and diastolic pressure retard lymphatic return. Increased capillary colloid osmotic pressure decreases the formation of lymph. Muscular contraction massages the lymph vessels of the lower extremity, facilitating lymph return.

12. b. The arterioles are the site of the greatest pressure drop and the greatest component of peripheral resistance to blood flow and of autonomic (sympathetic) control of arterial blood pressure.

13. b. QRS corresponds to ventricular depolarization (and therefore contraction). The T wave corresponds to repolarization, which is a physiologic activity that occurs in the absence of contraction. The P wave is associated with atrial activity.

14. a. Heart valve opening should be silent. Closure of the aortic and pulmonic valves causes S2. S3 and S4 sounds are not associated with valve opening or closure.

15. a. In its simplest terms, the Frank-Starling law is "more in, more out." Regardless of heart rate or stroke volume, the heart can only pump as much blood as is returned to it through the venous system.

16. a. Oxygen binding affinity for the oxygen transport molecules, adult and fetal hemoglobin, is lower than for the oxygen storage molecule myoglobin. Oxygen molecules bind strongest to heme molecules because of the lack of interference by the globin chains. Heme forms a "picket fence" with oxygen molecules sandwiching between every two heme molecules.

17. d. Anemia is characterized by a decrease in oxygen transport capacity of blood. Iron-protoporphyrin IX is heme and is the nonprotein, organic component of hemoglobin. Myoglobin is the oxygen storage protein in muscle tissue. The Hb alpha chain protein is well conserved across developmental stages.

18. d. Increases in cardiac force of contractions (inotropicity) and heart rate (chronotropicity) can increase cardiac output and thereby cause an increase in BP. The effect, however, is minimal. Conductance vessels facilitate flow of blood from the heart during systole and do not provide as much resistance to the flow of blood as do vessels with smaller diameter. The total cross-sectional diameter of the precapillary arterioles (peripheral vasculature) is far greater than that of blood vessels with larger diameters.

19. c. The myocardial sodium pump reestablishes the resting potential. Inhibiting the sodium pump prolongs the plateau phase of the cardiac action potential and allows for more exchange of intracellular Na^+ for extracellular fluid Ca^{2+}, thereby increasing intracellular Ca^{2+} concentration to cause positive inotropicity (increase in stroke volume and cardiac output). K^+ influx occurs during the repolarization phase.

20. b. CN X stimulation causes bradycardia by inhibiting automaticity of the SA node. Tachycardic effects are caused by inhibiting, not stimulating, the vagus. Cardiac rigor is a consequence of hypercalcemia and causes the heart to stop in systole.

21. a. Cardiac muscle experiences two loads during the contraction process. The preload is the load placed on cardiac muscle by the volume of blood in the ventricle prior to contraction. The preload is important because it determines the length-tension relationship and the force of contraction. The afterload is primarily determined by the pressure in the aorta. It is the load against which the ventricular muscle contracts.

22. c. The average cardiac output is 5 L/min. The ability to increase cardiac output is called cardiac reserve. Young healthy individuals should be able to increase cardiac output 5 to 6 times the average cardiac output.

23. b. Blood flow through the coronary circulation is primarily regulated by local metabolic control. The autonomic nervous system has little direct effect on coronary circulation. Of the metabolic mechanisms for control, the availability of oxygen seems to be the most significant.

24. a. Venous return and cardiac output equal the sum of all blood flows from the various peripheral tissue beds. Long-term regulation of cardiac output results from metabolic control of blood flow in the periphery.

25. d. The juxtaglomerular cells in medullary nephrons play a major role in regulating renal filtration pressure. A decrease in filtration pressure will stimulate the juxtaglomerular cells to release an enzyme renin. Renin activates the renin-angiotensin-aldosterone system. The renin-angiotensin-aldosterone system will increase plasma volume and peripheral resistance. These two actions will increase arterial blood pressure.

CHAPTER 19

Respiratory Physiology

CONTENT AREAS

- Mechanics of breathing
- Ventilation, lung volumes and capacities
- Regulation of respiration
- O_2 and CO_2 transportation
- Gaseous exchange

1. Which of the following statements is related to the Bohr effect?
   a. pressure-volume relationship
   b. effect of pH or plasma carbon dioxide partial pressure on the oxygen-hemoglobin dissociation curve
   c. diffusing capacity of the respiratory membrane
   d. effect of oxygen-hemoglobin binding on the transport of carbon dioxide

2. Which part of the respiratory center is the source of the "ramp" signal that is responsible for inspiration?
   a. dorsal respiratory group
   b. cerebral cortex
   c. ventral respiratory group
   d. chemosensitive area of the medulla

3. The force or energy that propels gases out of the lungs during expiration is:
   a. an upward contraction of the diaphragm
   b. atmospheric pressure
   c. elastic recoil of the tissues of the chest wall
   d. contraction of the intercostal muscles

4. Which of the following correctly describes lung surfactant?
   a. it increases the surface tension on the inner alveolar surfaces, thereby preventing collapse of the alveoli
   b. it is primarily a phospholipid
   c. it is secreted by type I pneumocyte of the alveolar epithelium
   d. it is not of any particular importance in fetal viability in the instance of premature parturition

5. The volume of air moved going from full forced expiration to full forced inspiration is known as which of the following?
   a. inspiratory capacity
   b. vital capacity
   c. total lung capacity
   d. inspiratory reserve volume

6. Which of the following accurately describes the Hering-Breuer reflex?
   a. efferent receptors are stretch receptors in the walls of the bronchi and bronchioles
   b. reflex activates a feedback response that "switches on" inspiration
   c. reflex is not activated until total lung capacity exceeds 1.5 liters
   d. reflex is a protective mechanism for preventing excessive lung inflation

7. The amount of a given gas dissolved in the blood is due to which of the following factors?
   a. it is directly proportional to the solubility of the gas
   b. it increases at higher altitudes
   c. the concentration of albumin
   d. it is described primarily by the law of Laplace

8. Which is TRUE of the affinity of hemoglobin for oxygen?
   a. it is greater than the affinity for carbon monoxide
   b. it is increased in methemoglobin
   c. it decreases as the height above sea level increases
   d. it is increased in response to metabolic alkalosis

9. Hyperventilation is compensatory mechanism in response to which of the following conditions?
   a. metabolic alkalosis
   b. respiratory alkalosis
   c. metabolic acidosis
   d. respiratory acidosis

10. The medullary respiratory center is stimulated by which of the following changes in the plasma?
    a. increase in pO_2
    b. increase in pCO_2
    c. decrease in pO_2
    d. decrease in pCO_2

Answers

1. b. The amount of carbon dioxide and hydrogen ions in blood plasma has a significant effect on the oxygen-hemoglobin dissociation curve. An increase in the carbon dioxide partial pressure or hydrogen ion concentration will shift the curve to the right and decrease the affinity that hemoglobin has for oxygen. A decrease in the plasma carbon dioxide partial pressure or hydrogen ion concentration will shift the curve to the left and increase the affinity that hemoglobin has for oxygen. The Bohr effect is very significant in oxygen-hemoglobin binding at the lung and the release of oxygen from hemoglobin at the tissue level.

2. a. Neurons associated with the dorsal respiratory group are responsible for the "ramp signal" that is responsible for respiratory motor control of inspiration. It is called a ramp signal because the intensity of the electrical activity gradually increases during inspiration and then abruptly ceases during expiration.

3. c. During normal resting respiration, inspiration requires muscular activity and expiration is passive.

4. b. Surfactant decreases surface tension in the alveoli, and it is the primary determinant of fetal viability in the survival of premature infants. It is produced by type II pneumocytes; type I pneumocytes are squamous cells that allow gas exchange between the blood and the atmosphere.

5. b. Inspiratory capacity is the volume of air moved going from normal expiration to full forced inspiration. Total lung capacity is the volume of air in the lung on full forced inspiration and cannot be measured on spirometry. Inspiratory reserve volume is the volume of air moved going from normal inspiration to full forced inspiration.

6. d. There is no such thing as an efferent receptor. The Hering-Breuer reflex represses inspiration when the tidal volume exceeds about 1.5 liters. Total lung capacity is not dynamic.

7. a. The amount of gas dissolved in the blood is proportional to the solubility of the gas in fluid and is proportional to the partial pressure of the gas.

8. d. Various factors cause a shift in the oxyhemoglobin dissociation curve. Alkalosis causes a leftward shift and, as a result, increases the affinity of hemoglobin for oxygen.

9. c. Hyperventilation causes plasma pH to increase due to loss of volatile acid (CO_2). It is triggered as a rapid compensatory mechanism against metabolic acidosis. Respiratory acidosis is caused by inspiratory/expiratory compromise as in COPD.

10. b. Cells in the respiratory nuclei in the medulla oblongata are most sensitive to changes in plasma CO_2 content. Increases in pCO_2 stimulate the center, while decreases provide a correspondingly lower stimulus.

Body Fluids and Renal Physiology

1. Which of the following is the protein component in plasma that is absent in serum?
    a. albumin
    b. gamma globulins
    c. fibrinogen
    d. angiotensinogen

2. Antidiuretic hormone helps conserve total body water by incorporating water channels in what part of the kidney tubular system?
    a. proximal convoluted tubule
    b. ascending Henle's loop
    c. distal convoluted tubule
    d. collecting duct

3. Which is the section of the tubular nephron that is also referred to as the diluting segment?
    a. descending Henle's loop
    b. ascending Henle's loop
    c. proximal convoluted tubule
    d. distal convoluted tubule

4. During normal blood circulation, water can migrate from the arterial side of the capillary beds to the interstitial fluids, as it is pushed through the fenestrations of the capillary walls via mechanical pressure. This water returns to the plasma of the circulatory system by:
    a. migrating through fenestrations of the venous capillary beds by being pushed through by mechanical pressure
    b. migrating through fenestrations of the venous capillary beds by being pushed through by osmotic pressure
    c. lymphatic drainage, which eventually reenters the bloodstream via the cisterna chyle
    d. active transport, as the brush border of the venous capillaries moves sodium from the interstitial fluids to the venous blood, creating a strong osmotic gradient that the water then follows

5. Which of the following can produce metabolic acidosis?
    a. vomiting
    b. decreased respiration
    c. hyperventilation
    d. diarrhea

6. Which of the following has no significant role in maintaining the acid-base balance in the blood?
    a. liver
    b. kidneys
    c. lungs
    d. adrenals

7. Which of the following substances has the greatest renal clearance rate?
    a. glucose
    b. serum albumin
    c. urea
    d. glycine

8. The cells located at distal tubules of the nephron secrete:
    a. aldosterone
    b. potassium
    c. sodium
    d. angiotensinogen

9. The kidney filters small molecules from the blood and then reabsorbs nutrients from the filtered fluids. In one area, called the brush border, the cells have been modified with thousands of microscopic microvilli to increase their surface area to make absorption more efficient. The brush border is located in the:
    a. glomerulus
    b. proximal convoluted tubule
    c. distal convoluted tubule
    d. collecting ducts

10. The tubular filtrate has the greatest osmolarity at what site?
    a. as it enters the proximal convoluted tubule
    b. as it enters the distal convoluted tubule
    c. at the tip of the loop of Henle
    d. as it exits the proximal convoluted tubule

11. Glomerular filtration would be decreased by which of the following conditions?
    a. increased plasma protein concentration
    b. increased glomerular filtrate protein concentration
    c. decreased glomerular hydrostatic pressure
    d. increased mean arterial pressure

12. Which of the following is true of diuretics?
    a. they decrease urine production
    b. they induce hypertension
    c. they often act on the proximal convoluted tubule
    d. they often act on the distal convoluted tubule

13. Which of the following is a major buffer in the kidney tubule lumen?
    a. sodium bicarbonate
    b. protein
    c. phosphate
    d. carbonic acid

14. Which of the following will increase sodium reabsorption in the cortical collecting ducts?
    a. decrease in renin secretion
    b. increase in antidiuretic hormone secretion
    c. decrease in angiotensin II secretion
    d. increase in aldosterone secretion

15. Of the following electrolytes, which is more abundant in the intracellular fluid compartment than in the extracellular fluid compartment?
    a. sodium ions
    b. potassium ions
    c. bicarbonate ions
    d. chloride ions

1. c. Plasma and serum are obtained by separating the cellular components from whole blood; the former in the presence of an anticoagulant and the latter after allowing blood to clot. All plasma proteins are present in plasma while fibrinogen is used up to form the clot.

2. d. The collecting duct is normally water impermeable. ADH promotes water conservation by stimulating the incorporation of water channel proteins in the collecting duct.

3. b. The thick, ascending limb of the loop of Henle is the site of active absorption of Na^+ and Cl^- from the filtrate into the medullary interstitium and is not accompanied by obligatory water movement with Na^+. Because only solute is absorbed, this segment is also known as the "diluting segment" of the tubular nephron.

4. b. Mechanical pressure in the venous capillaries is still higher than in the interstitial fluids. Lymphatic drainage is how large proteins or particles return to the blood stream. Choice "d" describes fluid movement through the kidneys.

5. d. Changes in respiration can cause changes in body fluid pH but would be responses to metabolic pH imbalance rather than a cause. Vomiting causes alkalosis (loss of stomach acid).

6. a. The adrenals influence serum pH through the secretion of aldosterone as it causes sodium retention, which in turn leads to hydrogen secretion. The kidneys influence pH through hydrogen secretion and the lungs through loss of bicarbonate in the form of CO_2.

7. c. Renal clearance is the equivalent volume of blood from which the kidneys completely remove all of a substance in 1 minute. Glucose and glycine are filtered but are actively reabsorbed. Serum albumin is not filtered. Urea is filtered and excreted.

8. b. The cells of the distal tubule secrete potassium and hydrogen into the urine, in exchange for sodium, under the control of aldosterone.

9. b. The introductory text says that the brush border is in the area where the most efficient absorption takes place. Most absorption occurs in the proximal tubule. The glomerulus is the site of filtration. The distal tubule and collecting ducts are important sites for regulation of the water content of body fluids.

10. c. Only water is reabsorbed as it passes from the proximal tubule down to and including the tip of the loop of Henle. As a result, the concentration of ions is the greatest here.

11. a. Any factor that would decrease the net fluid filtration across the glomerular capillaries would decrease GFR. Increased plasma proteins will do this as well as increase the rate of fluid reabsorption.

12. d. This area of the kidney is responsible for ionic reabsorption. Diuretics cause a decrease in reabsorption of these ions (e.g., sodium), thereby causing more loss of sodium in the urine. Water will follow sodium, causing a greater volume of urine to be produced.

13. c. The phosphate buffer system is not important as an extracellular buffer because the concentration is very low. Phosphate is an important buffer in the kidney because it becomes very concentrated in the nephron and also because the pK (6.8) is very close to the pH of urine.

14. d. Aldosterone is secreted by the zona glomerulosa cells of the adrenal cortex. Aldosterone increases sodium resorption and potassium secretion in the collecting ducts by stimulating the sodium-potassium ATPase pump.

15. b. Potassium and phosphates are more abundant in the intracellular fluid compartment, whereas sodium and chloride are more abundant in the extracellular fluid compartment.

CHAPTER 21

Gastrointestinal Physiology

CONTENT AREAS

- Ingestion
- Digestion
- Absorption
- Regulation of gastrointestinal function

1. Pernicious anemia may be due to damage to what structure?
   a. proximal ileum
   b. distal jejunum
   c. gastric mucosa
   d. erythropoietic tissues of the bone marrow

2. Nutrient absorption occurs after mastication and digestion. How are proteins absorbed from the intestinal lumen into the body?
   a. protein molecules are bound to specific receptors on the intestinal epithelium and enter the body through cotransport with sodium ions
   b. proteins are absorbed directly through the epithelial cell membranes by pinocytosis
   c. the hydrophobic portions of the peptide structure bind passively to lipid molecules, and these hydrophobic complexes then diffuse passively through the epithelial cell membrane
   d. proteins are not absorbed in the intestines

3. The hormone secretin is released in response to:
   a. cholecystokinin
   b. acidic chyme
   c. gastrin
   d. somatostatin

4. Which gastric cells secrete pepsinogen?
   a. chief cells
   b. oxyntic cells
   c. parietal cells
   d. mucous neck cells

5.   Which of the following occurs during the intestinal phase of gastric function?
   a.   the vagus nerve stimulates gastrin secretion
   b.   stomach distention stimulates acid secretion
   c.   vagal nuclei are stimulated by smelling food
   d.   gastric emptying is inhibited

6.   The majority of disaccharide hydrolysis occurs due to the action of which enzymes?
   a.   enzymes from the pancreatic juice
   b.   enzymes in the brush border of the small intestine
   c.   enzymes found in the saliva
   d.   enzymes in the gastric mucosa

7.   Ingested water is primarily absorbed through the mucosa of what part of the gastrointestinal tract?
   a.   oral cavity
   b.   stomach
   c.   small intestine
   d.   colon

8.   Amino acid absorption in the jejunum occurs via which mechanism?
   a.   simple diffusion
   b.   cotransport with glucose
   c.   facilitated diffusion
   d.   active transport

9.   Where are chylomicrons produced in the gastrointestinal tract?
   a.   gut lumen associated with bile salts
   b.   gastrointestinal tract enterocytes
   c.   liver
   d.   lymphatic system

10.   Which one of the following proteolytic enzymes is most important in the digestion of collagen?
   a.   pepsin
   b.   trypsin
   c.   carboxypeptidase
   d.   brush border peptidases

Answers

1. c. The gastric mucosa is the site of production of intrinsic factor, and pernicious anemia can result from chronic gastritis. Absorption is at the distal ileum, and damage to this area can cause pernicious anemia as well.

2. d. Choice "a" would be correct if the words "protein molecules" were replaced with "amino acids." If humans absorbed proteins without breaking them down first, they would probably develop allergies to everything. Additionally, if choice "c" were correct, then a fatty meal would allow the cellular proteins to leak out into the intestines.

3. b. Secretin is released when acidic stomach contents flow into the duodenum and mildly inhibits gastrointestinal motility. Cholecystokinin is released in response to fats within the duodenum. Gastrin stimulates parietal cells and is released in response to both chemical stimuli from food in the stomach and mechanical distention of the stomach. Somatostatin is a secretion of the hypothalamus/pituitary that inhibits secretion of both insulin and glucagons.

4. a. Oxyntic and parietal are synonyms with regard to the cells of the stomach, and are responsible for secretions of HCl. Mucous neck cells secrete mucus that protects the stomach lining.

5. d. Food in the small intestine releases hormones that decrease gastric emptying.

6. b. Enzymes responsible for the breakdown of disaccharides are located in the brush border.

7. d. The limited surface area of the oral mucosa does not allow for significant absorptive function. The stomach is the site of protein digestion and also has limited surface area for absorption. The small intestines are the site for lipid digestion, and most substances are absorbed due to the villi and microvilli affording a very large area. Water is predominantly absorbed across the colonic mucosa while forming the stools.

8. b. Amino acids are charged molecules and have low lipid solubility. Absorption of amino acids and dipeptides occurs as cotransport (symport) with glucose.

9. b. Micelles are formed in the lumen of the gastrointestinal tract in the presence of bile salts and lipids. Digested lipids are absorbed from the micelles into the enterocytes where lipids are resynthesized. A chylomicron is composed of reformed lipids and beta-lipoprotein. Chylomicrons are moved from the enterocyte to the lymphatic system via exocytosis.

10. a. Proteolytic enzymes are produced in the stomach and pancreas. Proteolytic enzymes are also associated with the intestinal brush border. Pepsin, which is secreted in the stomach, is the only proteolytic enzyme that will digest collagen.

CHAPTER 22

Reproductive Physiology

1. Which of the following hormones stimulates ovulation in the female?
   a. follicle-stimulating hormone
   b. growth hormone
   c. prolactin
   d. luteinizing hormone

2. Which hormone from the anterior pituitary stimulates spermatogenesis?
   a. FSH
   b. LH
   c. progesterone
   a. ACTH

3. As human gestation nears its conclusion, multiple hormones are involved in the functional development of breast tissue and the production of milk. Which of the following hormones is a stimulus to maternal mammary secretion?
   a. prolactin
   b. progesterone
   c. oxytocin
   d. estrogen

4. The secretory phase of the endometrium occurs when the ovary is in what phase?
   a. follicular
   b. luteal
   c. menstrual
   d. ovulatory

5. Ovulation occurs in response to a spike in the plasma concentration of which of the following hormones?
   a. estrogen
   b. luteinizing hormone
   c. follicle-stimulating hormone
   d. progesterone

Answers

1. d. During the preovulatory phase of menstrual cycle, follicle-stimulating hormone is the dominant hormone. The feedback mechanism of high levels of estradiol cause a midcycle surge in luteinizing hormone (LH). About 24 hours after the surge in LH, the follicle ruptures and ovulation occurs. LH also maintains the function of the corpus luteum in the postovulatory phase of the cycle.

2. a. FSH (follicle-stimulating hormone) is the same hormone in both genders and stimulates the formation of gametes in both genders. Progesterone is not a pituitary secretion but originates in the ovary and adrenal cortex. ACTH stimulates the adrenal cortex and can increase the circulating levels of sex hormones but does not directly influence gamete formation. In males, LH is also known as ICSH (interstitial cell–stimulating hormone) and results in testosterone release.

3. c. Prolactin, progesterone, and estrogen are all essential for the development of functional breast tissue and subsequent formation of milk. Oxytocin is necessary for expression of milk but not for breast development or milk production.

4. b. During the luteal phase in which the corpus luteum of the ovary is secreting progesterone, the endometrium is in its secretory phase in preparation for implantation.

5. b. Maturation of ovarian follicles is dependent upon FSH secretion. LH leads to ovulation, after which the follicle differentiates into the corpus luteum. The corpus luteum secretes progesterone to prepare the endometrium for implantation of the fertilized ovum.

Endocrine Physiology

1. Growth, body temperature, and oxygen consumption are all increased by which of the following lipophilic hormones?
   a. somatotropin
   b. corticotropin
   c. triiodothyronine
   d. testosterone

2. Aldosterone is secreted by which of the following endocrine structures?
   a. zona glomerulosa of the adrenal cortex
   b. parafollicular cells of the thyroid gland
   c. alpha cells of the pancreatic islets
   d. corticotrophs of the adenohypophysis

3. Erythropoietin is a hormone required for the production of red blood cells. It is produced primarily in the:
   a. kidney
   b. lung
   c. marrow
   d. liver

4. Which pair of glands represents a situation in which the first gland secretes a hormone in response to hormones released from the second gland?
   a. parathyroid/pituitary
   b. thyroid/pituitary
   c. pancreas/adrenal (cortex)
   a. pituitary/testes

5. Medullary suprarenal adenomas (pheochromocytomas) often exhibit constant, uncontrolled epinephrine secretion. Associated with this type of endocrine tumor are vascular changes that may lead to which of the following?
    a. thin, shiny skin (trophic changes)
    b. warm skin
    c. anhydrosis
    d. pallor

6. Overproduction of somatotropin in an individual with open skeletal physes will result in:
    a. osteogenesis imperfecta tarda
    b. acromegaly
    c. giantism
    d. achondroplasia

7. The actions of parathyroid hormones are antagonized by the actions of:
    a. vitamin D
    b. calcitonin
    c. estradiol
    d. insulin

8. Elevated concentrations of glucagon would result in:
    a. decreased lipolysis
    b. decreased glycogen synthesis
    c. increased gluconeogenesis
    d. increased lipogenesis

9. Which of the following is a function of parathyroid hormone?
    a. increased digestion in the gastrointestinal tract
    b. rapid reabsorption of calcium salts from bone
    c. control of thyroid function
    d. increased basal metabolic rate

10. Which of the following will increase with elevated thyroid hormones?
    a. basal metabolic rate
    b. fat stores
    c. body weight
    d. skin dryness

Answers

1. c. Growth hormone stimulates growth and development of somatic cells; adenocorticotrophic hormone (ACTH) stimulates the synthesis and secretion of glucocorticoids in the zona fasciculata of the adrenal cortex; T_3, derived by deiodination of T_4 in target tissues, stimulates mitochondrial oxygen consumption and stimulates metabolism and body heat generation; and testosterone stimulates development of the male secondary sexual characteristics.

2. a. Cells in the zona glomerulosa synthesize and secrete the sodium-retaining hormone aldosterone in response to decreases in extracellular fluid volume. Cells in the zona fasciculata synthesize and secrete glucocorticoids in response to adenohypophyseal ACTH, while those in the zona reticularis function as a secondary source of sex steroids. Parafollicular thyroid cells secrete calcitonin, alpha cells of the endocrine pancreas secrete glucagon, and the adenohypophyseal corticotrophs secrete ACTH.

3. a. Eighty percent to 90% of erythropoietin is formed in the kidney, with the remainder coming from the liver. Marrow responds to this hormone.

4. b. Thyroid-stimulating hormone from the pituitary causes release of thyroxine and triiodothyronine from the thyroid gland. There are a number of endocrine functions that are not under the control of the hypothalamus-pituitary axis. Among these are pancreatic function, parathyroid function, and release of calcitonin from the thyroid. While testicular secretions do affect the pituitary, that affect is inhibitory and does not stimulate pituitary secretion.

5. d. Dermal atrophy, excessive skin warmth, and loss of sweating are all associated with loss of sympathetic function. With epinephrine secretion, there is increased sympathetic activity, with resulting capillary vasoconstriction that may cause relative pallor.

6. c. Somatotropin (growth hormone) causes giantism before puberty and acromegaly after puberty. Osteogenesis imperfecta tarda and achondroplasia are forms of altered osseous formation due to genetic defects and are not due to hormonal causes.

7. b. Through negative feedback control, parathyroid hormone (PTH) will be decreased with increases in calcitonin.

8. b. Glucagon acts in an antagonistic manner to insulin. Glucagon is a catabolic hormone, not only causing glycogen breakdown but also decreasing its storage.

9. b. PTH stimulates osteoclast activity to cause the release of calcium and phosphates from bone. PTH also increases intestinal absorption of calcium and phosphate, decreases calcium excretion by the kidney, and increases phosphate excretion by the kidney.

10. a. The thyroid hormone increases the basal metabolic rate (BMR) in most cells in the body. The general effect of thyroid hormone is to increase nuclear transcription of many genes. The result is a significant increase in protein synthesis and cellular metabolic activity in the body. The BMR is related to the quantity of the hormone that is synthesized and released.

CHAPTER 24

Exercise and Stress Physiology

1. Which of the following is NOT related to chronic stress syndrome?
   a. osteoporosis
   b. increase in lean body mass
   c. decrease in wound healing
   d. thin fragile skin and thin fragile capillaries

2. Creatine supplementation best enhances performance involving which of the following muscle types?
   a. white skeletal
   b. red skeletal
   c. cardiac
   d. smooth

3. What is the most effective mechanism the body uses to maintain normal body temperature if the body has become chilled?
   a. shivering
   b. vasodilate cutaneous capillary beds
   c. vasoconstrict cutaneous capillary beds
   d. generate heat in the brown fat by activation of metabolic futile cycles

4. During periods of intense physical activity, many physiologic adaptations occur, especially in the circulatory system. Which of the following occurs during increased physical exertion?
   a. increased ventricular refilling, secondary to increased venomotor tone
   b. decreased cardiac output
   c. decreased stroke volume
   d. increased cardiac cycle time

5. During an isometric contraction, which type of mechanoreceptor is stimulated?
   a. Golgi tendon organ
   b. muscle spindle organ
   c. Pacinian corpuscle
   d. joint capsule

6. During exercise, how does glucose enter the muscle cells?
   a. via secondary active transport
   b. coupled with sodium
   c. via the GLUT-4 receptor
   d. via primary active transport

Answers

1. b. Cortisol stimulates the release of amino acids primarily from muscles. The amino acids are used for gluconeogenesis in the liver. Sustained high levels of cortisol associated with chronic stress syndrome will decrease total muscle mass.

2. a. Creatine supplementation facilitates rapid regeneration of ATP for enhanced contraction-relaxation cycles in the muscle type that has low capability for ATP synthesis. White (fast twitch) skeletal muscle is glycolytic (2 ATP molecules/glucose) compared with red skeletal muscle that synthesizes ATP molecules via oxidative-phosphorylation in mitochondria (32 to 38 ATP molecules/glucose). The cardiac muscle inherently has a higher creatine phosphate content to maintain ATP availability for normal functioning. Contraction-relaxation cycles in smooth muscles are regulated by changes in intracellular Ca^{2+} concentration.

3. a. Vasoconstriction of capillary beds in the extremities does help retain body heat, but shivering actually generates sufficient heat energy to increase core temperature. Brown fat is metabolically active but at very low levels compared with muscular contraction. Vasodilatation would cause loss of body heat.

4. a. Cardiac output and stroke volume both increase during exertion. Increased cardiac cycle time is just another way of saying the heart is beating slower, which is the opposite of what occurs with exertion.

5. a. The Golgi organ is stimulated by changes in the tension on a musculotendinous structure. The muscle spindle organ is stimulated by changes in the length of a muscle. Pacinian corpuscles in the skin respond to changes in skin tension overlaying the muscle. Joint capsules contain receptors remarkably like Pacinian corpuscles. All of the incorrect answers here are stimulated by changes in joint position but not by muscle tension.

6. c. Glucose transporter-4 is located in skeletal muscles, which responsible for the uptake of glucose.

Section Three Recommended Reading

Berne R, Levy M, Koeppen B, Stanton B, eds: *Physiology,* ed 5, St Louis, 2003, Mosby.

Ganong W: *Review of medical physiology,* ed 22, Stamford, Conn, 2005, Appleton & Lange.

Guyton A, Hall J: *Textbook of medical physiology,* ed 11, Philadelphia, 2005, WB Saunders.

McArdle W, Katch F, Katch V: *Exercise physiology: energy, nutrition, and human performance,* ed 5, Philadelphia, 2004, Lippincott Williams & Wilkins.

Chemistry

*Susan Boger-Wakeman, Geracimo Bracho,
Alan L. Campbell, Christian G. Linard, Richard Valente,
Michael R. Valentine*

Carbohydrates

1. Which pair of enzymes listed below is unique to gluconeogenesis?
   a. pyruvate kinase and pyruvate carboxylase
   b. phosphoenolpyruvate carboxykinase and pyruvate carboxylase
   c. fructose bisphosphatase and phosphofructokinase
   d. pyruvate dehydrogenase and glucose 6-phosphatase

2. Which two polysaccharides contain the same types of bonds?
   a. cellulose and amylose
   b. amylopectin and glycogen
   c. glycogen and cellulose
   d. amylose and amylopectin

3. Which glycolytic enzyme catalyzes a substrate-level phosphorylation?
   a. glucokinase
   b. phosphofructokinase
   c. phosphoglycerate kinase
   d. hexokinase

4. An example of a food that is an excellent source of soluble fiber is:
   a. wheat bran cereal
   b. brown rice
   c. whole wheat bread
   d. oatmeal

5. Which polysaccharide has the highest proportion of α-1,4 glycosidic linkages?
   a. starch
   b. amylopectin
   c. glycogen
   d. amylose

6. Which sugar has a C-2 carbonyl carbon?
   a. fructose
   b. galactose
   c. glucose
   d. mannose

7. Which molecule is not essential for the complete degradation of glycogen in muscle and liver?
   a. inorganic phosphate
   b. glycogen phosphorylase
   c. glycogenin
   d. glycogen debranching enzyme

8. Which glucose transporter is saturated or close to saturation only after a carbohydrate-rich meal?
   a. GLUT-1
   b. GLUT-2
   c. GLUT-3
   d. GLUT-4

9. Which of the following is NOT considered a reducing sugar?
   a. glucose
   b. fructose
   c. sucrose
   d. lactose

10. What are carbohydrates that consist of long disaccharide repeats and are important components of connective tissue called?
    a. peptidoglycan
    b. proteoglycans
    c. glycogen
    d. glycosaminoglycans

11. Conversion of glucose into carbon dioxide and passage of its electrons to molecular oxygen represents the complete _____ of the sugar.
    a. oxidation
    b. reduction
    c. phosphorylation
    d. destruction

12. The action of what enzyme during glycolysis directly produces one molecule of NADH per molecule of substrate?
    a. hexokinase D
    b. phosphofructokinase-1
    c. glyceraldehyde-3-phosphate dehydrogenase
    d. α-ketoglutarate dehydrogenase

13. An abundance of what substance will inhibit some of the enzymes of the citric acid cycle?
    a. adenosine diphosphate
    b. acetyl-coenzyme A
    c. NADH
    d. glucose

14. What is the major source of energy fuel in the average human diet?
    a. carbohydrates
    b. ethanol
    c. fats
    d. proteins

15. Starch is the most common digestible polysaccharide in plants and exists mainly as amylose and amylopectin. These polymers are composed of which basic residue?
    a. D-fructose
    b. D-galactose
    c. D-glucose
    d. D-ribose

16. Which of the following forms of dietary fiber is insoluble?
    a. cellulose
    b. gum
    c. mucilages
    d. pectin

17. The hydrolysis of lactose by lactase produces equimolar amounts of which two monosaccharides?
    a. fructose and glucose
    b. fructose and galactose
    c. galactose and glucose
    d. glucose and glucose

18. Which of the following describes glycogenin?
    a. it is a protein of muscular glycogen
    b. it has no enzymatic activity
    c. it is attached to the nonreductive end of glycogen
    d. it has an amylo-(1,4-1,6)-transglycosylase activity

19. Which of the following describes glycogen?
    a. it is a heteropolysaccharide
    b. it is a polymer of (α1-4)-linked subunits of glucose, with (α1-6) branches every 24 to 30 residues
    c. it has many more monosaccharide units than starch
    d. it is a form of stored energy in cytoplasmic vesicles

20. Which is true of UDP-glucose?
    a. it is a substrate of UDP-glucose pyrophosphorylase
    b. it contains one sugar with five carbons and one sugar with six carbons
    c. it is a substrate of the degradation of glycogen
    d. it is an allosteric activator of glycogen-branching enzyme

21. Which is true of glycogen phosphorylase?
    a. it is active in its *b* form (phosphorylase *b*)
    b. it is phosphorylated by phosphoprotein phosphatase
    c. when not phosphorylated, it is activated in the presence of glucose 6-phosphate in the liver
    d. when phosphorylated, it is inactive in the presence of glucose

22. Which of the following enzymes represents the step where the second high-energy phosphate is invested in glycolysis?
    a. pyruvate kinase
    b. 3-phosphoglycerate dehydrogenase
    c. phosphofructokinase
    d. pyruvate dehydrogenase
    e. hexokinase

23. The digestion of starch begins in what location?
    a. in the duodenum with pancreatic amylase
    b. in the mouth with salivary amylase
    c. in the jejunum with maltase
    d. in the colon with absorption of water

24. In the formation of a proteoglycan, which trisaccharide is used to attach the carbohydrate to the protein?
    a. xylose–galactose–galactose
    b. rhamnose–galactitol–galactitol
    c. arabinose–glucose–glucose
    d. trehalose–fucose–fucose

25. Which of the following GLUT transporters brings in fructose?
    a. GLUT-2
    b. GLUT-3
    c. GLUT-4
    d. GLUT-5

Answers

1. b. Gluconeogenesis is a pathway that converts pyruvate to glucose. Two reactions catalyzed by pyruvate carboxylase and phosphoenolpyruvate carboxykinase are required to bypass the irreversible reaction catalyzed by pyruvate kinase in the glycolytic pathway. Pyruvate carboxylase converts pyruvate to oxaloacetate and then phosphoenolpyruvate carboxykinase converts oxaloacetate to phosphoenolpyruvate.

2. b. Amylopectin, a branched glucose polymer present in starch, has chains of d-glucose residues connected by (α1-4) glycosidic bonds with branch points occurring every 24 to 30 residues that have (α1-6) linkages. Glycogen, the main storage polysaccharide of animal cells, is more highly branched, with branch points occurring every 8 to 12 glucose residues.

3. c. Directly transferring a high-energy phosphate group from the substrate to adenosine diphosphate (ADP) in the formation of adenosine triphosphate (ATP) is called a substrate-level phosphorylation. There are two substrate-level phosphorylations that occur in the glycolytic pathway. Phosphoglycerate kinase transfers the high-energy phosphoryl group from the carboxyl group of 1,3-bisphosphoglycerate to ADP, forming ATP and 3-phosphoglycerate.

4. d. Dietary fiber can be classified based on solubility. Cellulose, lignin, and most hemicelluloses are not soluble in water. Most gums, pectins, and other polysaccharides such as mucilages are water soluble. Oats, as in oatmeal, is a soluble fiber, whereas wheat bran cereal, brown rice, and whole wheat bread are sources of insoluble fibers.

5. d. Amylose is the only listed polysaccharide that is entirely linear, containing 100% of α-1,4 glycosidic linkages. Both glycogen and amylopectin are branched polysaccharides, containing (α-1,4) and (α-1,6) linkages. Starch contains amylose and amylopectin.

6. a. Fructose is a ketohexose, having a ketone functional group at carbon 2. The other three sugars are all aldo-hexoses, with an aldehyde functional group at carbon 1.

7. c. Glycogenin is involved in the synthesis of glycogen, not in its degradation. It is needed for the synthesis of a glycogen primer. Inorganic phosphate is a substrate for the reaction catalyzed by glycogen phosphorylase (phosphorolysis), which is the key enzyme in the degradation of glycogen. Glycogen debranching enzyme participates in the degradation of glycogen by removing glucoses attached by α-1,6 glycosidic linkages (branches).

8. d. GLUT-4 is the insulin-dependent glucose transporter that is mostly localized on muscle and fat cells and recruited to the plasma membrane of those cells when insulin is elevated in blood due to high blood glucose from the carbohydrate-rich meal. The K_m for GLUT-4 is about 5 mM. Blood glucose can reach 10 mM or slightly higher, depending on the amount of glucose in the meal, allowing for near-saturation or complete saturation of GLUT-4. GLUT-1 and GLUT-3 are present in most cells and are saturated or close to saturation even under fasting conditions because of their low K_m (about 1 mM). GLUT-2 is found in liver, pancreas, and intestinal cells and has a K_m of at least 20 mM. The concentration of blood glucose is unlikely to reach this high after a carbohydrate-rich meal under normal, healthy conditions. It is unlikely, therefore, that GLUT-2 will be saturated or near-saturation.

9. c. The hydroxyl group of the reducing end (hemiacetal or hemiketal) of a sugar must be free to reduce a weak oxidizing agent such as Benedict's reagent. In sucrose, those groups are involved in the glycosidic bond between glucose and fructose.

10. d. Glycosaminoglycans like chondroitin sulfate are long-chain disaccharide repeats that are abundant in connective tissue. Peptidoglycan is a component of bacterial cell walls, glycogen consists of monosaccharide repeats, and proteoglycans are more complex, also involving core proteins.

11. a. Glycolysis, the citric acid cycle, and oxidative phosphorylation are oxidative processes. Reduction is the opposite of oxidation. Some intermediates of glycolysis are phosphorylated, but those phosphates get transferred to ADP. Destruction of glucose would be a violation of the first law of thermodynamics.

12. c. Production of NADH from NAD⁺ is half of an oxidation-reduction reaction. Such reactions are catalyzed by oxidoreductases. All dehydrogenases are oxidoreductases. This is the sixth reaction of the pathway of glycolysis.

13. c. The enzymes of a pathway that are subject to allosteric regulation tend to be activated by the substrates of the pathway and inhibited by its products. NADH is a product of the citric acid cycle, while none of the other choices are. Thus, NADH must be the inhibitor.

14. a. The ADA recommends an intake of approximately 50% to 55% of calories from carbohydrates, 10% to 20% of calories from protein, and fewer than 30% of calories from fat for most individuals. The emphasis here is the average human diet. Dieters following a low-carb diet, epileptics on a ketogenic diet, or chronic alcoholics will invariably have altered energetic profiles emphasizing proteins, fats, and ethanol, respectively.

15. c. The polyglucoses found in starch and glycogen are the major storage forms of carbohydrate in plants and animals, respectively.

16. a. Dietary fiber can be classified as soluble or insoluble based on its solubility in hot water. Foods high in cellulose include bran, legumes, root vegetables, and vegetables of the cabbage family. Mucilages, gum, and pectin are soluble, whereas cellulose and lignin are insoluble. Hemicelluloses can be either soluble or insoluble.

17. c. The enzymatic hydrolysis products of the three main disaccharides are as follows:
lactose becomes galactose and glucose
maltose becomes glucose and glucose
sucrose becomes fructose and glucose

18. a. Glycogenin acts as the primer to which the first glucose residue is attached, and also as the catalyst for synthesis of a nascent glycogen molecule with up to eight glucose residues. The first step in glycogen synthesis is the covalent attachment of a glucose residue to the Tyr194 OH group of glycogenin by the protein's glucosyltransferase activity. Each glycogen granule, which contains a single glycogen molecule, has but one molecule each of glycogenin and glycogen synthase.

19. c. Glycogen is the main storage polysaccharide in the cytosol of animal cells. Glycogen is a homopolysaccharide. Glycogen is a polymer of (α1-4)-linked subunits of glucose, with (α1-6)-linked branches, but glycogen is more extensively branched (branches occur every 8 to 12 residues) and is more compact than starch.

20. b. UDP-glucose (uridine-5′-diphosphate-glucose) contains one pentose (five carbons) and one glucose (six carbons). UDP-glucose is the immediate donor of glucose residues in the enzymatic formation of glycogen by the action of glycogen synthase. Glucose binding to an allosteric site in liver glycogen phosphorylase *a* induces a conformational change that exposes the phosphorylate Ser14 residues to the action of phosphorylase *a* phosphates, which converts phosphorylase *a* to *b*, reducing its activity in response to high blood glucose.

21. d. Glycogen phosphorylase occurs in two forms: the active form is phosphorylase *a* and the relatively inactive form is phosphorylase *b*. Phosphorylase *a* has two subunits, each with a specific serine residue that is phosphorylated at its hydroxyl group by the phosphorylase kinase.

22. c. In the glycolytic pathway, phosphofructokinase is the enzyme that utilizes the second high-energy phosphate from ATP. Hexokinase is the enzyme where the first ATP is utilized. All other choices are far removed from the correct answer.

23. b. Digestion of starch starts in the oral cavity with salivary amylase. Pancreatic amylase is not the correct answer because some digestion does occur in the oral cavity. Maltase in the jejunum is incorrect as its target is only maltose, not starch.

24. a. Proteoglycans are produced by joining glycosaminoglycans to a protein spine. All other answers are not observed in any proteoglycan analyzed.

25. d. Fructose transport occurs by the GLUT-5 transporter. All other transporters work with glucose.

Lipids

1. Which of the following lipids is NOT found in eukaryotic membranes?
   a. phosphatidyl inositol
   b. triglycerides
   c. cholesterol
   d. gangliosides

2. Which of the following is true of Tay-Sachs disease?
   a. it is provoked by a sphingomyelinase deficiency
   b. it is transmitted by the mother
   c. it promotes a specific ganglioside accumulation, mainly in the brain and spleen
   d. it is an autosomal dominant disease

3. Which is TRUE of cholesterol?
   a. it is present in prokaryotic membranes
   b. it has a hydroxyl on its number 3 carbon
   c. in the serum, it is eliminated by the kidneys
   d. it is transported in blood by albumin

4. Which of the following is TRUE of chylomicrons?
   a. they are always present in the lymphatic circulation
   b. they are synthesized by the liver
   c. they are enriched in esterified cholesterol and free fatty acid
   d. in the serum, they carry apolipoproteins A, B-48, CII, and E

5. Which is TRUE of nascent high-density lipoprotein (HDL)?
   a. it contains lecithin-cholesterol acyl transferase
   b. it principally functions as storage for apolipoproteins A and E
   c. it is rich in triglycerides
   d. it is synthesized only by the liver

6. If blood plasma levels are extremely high in arachidonic acid, which type of supplement listed would be useful in increasing eicosapentanoic acid (EPA) and docosahexanoic acid (DHA) levels?
   a. glucosamine and chondroitin
   b. B complex with B6, B12, and folate
   c. cold water fish oil supplement
   d. ADEK, the fat-soluble vitamins

7. Which of the following is the carrier for fatty acids into the inner mitochondria?
   a. CoA
   b. FAD
   c. carnitine
   d. fatty acetyl-CoA

8. Odd chain fatty acid degradation leads to the production of acetyl-CoA and what other compound?
   a. propionyl-CoA
   b. malonyl-CoA
   c. acetoacetyl-CoA
   d. β-hydroxybutyrate

9. Which of the following unsaturated fatty acids is one that can be synthesized by the liver?
   a. linoleic acid
   b. linolenic acid
   c. oleic acid
   d. arachidonic acid

10. What is the end product of β-oxidation of fatty acids, which feeds into the TCA cycle?
    a. pyruvate
    b. oxaloacetate
    c. α-ketoglutarate
    d. acetyl-CoA

11. Which lipids are NOT charged at physiologic pH?
    a. glycerophospholipids
    b. cholesteryl esters
    c. sphingomyelins
    d. fatty acids

12. Which molecule is NOT derived from cholesterol?
    a. vitamin D
    b. cortisol
    c. leukotriene A_4
    d. taurocholate

13. Which condition accelerates the mobilization of fat from adipocytes?
    a. activation of lipoprotein lipase
    b. activation of phospholipase A_2
    c. activation of hormone-sensitive lipase
    d. activation of acetyl-CoA carboxylase

14. Which fatty acid process/cell location is a correct match?
    a. fatty acid activation/cytosol
    b. fatty acid oxidation/endoplasmic reticulum
    c. fatty acid desaturation/nucleus
    d. fatty acid synthesis/mitochondria

15. Which condition stimulates the highest rate in the synthesis of ketone bodies?
    a. feasting
    b. physical activity
    c. overnight sleep
    d. starvation

16. Which of the following foods contains no cholesterol?
    a. roast beef
    b. bacon
    c. ice cream
    d. baked potato

17. What disease is caused by a genetic defect in the enzyme sphingomyelinase leading to the accumulation of sphingomylin in the brain, liver, and spleen?
    a. Niemann-Pick disease
    b. sudden infant death syndrome (SIDS)
    c. Tay-Sachs disease
    d. maple syrup urine disease

18. Which of the following is an example of an omega-3 polyunsaturated fatty acid?
    a. eicosapentaenoic acid, 20:5 (Δ5,8,11,14,17)
    b. arachidonic acid, 20:4 (Δ5,8,11,14)
    c. linoleic acid, 18:2 (Δ9,12)
    d. docosahexanoic acid, 22:4 (Δ7,10,13,16)

19. In the transportation of fatty acids into the mitochondria, fatty acyl-CoA needs a carrier to cross the inner membrane of the mitochondria. What is the name of this carrier?
    a. creatine
    b. lipoate
    c. acetyl-CoA
    d. carnitine

20. What is the name of the enzyme present in the capillaries of muscle and adipose tissue that is activated by apolipoprotein CII to hydrolyze triacylglycerols to fatty acids and glycerol?
  a. pancreatic lipase
  b. lipoprotein lipase
  c. hormone-sensitive lipase
  d. lingual lipase

21. Which is the best source of oleic acid?
  a. corn oil
  b. olive oil
  c. safflower oil
  d. soybean oil

22. Which of the following dietary lipids has the most influence on raising total blood cholesterol levels?
  a. cholesterol
  b. saturated fatty acids
  c. polyunsaturated fatty acids
  d. monounsaturated fatty acids

23. Which is the preferred polyunsaturated fatty acid source for the production of the series 3 prostaglandins?
  a. borage oil
  b. corn oil
  c. linseed oil
  d. salmon oil

24. A high omega-6:omega-3 fatty acid ratio in the diet favors the synthesis of which eicosanoid via the $\Delta5$-desaturase enzyme?
  a. 1-series prostaglandins
  b. 2-series prostaglandins
  c. 3-series thromboxanes
  d. 5-series leukotrienes

25. Hydrogenation of polyunsaturated fatty acids produces which of the following products that are particularly atherogenic?
  a. α-linolenic acids
  b. cis-fatty acids
  c. γ-linolenic acids
  d. *trans*-fatty acids

26. Triglycerides consist of three fatty acids attached to a backbone made of which of the following?
    a. glyceraldehyde
    b. glycerol
    c. sphingosine
    d. glycogen

27. Triglycerides contain more energy per gram than carbohydrates because of what reason?
    a. they are denser
    b. they are in a more oxidized form
    c. they are in a more reduced form
    d. they are more hydrophobic

28. Which of the following is a lipid that functions as a chemical messenger at or near the site of its production and is directly derived from arachidonic acid?
    a. steroid hormone
    b. prostaglandin
    c. peptide hormone
    d. second messenger

29. Each round of β-oxidation of fatty acids produces one molecule each of which of the following?
    a. $FADH_2$, NADH, and acetyl-CoA
    b. $FADH_2$, NADPH, and acetyl-CoA
    c. FAD, NAD^+, and acetyl-CoA
    d. FAD, $NADP^+$, and acetyl-CoA

30. The reaction catalyzed by which enzyme (the target of the statin drugs) is the rate-limiting step in cholesterol biosynthesis?
    a. desmolase
    b. hydroxymethylglutaryl-CoA reductase
    c. squalene epoxidase
    d. cyclase

Answers

1. b. The main lipids in mammalian membranes are phospholipids (as phosphatidyl inositol), glycosphingolipids (as cerebrosides and gangliosides), and cholesterol. The triglycerides (or triacylglycerols) are nonpolar, hydrophobic molecules that are essentially insoluble in water and thus are not found in biologic membranes.

2. c. Tay-Sachs disease is a condition in which a specific ganglioside accumulates in the brain and spleen owing to the lack of the lysosomal enzyme hexosaminidase A. The defective gene is transmitted through a recessive mode.

3. b. Cholesterol, the major sterol in animal tissues, is amphipathic, with a polar head group (the hydroxyl group at C-3) and a nonpolar hydrocarbon body (the steroid nucleus and the hydrocarbon side chain at C-17). It is carried in the blood by lipoprotein and is eliminated in the form of bile acids.

4. d. Chylomicrons, rich in triacylglycerols, are synthesized by the small intestine following the absorption of dietary triglycerides and are liberated into the lymphatic circulation prior to being returned to the blood. In the blood, they acquire apolipoproteins A, B-48, CII, and E.

5. a. The liver and intestines synthesize and secrete HDL. An important function of HDL is to serve as storage for apoproteins C and E, which are indispensable in the metabolism of chylomicrons and VLDL. They are rich in proteins and phospholipids.

6. c. High relative levels of arachidonic acid in the blood indicate a diet high in omega-6–containing lipids. Cold water fish contain high levels of omega-3 lipids that relate directly to the lipids called eicosapentanoic acid and docosahexanoic acid. All of these long-chain fatty acids relate to overall health through their effects on levels of various eicosanoid hormones within the body. All other answers will not have the desired effect.

7. c. Carnitine is the carrier of fatty acids from the cells cytosol through the outer and inner membrane of the mitochondria.

8. a. Odd chain fatty acids in the last round of β-oxidation produce one molecule of acetyl-CoA and a three-carbon intermediate called propionyl-CoA.

9.   c.   Oleic acid is the only unsaturated fatty acid synthesized by the human liver, which has a desaturase for direct synthesis. Other components listed are all ones that must be ingested.

10. d.   The β-oxidation pathway for fatty acids produces large amounts of acetyl-CoA. None of the other components are produced from this pathway.

11. b.   Typical esters are derived from the condensation of a carboxylic acid with an alcohol and are not charged. Glycerophospholipids and sphingomyelins contain a charged phosphate and can also contain a charged alcohol attached to the phosphate molecule. Fatty acids contain a carboxylic acid functional group at carbon 1 that is completely dissociated at physiologic pH because of its relatively low pK_a (4 to 5).

12. c.   Eicosanoids such as leukotriene A_4 regulate many processes and are derived from membrane phospholipids by the action of phospholipase A_2 and lipoxygenase. Vitamin D is a lipid-vitamin that regulates blood calcium and is derived from cholesterol by reactions in the skin, liver, and kidneys. Cortisol is a glucocorticoid (regulates blood glucose) made from cholesterol in the adrenal glands. Taurocholate is a typical bile salt essential for the digestion of dietary lipids that is synthesized from cholesterol in the liver.

13. c.   Fat is hydrolyzed (mobilized) in adipocytes during normal fasting and/or during physical activity to provide fatty acids for energy and glycerol for gluconeogenesis. This is accomplished via hormone-sensitive lipase, which is activated by glucagon and epinephrine. Lipoprotein lipase modifies blood lipoproteins (chylomicrons and VLDL) by mostly removing triacylglycerols that are taken up by peripheral tissues. Phospholipase A_2 hydrolyzes the fatty acid at carbon 2 of glycerophospholipids (mostly) and sphingomyelins to generate a free fatty acid precursor of eicosanoids. Acetyl-CoA carboxylase catalyzes the conversion of acetyl-CoA to malonyl-CoA, the key reaction in the synthesis of fatty acids.

14. a.   Activation of fatty acids takes place in the cytosol of cells that can oxidize them for energy even though the oxidation reactions actually take place in the mitochondria or in the peroxisomes but not in the endoplasmic reticulum. The nucleus is not involved in fatty acid metabolism. Fatty acid desaturation takes place in the endoplasmic reticulum. Fatty acid synthesis takes place in the cytosol of liver cells (mostly) and of fat cells.

15. d. There is some synthesis of ketone bodies during normal fasting—that is between meals and overnight sleep—but the highest rate of synthesis occurs during long fasting (starvation). This acceleration is due to the lack of glucose for energy, which in turn causes accumulation of acetyl-CoA in liver mitochondria from the incomplete oxidation of fatty acids. Excess acetyl-CoA that is not oxidized by the Krebs cycle is converted to ketone bodies. Physical activity accelerates the rate of glycolysis and fatty acid oxidation. Under normal, healthy conditions, there is no synthesis of ketone bodies when there are ample amounts of dietary glucose from feasting.

16. d. Cholesterol is a type of lipid present only in foods containing animal products; it is not present in any plant sources of food. Ice cream is made from cream and milk obtained from dairy cattle, and roast beef and bacon are animal products.

17. a. The polar membrane lipid sphingomylin is normally degraded to phosphocholine and ceramide by the enzyme sphingomyelinase. When there is a defect or absence of sphingomyelinase, the resulting build-up of sphingomyelin can cause mental retardation and early death.

18. a. Greek letters are used to refer to the placement of the carbons in the fatty acid. Omega (ω) refers to the last carbon in the fatty acid. In an omega-3 fatty acid, the first carbon-carbon double bond has to occur three carbons from the methyl terminus of the fatty acid. Arachidonic acid, linoleic acid, and docosatetrenoic acid are all examples of omega-6 fatty acids. The first double bond occurs six carbons from the methyl (omega) terminus.

19. d. Fatty acids destined for mitochondrial oxidation have to move from the cytoplasm into the mitochondria crossing over the mitochondrial membrane. The fatty acid is cleaved from coenzyme A by the enzyme carnitine acyltransferase I and attached to the hydroxyl group of carnitine. Carnitine transports the fatty acid through the inner membrane into the matrix of the mitochondria. Carnitine acyltransferase II catalyzes the removal of carnitine from the fatty acid and regenerates the fatty acyl-CoA.

20. b. Apolipoprotein CII (apoCII) is a lipid-binding protein present in the outer surface of two lipoproteins called chylomicrons and very low density lipoproteins. These two lipoproteins transport triacylglycerols to the muscle and adipose tissue. Lipoprotein lipase is activated by apoCII in the capillaries of the muscle and adipose tissue to convert the triacylglycerols to fatty acids and glycerol.

21. b. All of these oils contain a mixture of monounsaturated fatty acids (MUFAs) and polyunsaturated fatty acids (PUFAs); however, olive oil is the richest source, consisting of about 77% MUFA or oleic acid. Diets rich in MUFA decrease the risk of coronary vascular disease by decreasing the LDL/HDL ratio.

22. b. Dietary cholesterol, contrary to popular belief, has only a minor impact on blood cholesterol levels in most people. MUFAs and PUFAs lower blood cholesterol levels.

23. d. Borage oil and corn oil are from the omega-6 family of fatty acids, which can be used to synthesize prostaglandins of 1-series. Linseed oil consists mainly of α-linolenic acid, which must be converted to eicosapentanoic acid (EPA) and then to prostaglandins of the 3-series. However, this enzymatic process is sluggish, with less than 20% of the α-linolenic acid being converted to EPA.

24. b. Excess omega-6 fatty acids positively modulate the Δ5-desaturase enzyme forming arachidonate, a precursor to the proinflammatory prostaglandins of the 2-series. The 1-series prostaglandins are associated with normal levels of omega-6 fatty acids. The 3-series thromboxanes and the 5-series leukotrienes are associated with the omega-3 eicosanoid pathway.

25. d. Some authors believe *trans*-fatty acids to be more atherogenic than saturated fatty acids (SFAs). Not only do *trans*-fatty acids raise total cholesterol and LDL, but unlike SFA, they lower HDL.

26. b. Triacylglycerols is another name for triglycerides. Thus, the backbone is derived from glycerol.

27. c. Energy is released from biochemical molecules mainly through oxidative processes, β-oxidation in the case of fatty acids. Molecules in more reduced forms can undergo more oxidation, releasing more energy.

28. b. Steroid hormones are derived from cholesterol and tend to have their effects far from their site of production. Peptide hormones are not lipids. Second messengers can be lipids, but they are not directly synthesized from arachidonic acid.

29. a. NADPH is the electron donor for fatty acid synthesis, and NAD^+ is the electron acceptor for β-oxidation. In β-oxidation, the fatty acid is oxidized, and NAD^+ and FAD are reduced to NADH and $FADH_2$.

30. b. Desmolase catalyzes the first step in steroid hormone synthesis. Squalene epoxidase and cyclase are not the rate-limiting enzymes in cholesterol biosynthesis.

Proteins, Amino Acids, and Peptides

1. Which of the following amino acids can be used to produce pyruvate?
   a. isoleucine
   b. arginine
   c. methionine
   d. serine

2. Which of the following amino acids is the precursor to dopamine?
   a. tyrosine
   b. phenylalanine
   c. lysine
   d. tryptophan

3. The amino acid alanine can give rise to what compound by transamination?
   a. phosphoenolpyruvate
   b. pyruvate
   c. oxaloacetate
   d. fumarate

4. Which of the following amino acids is the one normally found in globular proteins?
   a. glutamine
   b. serine
   c. tyrosine
   d. valine

5. Which is true of 2,3-bisphosphoglycerate (BPG)?
   a. it is formed from an intermediate of the pentose phosphate pathway
   b. its concentration is four times that of hemoglobin A
   c. it weakly attaches to hemoglobin F
   d. it is not present in the fetus

6. Which is true of the O_2-saturation curve of hemoglobin A?
    a. it is displaced toward the right in the presence of an increased hydrogen ion (H^+) concentration
    b. it is not influenced by 2,3,-bisphophoglycerate (BPG)
    c. it is a simple hyperbolic curve
    d. it is influenced by nitrogen (N_2)

7. Which amino acid is utilized in the synthesis of serotonin?
    a. histidine
    b. phenylalanine
    c. tryptophan
    d. tyrosine

8. Purines are oxidized in the liver to yield which product?
    a. acetic acid
    b. oxalic acid
    c. glutamic acid
    d. uric acid

9. Legumes are an incomplete source of protein because they lack which essential amino acid?
    a. lysine
    b. methionine
    c. threonine
    d. tryptophan

10. α-Helices and β-pleated sheets represent aspects of what structure in proteins?
    a. primary
    b. secondary
    c. tertiary
    d. quaternary

11. Which of the following is an exclusively ketogenic amino acid?
    a. valine
    b. glycine
    c. aspartate
    d. lysine

12. Which of the following is a peptide hormone?
    a. thyroxine
    b. cortisol
    c. glutathione
    d. glucagon

13. What are the isoflavones in soy protein called?
    a. genistein, daidzein, and glycitein
    b. estrogen and testosterone
    c. indoles and isothiocyanates
    d. chymotrypsin and trypsin

14. Which of the following is associated with the presence of edema in kwashiorkor?
    a. inadequate intake of water
    b. high plasma albumin levels
    c. low plasma albumin levels
    d. excessive intake of dietary protein

15. What is the name of the uncoupler protein present in brown fat mitochondria?
    a. glycogenin
    b. thermogenin
    c. lipogenin
    d. chymotrypsinogen

16. Which amino acid is NOT aromatic?
    a. tyrosine
    b. phenylalanine
    c. histidine
    d. tryptophan

17. Which of these molecules is the smallest?
    a. insulin
    b. glucagon
    c. glutathione
    d. myoglobin

18. Which protein is mostly triple-helical and practically insoluble in water?
    a. elastin
    b. collagen
    c. myoglobin
    d. trypsin

Answers

1. d. Serine is the amino acid from this list that is easily converted to pyruvate.

2. a. Tyrosine is converted to dopamine. Tryptophan can be converted to serotonin. Others are incorrect as only tyrosine runs directly into dopamine synthesis.

3. b. Alanine can lead to pyruvate directly by a transamination reaction. Both have three carbons. Oxaloacetate and fumarate have four carbons. Phosphoenolpyruvate has a complex structure and can be ruled out because it could not be produced by a simple transamination reaction.

4. d. Valine has a nonpolar side chain. Hydrophobic residues must be buried in the protein interior and away from water.

5. c. BPG is synthesized from an intermediate of glycolysis. Its concentration in red blood cells is about equal to the concentration of hemoglobin. BPG, by binding to deoxyhemoglobin, stabilizes hemoglobin in this deoxygenated form. The effect is to shift the O_2-saturation curve to the right.

6. a. As the concentration of H^+ rises, protonation of His HC3 of the β subunits of HbA promotes release of oxygen by favoring a transition to the T state. The T state of HbA provokes the release of oxygen.

7. c. Tryptophan is converted to 5-OH tryptophan and then to 5-OH tryptamine (serotonin). Phenylalanine and tyrosine can be used to synthesize catecholamines (dopamine, norepinephrine, and epinephrine).

8. d. The progressive oxidation of purines forms hypoxanthine, xanthine, and uric acid, which is excreted in the urine. Accumulation of uric acid, from a high purine diet (i.e., anchovies, organ meats, and shrimp), can lead to gout and renal calculi.

9. b. Lysine, threonine, and tryptophan are amino acids that tend to be lacking in grains such as wheat, rice, and corn.

10. b. Primary structure refers to the amino acid sequence of a protein, tertiary structure refers to three-dimensional folding, and quaternary structure is the interaction of multiple subunits.

11. d. Valine is degraded to succinyl-CoA, so it is glucogenic. Glycine is degraded to pyruvate that can be converted to either oxaloacetate or acetyl-CoA, so it is both glucogenic and ketogenic. Aspartate is degraded to oxaloacetate and is therefore glucogenic. Lysine and leucine are the only exclusively ketogenic amino acids.

12. d. Thyroxine is an amino acid derivative, cortisol is a steroid, and glutathione is a peptide but not a hormone.

13. a. Isoflavones are a phenol subclass of phytochemicals found in soybeans, beans, and other legumes. Genistein, daidzein, and glycitein are the major isoflavones present in soy protein.

14. c. Kwashiorkor is common in children due to a diet that may be adequate in total kilocalories but low in dietary protein. Synthesis of visceral proteins such as albumin by the liver is decreased in severe protein deficiency, resulting in decreased colloidal osmotic pressure. This causes an abnormal fluid shift from the plasma to the interstitial space resulting in edema, ascites, or anasarca.

15. b. Newborn infants have a type of adipose tissue called brown fat where fuel oxidation functions to generate heat rather than ATP to help keep the infant warm. Thermogenin is an uncoupler protein that provides a channel for protons to return to the mitochondrial matrix without passing through the ATP synthase complex (FoF1). The energy of oxidation is dissipated as heat rather than utilized for ATP synthesis.

16. c. All four amino acids contain rings, but the imidazole ring in histidine is not aromatic and the rings in the other amino acids are aromatic.

17. c. Glutathione is a blood tripeptide antioxidant. Insulin and glucagon are pancreatic peptide hormones containing 51 and 29 amino acids, respectively. Myoglobin is an O_2-binding protein with more than 150 amino acids.

18. b. Both elastin and collagen are typical fibrous proteins practically insoluble in water, but elastin is characterized by having a random conformation that goes from relaxed to stretched. The best-known collagens form fibers with triple helices formed with α-chains.

Enzymes

1. What condition applies to an enzyme-catalyzed reaction when $[S] > K_m$?
    a. velocity is half of Vmax
    b. velocity is directly proportional to [S]
    c. velocity depends on [E] and [S]
    d. velocity is near Vmax

2. What is the name of the inactive precursor of a protein that is regulated by proteolytic cleavage?
    a. phosphatase
    b. zymogen
    c. apoprotein
    d. peptide

3. The enzyme trypsin is classified as which of the following?
    a. oxidoreductase
    b. lyase
    c. hydrolase
    d. ligase

4. Individuals with lactose intolerance are often capable of tolerating small quantities of lactose found in which of these dairy products?
    a. buttermilk
    b. ice cream
    c. milk
    d. yogurt

5. In a catalyst reaction by an enzyme, the maximum initial velocity Vmax is which of the following?
    a. it is achieved when the enzyme is saturated by a substrate
    b. it is equal to two times the Michaelis-Menten constant K_m
    c. it is diminished in the presence of a competitive inhibitor
    d. it is independent of the concentration of the enzyme utilized

6. Enzymes that utilize coenzymes that are reversibly oxidized and reduced are in what class of enzymes?
    a. oxidoreductases
    b. transferases
    c. hydrolyses
    d. isomerases

Answers

1. d. At high substrate concentration ($[S] \geq 100\ K_m$), the enzyme is virtually saturated with substrate, the velocity of the reaction is near maximum, and a further increase in [S] has little effect on this velocity. The direct proportionality between velocity and [S] only applies early in the reaction when [S] is very low. Reaction velocity always depends on [E] and [S], except when the enzyme is already saturated with substrate at high [S]. Half-Vmax is reached when $[S] = K_m$.

2. b. The inactive precursor of an enzyme that is regulated by proteolytic cleavage is called a zymogen. The specific cleavage causes a conformational change that exposes the enzyme's active site. One example of a zymogen is trypsinogen. An enteropeptidase cleaves the last six amino acid residues from the amino terminus of the protein to yield trypsin; the active form of the enzyme.

3. c. Peptide bonds are broken with the addition of a molecule of water. This type of reaction is catalyzed by hydrolases. Oxidoreductases, lyases, and ligases catalyze oxidation-reduction reactions, bond breaking without addition of water, and bond making respectively.

4. d. Much of the lactose content in yogurt is metabolized for energy purposes by the bacteria.

5. a. At high [S], where $[S] > K_m$, the K_m term in the denominator of the Michaelis-Menten equation becomes insignificant, and the equation simplifies to V0 = Vmax. This is consistent with the plateau observed at high [S].

6. a. All oxidoreductases utilize coenzymes, which are reversibly oxidized and reduced. None of the other enzymes classes do this sort of reaction.

Hormones

1. Which of the following atoms is added to the structure of T_3 and T_4?
   a. selenium
   b. copper
   c. iodine
   d. magnesium

2. Which of these enzymes causes release of arachidonic acid from membrane phospholipids?
   a. phospholipase A_2
   b. phospholipase A_1
   c. phospholipase C
   d. phospholipase D

3. Which hormone is derived from an amino acid?
   a. insulin
   b. epinephrine
   c. retinoic acid
   d. calcitriol

4. Which is NOT a normal response to high blood insulin?
   a. ↑ glycolysis
   b. ↑ fatty acid synthesis
   c. ↓ glycogen degradation
   d. ↓ glucose uptake

5. Which of the following is true of Graves' disease?
   a. it promotes a hypothyroid state in the affected person
   b. it is provoked by the presence of antibody, which inhibits the TSH receptor
   c. it is characterized by a weak concentration of serum TSH
   d. it is characterized by destruction of the thyroid gland

6. Which is true of triiodothyronine (T$_3$)?
    a. it is a peptide hormone
    b. it is recognized by a membrane receptor on a target cell
    c. it is elevated in the serum in goiter caused by deiodase deficiency
    d. at high blood concentrations, it inhibits protein synthesis and produces a negative nitrogen balance

7. Leptin, which functions to decrease appetite, is synthesized in what tissue?
    a. liver
    b. adipose tissue
    c. muscle
    d. hypothalamus

8. Glucagon and epinephrine activate adenylyl cyclase present in the adipocyte cell membrane that initiates the intracellular second messenger cascade, which activates which enzyme?
    a. hormone-sensitive lipase
    b. lipoprotein lipase
    c. pancreatic lipase
    d. lingual lipase

9. The main function of iodine is for the synthesis of which type of hormone?
    a. catecholamine
    b. glucocorticoid
    c. parathyroid
    d. thyroid

10. Which hormone stimulates calcitriol synthesis in the kidneys?
    a. aldosterone
    b. calcitonin
    c. parathyroid hormone
    d. thyroxine

11. Which of the following hormones will stimulate gluconeogenesis?
    a. insulin
    b. glucagon
    c. aldosterone
    d. vasopressin

12. Hormones can be members of the all of the following classes of molecules EXCEPT for which one?
    a. peptides
    b. lipids
    c. carbohydrates
    d. amino acid derivatives

Answers

1. c. T_3 (triiodothyronine) and T_4 (thyroxine) require iodine be added to their structure so they can be fully functional.

2. a. Phospholipase A_2 releases the very long chain unsaturated fatty acids like arachidonic acid. These fatty acids are typically attached to the glycerol backbone of phospholipids at the middle of the glycerol, and this is where phospholipase A_2 lyses. All the others release different component parts of the phospholipids.

3. b. Epinephrine is made from tyrosine in the adrenal glands. Insulin is a pancreatic peptide hormone of 51 amino acids. Retinoic acid and calcitriol are active forms of the lipid-vitamins A and D, respectively.

4. d. Under normal healthy conditions, elevation of blood insulin after a meal should stimulate the rate of glycolysis, fatty acid synthesis, glycogen synthesis (and inhibition of glycogen degradation), and the uptake of glucose by cells, particularly in muscle, fat, liver, and pancreas cells.

5. c. Graves' disease is provoked by the production of IgG stimulating the thyroid, which activates the TSH receptor. It is followed by diffuse hypertrophy of the thyroid gland and excessive production (uncontrollable) of T_3 and T_4 with diminished serum TSH.

6. d. T_3 is synthesized as a tyrosyl residue of thyroglobulin. The thyroid hormones bind on the specific receptors present in the nucleus of the target cell. In the absence of deiodase, T_4 cannot be transformed into T_3. The very high concentrations of T_3 inhibit protein synthesis and produce a negative nitrogen balance.

7. b. Leptin is a small protein (167 amino acids) that is produced in the adipocytes. It acts on receptors of the arcuate nucleus of the hypothalamus to decrease the stimulation of the orexigenic (appetite-stimulating) neurons that synthesize and secrete neuropeptide Y (NPY) and increase the release of the anorexigenic peptides (inhibit appetite) in an effort to regulate energy intake. The level of leptin production and secretion increases with the number and size of adipocytes.

8. a. Glucagon and epinephrine are secreted in response to low blood glucose levels and signal the need for metabolic energy. They initiate the activation of hormone-sensitive lipase, which is present in the cytosol of adipocytes. Hormone-sensitive lipase functions to begin hydrolyzing triacylglycerols into free fatty acids (for oxidation) and glycerol (for gluconeogenesis).

9. d. Iodine deficiency causes an underactive thyroid gland and can lead to goiter.

10. c. The kidney is where vitamin D3 is converted to its biologically active form, calcitriol. Calcitriol, along with PTH, increases serum calcium levels by influencing its renal reabsorption, intestinal uptake, and bone resorption. The reabsorption of sodium is under the influence of aldosterone. Calcitonin lowers serum calcium levels.

11. b. Glucagon is produced in response to low blood sugar and functions to increase blood sugar. Thus, it stimulates pathways that produce glucose, such as gluconeogenesis.

12. c. Hormones like insulin and glucagon are peptides, the steroid hormones are lipids, and thyroxine is an amino acid derivative.

Nucleotides and Nucleic Acids

1. Which is a final degradation product of the purine nucleotides in humans?
   a. β-alanine
   b. xanthine
   c. urea
   d. uric acid

2. Which is a structural difference between DNA and RNA?
   a. DNA contains thymine instead of uracil
   b. DNA contains ribose instead of deoxyribose
   c. DNA contains uracil instead of thymine
   d. DNA contains guanine instead of cytosine

3. Which is the ring structure in pyrimidine biosynthesis that is placed onto the ribose phosphate using PRPP?
   a. uracil
   b. orotate
   c. cytosine
   d. thymine

4. Which of the following is a high-energy intermediate utilized in the salvage of a free nitrogenous base to elevate it to the monophosphate nucleotide level?
   a. 5′-phosphoribosylamine
   b. 5′-phosphoribosyl-1′-pyrophosphate
   c. methenyl-tetrahydrofolate
   d. formyl-tetrahydrofolate

5. Activated ribose (PRPP) is a key intermediate for the synthesis of nucleotides and some amino acids. Which reaction represents the activation of ribose?
   a. ribose 1-phosphate + ATP $\rightarrow$ PRPP + AMP
   b. ribose 2-phosphate + ATP $\rightarrow$ PRPP + AMP
   c. ribose 3-phosphate + ATP $\rightarrow$ PRPP + AMP
   d. ribose 5-phosphate + ATP $\rightarrow$ PRPP + AMP

6.   Which base is missing in DNA?
     a.   adenine
     b.   guanine
     c.   uracil
     d.   thymine

7.   Among the choices below, which one does not play a role in the replication of a bacterial chromosome?
     a.   UTP (uridine 5′-triphosphate)
     b.   reverse transcriptase
     c.   DNA polymerase I
     d.   helicases

8.   Regarding *E. coli,* the proofreading of DNA is performed by what enzyme?
     a.   3′-5′ exonuclease activity of RNA polymerase
     b.   5′-3′ polymerase activity of DNA polymerases I and III
     c.   3′-5′ exonuclease activity of DNA polymerases I, II, and III
     d.   5′-3′ exonuclease activity of DNA polymerase III

9.   Which sugar is involved in the synthesis of nucleic acids?
     a.   mannose
     b.   galactose
     c.   ribose
     d.   xylose

10. The synthesis of this nucleotide is derived from vitamin B2.
     a.   DNA
     b.   FAD
     c.   NAD
     d.   RNA

11. What is the name of the linkage (bond) that forms the covalent backbone of DNA and RNA?
     a.   ester linkage
     b.   phosphodiester linkage
     c.   hydrogen bond
     d.   glycosidic bond

12. What is the name of the disease that is caused by an elevated concentration of uric acid in the blood and tissues that causes joints to become inflamed, painful, and arthritic?
    a. Lyme disease
    b. gout
    c. Parkinson's disease
    d. rheumatoid arthritis

Answers

1. d. β-alanine is the degradation product of pyrimidines, xanthine is an intermediate in purine degradation, and urea is a degradation product of amino acids and purines in some lower animals.

2. a. RNA contains ribose and uracil, and both DNA and RNA contain guanine and cytosine.

3. b. Orotate is the pyrimidine structure attached first to ribose 5-phosphate.

4. b. The intermediate 5′-phosphoribosyl-1′-pyrophosphate (PRPP) is used by enzymes called phosphoribosyl transferases. These enzymes are important to the process of the salvage of nitrogenous bases. This offers the body a tremendous energy savings as de novo synthesis is energetically expensive. None of the other intermediates listed can fulfill this function.

5. d. PRPP is formed by ribose phosphate pyrophosphokinase by attachment of pyrophosphate from ATP to carbon-1 of ribose 5-phosphate.

6. c. Both DNA and RNA contain the purine bases adenine and guanine and the pyrimidine base cytosine but differ in the other pyrimidine base they contain. DNA contains thymine, and RNA contains uracil.

7. b. Reverse transcriptase (RNA-directed DNA polymerase) catalyzes the synthesis of a DNA strand complementary to the viral RNA. The same enzyme degrades the RNA strand in the resulting RNA-DNA hybrid and replaces it with DNA.

8. c. During the replication and repair of DNA, the DNA polymerases can remove the mispaired nucleotide, and the polymerase begins again. This activity is termed proofreading.

9. c. Ribose and deoxyribose form part of the molecular structures of RNA and DNA, respectively.

10. b. Riboflavin (B2) is a constituent of flavin adenine dinucleotide (FAD). Niacin (B3) is necessary for nicotinamide adenine dinucleotide (NAD) synthesis. These nucleotides play important roles in energy production. DNA and RNA are nucleic acids.

11. b. The nucleotides of both DNA and RNA are covalently linked where the 5′-phosphate group of one nucleotide unit is joined to the 3′-hydroxyl group of the next nucleotide, creating a phosphodiester linkage. These successive linkages form the backbone of the nucleotides similar to the sides of a stepladder.

12. b. Normal degradation of the purines, adenine and guanine, is the formation of uric acid. Gout often occurs due to the underexcretion of urate, which leads to abnormal deposition of sodium urate crystals in the joints and sometimes in the kidney tubules.

Vitamins and Minerals

1. A deficiency in which vitamin is associated with bleeding gums?
   a. vitamin A
   b. vitamin B6
   c. vitamin C
   d. vitamin D

2. Which vitamin is not an antioxidant?
   a. vitamin A
   b. vitamin C
   c. vitamin E
   d. vitamin K

3. Which of the following iron-containing foods contains the most absorbable form of dietary iron?
   a. red meat
   b. pasta
   c. milk
   d. spinach

4. What is the RDA for vitamin C?
   a. 60 mg/day
   b. 120 mg/day
   c. 500 mg/day
   d. 1,200 mg/day

5. Which of the following is a disease marked by accumulation of copper in the liver, brain, kidneys, and eye?
   a. Menke's disease
   b. hemochromatosis
   c. goiter
   d. Wilson's disease

6. What is the recommended daily intake for sodium?
   a. 1,000 mg/day
   b. 2,400 mg/day
   c. 5,000 mg/day
   d. 10,000 mg/day

7. The dietary precursor in mammals of coenzyme A is which of the following?
   a. pyridoxine
   b. niacin
   c. biotin
   d. pantothenic acid

8. Which is true of thiamine (vitamin B1)?
   a. it is a lipid-soluble vitamin
   b. it is necessary in humans because a deficiency may cause pellagra
   c. it is a coenzyme that participates in oxidative decarboxylation of α-keto acids
   d. it is made up of two nitrogen bases, two sugars, and two phosphates

9. Tetrahydrofolate is a coenzyme that permits the transfer of what substances?
   a. amine groups
   b. CO_2 (or bicarbonate)
   c. monocarbon groups other than CO_2
   d. multicarbon groups

10. Which vitamin is NOT required for the function of the pyruvate dehydrogenase complex?
    a. thiamine
    b. niacin
    c. pyridoxine
    d. pantothenic acid

11. Niacin deficiency is associated with which disease?
    a. rickets
    b. pellagra
    c. xerophthalmia
    d. scurvy

12. The RDA for what mineral in women of child-bearing age is more than double the RDA for men?
    a. calcium
    b. magnesium
    c. zinc
    d. iron

13. Phylloquinones and menaquinones are natural forms of which vitamin?
    a. vitamin A
    b. vitamin D
    c. vitamin E
    d. vitamin K

14. In what organ does the enzyme α-1-hydroxylase hydroxylate vitamin D3 (cholecalciferol) to its fully active hormonal form?
    a. liver
    b. kidney
    c. pancreas
    d. intestines

15. Which of the following foods is a good source of provitamin A carotenoids?
    a. pears
    b. roast beef
    c. cantaloupe
    d. cauliflower

16. Which vitamin/mineral pair is essential for glycolysis?
    a. riboflavin/calcium
    b. niacin/magnesium
    c. niacin/calcium
    d. riboflavin/magnesium

17. The pyruvate dehydrogenase complex catalyzes the conversion of pyruvate to acetyl-CoA in mitochondria. Which vitamin is NOT needed for this reaction?
    a. thiamine
    b. pantothenate
    c. pyridoxine
    d. riboflavin

18. Which condition/vitamin deficiency is NOT a correct match?
    a. night blindness/vitamin A
    b. hemolysis of red blood cells/vitamin D
    c. hemorrhage/vitamin K
    d. pellagra/niacin

Answers

1. c. Intakes of less than 10 mg/day of vitamin C can result in scurvy. Bleeding gums are one of the first signs, leading ultimately to loose and decaying teeth. Other signs and symptoms include petechiae, ecchymosis, arthralgia, and hyperkeratosis of hair follicles.

2. d. Antioxidant vitamins include vitamins A, C, and E and beta-carotene.

3. a. Heme iron, derived mainly from hemoglobin and myoglobin, is found in meat, fish, and poultry. Unlike nonheme iron, heme iron does not have to be enzymatically liberated and is absorbed intact by the enterocyte. Furthermore, the other choices contain inhibitors of iron absorption such as calcium (milk), oxalates (spinach), and phytates (pasta).

4. a. The RDA for vitamin C is set at 60 mg/day as this is sufficient to prevent scurvy and to allow for sufficient synthesis of catecholamine neurotransmitters.

5. d. Wilson's disease is the disease described here. Accumulation of iron would be called hemochromatosis.

6. b. The recommended daily intake for sodium is set at 2,400 mg/day. No other numbers seen here would be health promoting, and each would be associated with signs of illness.

7. d. Pantothenic acid is the dietary precursor of Coenzyme A.

8. c. Thiamine, formed from a nitrogen base and a thiazolium ring, is a water-soluble vitamin. The absence of vitamin B1 in the human diet leads to the condition known as beriberi. Thiamine pyrophosphate plays a role in chemical rearrangements involving transfer of an activated aldehyde group from one carbon to another.

9. c. Tetrahydrofolate (H4 folate) is synthesized in bacteria, and its precursor, folate, is a vitamin for mammals. The different forms of tetrahydrofolate are interchangeable and serve as donors of one-carbon units, such as methyl, methylene, methenyl, formyl, or formimino groups, in a variety of biosynthetic reactions.

10. c. Thiamine is required for pyruvate decarboxylase/dehydrogenase. Electrons are passed from pyruvate to lipoic acid, to FAD, and finally to NAD^+, a derivative of niacin. The acetyl group of pyruvate is passed to coenzyme A, which is derived from pantothenic acid. Pyridoxine (B6) is a precursor to pyridoxal phosphate, which is required for the function of many other enzymes.

11. b. Niacin forms the coenzymes NAD and NADP, which are used in oxidation-reduction reactions. Deficiency of niacin causes pellagra, which leads to dementia, diarrhea, and dermatitis.

12. d. Iron is one of the few nutrients require in larger quantities by women, owing to loss of iron through menstruation.

13. d. Phylloquinones (the vitamin K1 series) are synthesized by green plants, and the menaquinones (the vitamin K3 series) are synthesized by bacteria. The synthetic form of vitamin K (menadione) is twice as potent biologically as the naturally occurring forms of K1 and K2.

14. b. Cholecalciferol (vitamin D3) is produced in the skin by UV irradiation of 7-dehyrocholesterol. To become fully active as a hormone, vitamin D3 has to undergo two sequential hydroxylations. The first occurs in the liver and forms 25-hydroxyvitamin D3 (25-hydroxycholecalciferol). The second hydroxylation is performed by the enzyme α-1 hydroxylase in the kidney, which yields the most active form.

15. c. Preformed vitamin A exists only in foods of animal origin. Provitamin A carotenoids are found in dark green leafy and yellow-orange fruits and vegetables. Carrots, greens, orange juice, sweet potatoes, and cantaloupe are excellent sources of provitamin A.

16. b. Niacin is only vitamin that is essential in glycolysis. It is the precursor of NAD^+; a cosubstrate coenzyme in the only redox reaction of glycolysis catalyzed by glyceraldehyde 3-phosphate dehydrogenase. Magnesium is also essential in glycolysis. There are four reactions in glycolysis catalyzed by kinases; enzymes that always require magnesium and sometimes other minerals. The real substrate for kinases, and other enzymes that catalyze chemical reactions in which ATP/ADP is involved, is Mg-ATP or Mg-ADP.

17.   c.   The pyruvate dehydrogenase complex is a beautiful example of the role of vitamins in metabolism. This enzyme needs five coenzymes to convert pyruvate into acetyl-CoA, and four of these coenzymes are derived from vitamins: thiamine pyrophosphate (thiamine), coenzyme A (pantothenate), NAD^+ (niacin), and FAD (riboflavin). The other cofactor is lipoic acid; a metabolite-derived coenzyme made in ample amounts by humans. Pyridoxine (vitamin B6) does not participate in this reaction.

18.   b.   Hemolysis of RBCs could occur under conditions of deficiency or lack of vitamin E, not vitamin D, especially during periods of oxidative stress. Vitamin D regulates blood calcium. Vitamin A is essential for normal night and color vision. Vitamin K is essential for normal coagulation of blood. Pellagra could result from a lack of niacin in the diet.

Biochemical Energetics

1. What makes enzymes effective catalysts?
   a. they increase the energy released during a reaction
   b. they increase the activation energy required for a reaction
   c. they decrease the equilibrium of the reaction
   d. they decrease the activation energy required for a reaction

2. What type of reversible inhibitor competes with the substrate for the active site of an enzyme?
   a. noncompetitive inhibitor
   b. competitive inhibitor
   c. uncompetitive inhibitor
   d. mixed inhibitor

3. For this reaction, A → B, the $\Delta G'^{\circ} = 5.7$ kJ/mol at 25° C. Which is correct at equilibrium?
   a. $[B] = [A]$
   b. $Keq = 100$
   c. $[B] > [A]$
   d. $10[B] = [A]$

4. Which is a characteristic of a near-equilibrium cellular reaction?
   a. Keq and Q differ by several orders of magnitude
   b. ΔG is large and negative
   c. the reaction is potentially a regulatory point
   d. the reaction is reversible

5. A cereal breakfast bar containing 3 g of fat, 2 g of protein, and 30 g of carbohydrates has approximately how many calories?
   a. 140
   b. 150
   c. 155
   d. 290

6. Which vitamin-derived nucleotide is NOT involved in energy production within the Krebs cycle or the electron transport chain?
    a. NADPH
    b. FMN
    c. FAD
    d. NAD

7. Biochemical reactions are considered to be reversible if their $\Delta G'^{\circ}$ is which of the following?
    a. large and positive
    b. large and negative
    c. close to zero
    d. equal to $\Delta H0'$

8. A biochemical reaction taking place in a healthy human with a large positive ΔG can proceed in the forward direction only if which of the following is TRUE?
    a. it is catalyzed by an enzyme
    b. it is coupled with a reaction with a larger negative ΔG
    c. the temperature is increased
    d. the activation energy is lowered

9. The functional electron transport systems can be formed in vitro from purified components of the respiratory chain and vascular membranes. Assuming the presence of O_2, succinate, ubiquinone (UQ), cytochrome c, and complexes III and IV, the final electron receptor is which of the following?
    a. succinate
    b. complex III
    c. complex IV
    d. H_2O

10. Which of the following is TRUE of the Krebs cycle?
    a. it is implicated in the synthesis of glucose from acetyl-CoA
    b. it can function equally well aerobically and anaerobically
    c. it requires pyridoxal phosphate and lipoic acid for its activity
    d. it is inhibited by an elevated intracellular level of ATP, NADH, and citrate

11. The passage of a high-energy phosphate from one organic structure to another and facilitated by an enzyme is given what term?
    a. oxidative phosphorylation
    b. oxidase phosphorylation
    c. redox phosphorylation
    d. substrate-level phosphorylation

12. The majority of the energy conserved in the TCA cycle is by the harvesting of which of the following?
    a. high-energy phosphates
    b. high-energy esters
    c. high-energy thioesters
    d. high-energy electrons

1. d. Enzymes lower the activation energy for a reaction, which enhances the reaction rate. Covalent and noncovalent interactions between the enzyme and the substrate provide a lower-energy reaction path. Formation of noncovalent (weak) interactions in the enzyme-substrate complex results in the release of a small amount of free energy, which is a major source of free energy used by enzymes to lower the activation energies of reactions.

2. b. A competitive inhibitor competes for the active site of an enzyme, while the mixed inhibitor and uncompetitive inhibitor (noncompetitive inhibitor) bind to a site other than the active site of the enzyme.

3. d. The relationship between the equilibrium constant of a chemical reaction (Keq) and its standard free energy ($\Delta G'^{\circ}$) is established by this equation, $\Delta G'^{\circ} = -5.7\log$ Keq. The equilibrium constant (Keq) for this reaction is 0.1 (Keq = [B]/[A] = [B]/10[B] = 1/10). The log of 0.1 is equal to -1, therefore, $\Delta G'^{\circ} = -5.7\log$ Keq = $(-5.7)(-1) =$ 5.7 kJ/mol.

4. d. Cellular chemical reactions are divided into near-equilibrium reactions and far-from equilibrium reactions. This classification depends on the magnitudes of Keq and Q. Keq is the equilibrium constant calculated using in vitro or standard conditions (equilibrium conditions), whereas Q is the equilibrium constant using in vivo or cellular conditions (steady-state conditions). Near-equilibrium reactions are characterized by the following: (1) the magnitudes of Keq and Q are similar, (2) ΔG is a positive value or a small negative value, and (3) reaction is easily reversible, where the same enzyme catalyzes the forward and the reverse reaction.

5. c. 3 g (9 kcal/g) + 2 g (4 kcal/g) + 30 g (4 kcal/g) = 155 kcal. Although commonly expressed as calories, "kilocalories" is the technically correct unit of measurement.

6. a. NADPH acts as a reducing agent in many biosynthetic pathways, including fatty acid, cholesterol, and DNA synthesis.

7. c. $\Delta G'^\circ$ refers to the case where the concentration of all reaction components is 1 M and pH = 7. ΔG can be shifted away from $\Delta G'^\circ$ by altering the ratio of the concentrations of products and substrates. When $\Delta G'^\circ$ is close to 0, these adjustments to ΔG can change its sign, so these reactions can go forward or backward, depending on the concentrations of products and substrates.

8. b. The ΔG for coupled reactions is equal to the sum of the ΔGs for the reactions involved. Thus, if the negative ΔG is larger, the overall ΔG will be negative and the coupled reactions will be spontaneous.

9. a. Electrons of succinate reach O_2 through complex II, ubiquinone (UQ), complex III, cytochrome c, complex IV, and finally O_2 to form with $2H^+$ to make one H_2O molecule. In the absence of complex II, the electrons will remain on the succinate.

10. d. ATP inhibits the pyruvate dehydrogenase complex, citrate synthase, and isocitrate dehydrogenase. NADH inhibits the pyruvate dehydrogenase complex, citrate synthase, and α-ketoglutarate dehydrogenase. Citrate inhibits citrate synthase.

11. d. Passage of high-energy phosphate from one organic structure to another that is facilitated by an enzyme-catalyzed reaction is defined as substrate level phosphorylation. Oxidative phosphorylation is the name given to ATP produced from ADP and inorganic phosphate based on the work done by a transmembrane gradient of H^+ flowing through an ATP synthase. The rest of the answers are incorrect.

12. d. High-energy electrons of $NADH^+$, H^+, and $FADH_2$ represent the major sources of energy gathered in the TCA cycle. These high-energy electrons are used to pump protons across the inner membrane of the mitochondrion, and the H^+ subsequently trapped is utilized to drive the ATP synthase. While substrate-level phosphorylation does occur in the TCA, it is not the majority of the energy gained through the oxidation of the carbon structures of the cycle.

Section Four Recommended Reading

Champe P, Harvey R, Ferrier D: *Lippincott's illustrated reviews: biochemistry*, ed 3, Baltimore, 2004, Lippincott Williams & Wilkins.

Devlin T, ed: *Textbook of biochemistry with clinical correlations*, ed 6, New York, 2005, Wiley-Liss.

Mahan LK, Escott-Stump S, eds: *Krause's food, nutrition & diet therapy*, ed 11. Philadelphia, 2003, WB Saunders.

Murray R, Granner D, Mayes P, Rodwell V: *Harper's illustrated biochemistry*, ed 26, Stamford, Conn, 2003, Appleton & Lange.

Nelson D, Cox M: *Lehninger principles of biochemistry*, ed 4, New York, 2004, WH Freeman.

Nix S: *Williams' basic nutrition and diet therapy*, ed 12, St Louis, 2005, Mosby.

Smith C, Marks A, Lieberman M: *Marks' basic medical biochemistry: a clinical approach*, ed 2, Baltimore, 2004, Lippincott Williams & Wilkins.

Stipanuk M: *Biochemical and physiological aspects of human nutrition*, Philadelphia, 1999, WB Saunders.

Voet D, Voet J, *Biochemistry*, ed 3, Hoboken, NJ, 2004, Wiley.

Pathology

*Jill M. Davis, J. Michael Perryman, Seva Philomin,
Djamel Ramla, Virgil Stoia, Vrajlal H. Vyas*

Fundamentals of Pathology

1. What is the type of necrosis in which denaturation of proteins is the primary pattern?
   a. liquefactive necrosis
   b. coagulative necrosis
   c. fat necrosis
   d. caseous necrosis

2. Which of the following can be described as a change in tissue type from one adult form to another due to an adaptation to stress?
   a. transformation
   b. hyperplasia
   c. agenesis
   d. metaplasia

3. A loss of arterial blood flow to a tissue is best described by which term?
   a. hypoxia
   b. ischemia
   c. hypercapnia
   d. dyspnea

4. Which of the following is NOT a characteristic of apoptosis?
   a. reduced cell size
   b. nucleus fragmentation
   c. intact plasma membrane
   d. inflammation

5. Which of the following is LEAST likely to be present or associated with the early stage of acute inflammation?
   a. hyperemia
   b. fibroblastic proliferation
   c. increased neutrophils
   d. tissue exudates

6. What type of necrosis is MOST often associated with the granulomatous changes seen in pulmonary tuberculosis?
   a. fibrinoid
   b. gummatous
   c. liquefactive
   d. caseous

7. Which of the following changes in cellular morphology is considered irreversible?
   a. karyolysis
   b. mitochondrial swelling
   c. presence of surface membrane blebs
   d. clumping of nuclear chromatin

8. The most serious complication of lower extremity thrombophlebitis is which of the following?
   a. cerebral infarction
   b. pulmonary infarction
   c. myocardial infarction
   d. kidney infection

9. Pedal edema is a prominent feature of which condition?
   a. cirrhosis
   b. nephrotic syndrome
   c. kwashiorkor
   d. right heart failure

10. Which of the following is the earliest event that occurs in acute inflammation?
    a. leukocytic margination
    b. vasodilation
    c. increased permeability
    d. stasis

11. The morphologic features of chronic inflammation include all EXCEPT which of the following?
    a. mononuclear infiltration
    b. fibrosis
    c. angiogenesis
    d. neutrophilic infiltration

12. Red infarcts are found in all of the tissues EXCEPT which one of the following?
    a. heart
    b. liver
    c. lung
    d. intestine

13. An amyloidosis lesion corresponds to which of the following descriptions?
   a. it is an intracellular cytokeratin disorder resulting in Mallory bodies
   b. extracellular glycogen deposits occur in the liver
   c. it contains intercellular Congo red–stained protein deposits
   d. it contains intracellular transthyretin protein deposits

14. Karyorrhexis corresponds to which characteristic morphologic alteration of the nuclei?
   a. reversible cell degeneration
   b. chromatin fragmentation
   c. pyknosis of chromatin
   d. formation of apoptotic bodies

15. Transudates are characterized by which of the following conditions?
   a. increased active capillary endothelial permeability
   b. polymorphonuclear leukocytesand fibrinogen afflux out of the vessel
   c. high-gravity protein-rich fluid extravasation
   d. passive extravasation of plasmatic fluid

16. Which description BEST characterizes severe squamous epithelium dysplasia?
   a. well-differentiated in situ carcinoma
   b. abnormal mitoses, tetraploidy, and anisocytosis
   c. poorly differentiated metastatic tumor
   d. anaplastic, locally aggressive tumor

17. Which of the following characteristics is NOT consistent with ante mortem thrombus description?
   a. dry and crumbly aspect, migration in the bloodstream
   b. firmly adherent to the underlying vessel or heart wall
   c. easily detachable thrombi, without endocardiac alteration
   d. typical laminations corresponding to lines of Zahn

18. An enlargement of tissues or organs as a result of an enlargement of individual cells is the definition of what term?
   a. hypertrophy
   b. hyperplasia
   c. dysplasia
   d. metaplasia

19. This cellular adaptation is characterized by a disorderly arrangement of cells and nuclear atypia.
     a. hypertrophy
     b. hyperplasia
     c. dysplasia
     d. metaplasia

20. An enlargement of tissues or organs as a result of an increase in the number of cells is the definition of what term?
     a. hypertrophy
     b. hyperplasia
     c. dysplasia
     d. metaplasia

21. What is the pathogenetic mechanism of ischemia?
     a. anemia
     b. reduced arterial blood flow
     c. carbon monoxide poisoning
     d. cardiorespiratory failure

22. What is NOT part of distinct interrelated steps involved in phagocytosis of dead cells?
     a. recognition
     b. opsonization
     c. chemotaxis
     d. degradation

23. Which of the following statements is NOT a characteristic of chronic inflammation?
     a. tissue destruction
     b. infiltration with mononuclear cells
     c. increased vascular permeability
     d. connective tissue replacement of damaged tissue

24. If a patient survives the immediate effects of a thrombotic vascular obstruction, what is NOT the subsequent fate of the thrombus?
     a. organization
     b. consumption coagulopathy
     c. embolization
     d. propagation

Answers

1. b. In necrosis, there is intracellular acidosis; there is denaturation of structural proteins and enzymes, thus blocking proteolysis of the cell. This type of necrosis, termed coagulative necrosis, is typical of hypoxic cell death in all tissues except the brain. Liquefactive necrosis is the result of enzymatic digestion. Caseous necrosis is characteristic of tuberculosis infection. Fat necrosis is seen in pancreatitis, where pancreatic lipases are released.

2. d. An example of metaplasia is seen in patients with GERD (gastroesophageal reflux disease) in which stomach acid repeatedly irritates the lower esophagus, causing the mucosal epithelium to change from squamous to columnar (Barrett esophagus).

3. b. Ischemia refers to a decrease in blood flow. Hypoxia refers to a lack of oxygen in a tissue. It is true, however, that ischemia leads to hypoxia. Hypercapnia refers to an increase in carbon dioxide in the blood. Dyspnea refers to the feeling of breathlessness.

4. d. Apoptosis, or programmed cell death, is an orderly death of cells that is distinguished from necrosis by the lack of inflammation, cell membrane disruption, and pyknosis of the nucleus. Apoptosis is induced by a lack of growth factors or hormones, stimulation of death receptors, or DNA damage.

5. b. Fibroblastic proliferation is a feature of granulation tissue formation, longstanding or chronic inflammation. Hyperemia, neutrophilia, and exudative tissue swelling are early features of acute inflammation.

6. d. Caseous necrosis is a term derived from the white cheesy appearance of lesions associated with tuberculosis on gross examination. Gummas are rubber-like lesions associated with tertiary syphilis. Liquefaction is associated with abscesses and brain lesions.

7. a. Karyolysis results from the enzymatic breakdown of DNA following cell death. Other features are considered reversible if initiating factors are removed.

8. b. Thromboembolus formation is a common complication of thrombophlebitis in lower leg veins. Thrombi can pass through the heart and obstruct major pulmonary arteries.

9. d. At the sites of highest hydrostatic pressures, edema distribution is typically influenced by gravity (e.g., legs when standing) which is best seen in right heart failure. In cirrhosis (as ascites), nephrotic syndrome (as periorbital edema), and kwashiorkor (as generalized), the edema is due to decreased oncotic pressure.

10. b. Vasodilation is the earliest manifestation of inflammation resulting in increased blood flow, which then leads to heat and redness.

11. d. Neutrophilic infiltration is the hallmark of acute inflammation.

12. a. Red infarcts are found in tissues that have a double blood supply (such as the liver and lung) or that have collateral vessels (such as in the intestine), whereas white infarct occurs in the heart.

13. c. Amyloidosis is an intercellular congophilic proteinaceous substance deposit. Mallory bodies consist of hepatocyte intracellular cytokeratin acidophilic inclusions, which occur in chronic alcoholism. Glycogen deposits are encountered in glycogenesis disorders.

14. b. Karyorrhexis is a state of irreversible chromatin fragmentation, present in the necrosis process. Pyknosis consists of chromatin condensation. Apoptotic bodies are bleb-composed, tightly packed organelles, with or without nuclei, observed in apoptosis.

15. d. Transudate results from passive extravasation of plasmatic fluid through normal blood vessel endothelium, that is, vascular permeability is normal. Transudate is a low-gravity fluid, with no cells, fibrinogen, or leukocytes.

16. a. Severe squamous epithelial dysplasia corresponds to a well-differentiated in situ carcinoma. The remaining characteristics are compatible with anaplastic tumors.

17. c. Ante mortem thrombus is firmly adherent to altered heart walls. It is characterized by a dry, crumbly aspect, Zahn line formation with a succession of thrombocytes, fibrin, and red blood cell layers.

18. a. Hypertrophy is an enlargement of cells or tissue but not an increase in cell number. There is an increase in the number of organelles within the cell, however. Hypertrophy may be physiologic or pathologic.

19. c. Dysplasia is abnormal arrangement of cells with atypical nuclei being a common finding. Dysplasia is considered precancerous in soft tissue.

20. b. Hyperplasia is an increase in the number of cells that may result in enlargement of the organ involved.

21. b. Ischemia is caused by reduced arterial blood flow compromising the supply not only of oxygen but also of metabolic substrates like glucose. Anemia and carbon monoxide poisoning result in hypoxia due to reduced oxygen carried in the blood. Cardiorespiratory failure also results in hypoxia due to inadequate oxygenation of blood.

22. c. Chemotaxis is a process involved in acute inflammation that occurs before phagocytosis and after leukocyte emigration. Phagocytosis involves three distinct steps in the following order: recognition of an antigen, opsonization of an antigen, and degradation of an antigen by cytoplasmic biochemical processes of a phagocyte.

23. c. Increased vascular permeability is characteristic of acute inflammation that facilitates leukocyte exudation and precedes leukocytic events such as chemotaxis and phagocytosis. Continued phagocytic function is performed by mononuclear cells like monocytes and macrophages. These mononuclear cells also promote tissue destruction followed by initiation of connective tissue replacement of damaged tissue.

24. b. Consumption coagulopathy is a rapid consequent clinicopathologic outcome of disseminated intravascular coagulation, not the fate of a single thrombus. Propagation, embolization, and organization are the possible subsequent outcomes of single thrombus.

Genetic and Congenital Disorders

1. Marfan's syndrome is characterized by:
   a. a genetic defect in a receptor-mediated transport system
   b. an inherited defect in an extracellular glycoprotein called fibrillin-1
   c. some defect in the synthesis or structure of fibrillar collagen
   d. inherited deficiency of serum alpha-1 antitrypsin

2. Which one of the following is associated with the greatest likelihood of the development of a Wilms tumor?
   a. WAGR syndrome
   b. Denys-Drash syndrome
   c. Beckwith-Weidemann syndrome
   d. Behçet's syndrome

3. In which of the following is macroglossia likely?
   a. WAGR
   b. Denys-Drash syndrome
   c. Beckwith-Weidemann syndrome
   d. Becker muscular dystrophy

4. Marfan's disease is a hereditary autosomal dominant syndrome characterized by which of the following?
   a. arachnodactyly and joint ankylosis
   b. fibrillin-1 gene dysfunction
   c. crystalline ectopy and aortic stenosis
   d. collagen gene dysfunction

5. Which is the most common Mendelian (single-gene) disorder?
   a. retinoblastoma
   b. familial hypercholesterolemia
   c. cystic fibrosis
   d. colonic polyposis

6. An individual who is phenotypically female complains of amenorrhea and infertility. On examination, it is noted that she is abnormally short in stature and has a webbed neck. Which of the following is the most likely diagnosis for this individual?
    a. Turner's syndrome
    b. Cri-du-chat syndrome
    c. Down syndrome
    d. Klinefelter's syndrome

7. Multiple neural tumors, café au lait spots, and Lisch nodules are characteristic of which disease?
    a. neurofibromatosis
    b. multiple myeloma
    c. amyloidosis
    d. alkaptonuria

Answers

1. b. Marfan's syndrome is a connective tissue disorder with a defect in extracellular glycoprotein called as fibrillin-1. A defect in a receptor-mediated transport system is seen in familial hypercholesterolemia. A defect in the synthesis or structure of fibrillar collagen is seen in Ehlers-Danlös syndrome. A deficiency of serum alpha-1 antitrypsin is seen in emphysema.

2. b. The order of occurrence of Wilms tumor is Denys-Drash syndrome followed by WAGR syndrome and then Beckwith-Weidemann syndrome. Behçet's syndrome is not associated with Wilms tumor.

3. c. Although the first three choices are associated with an increased risk of developing Wilms tumor, only Beckwith-Weidemann syndrome is associated with macroglossia.

4. b. Marfan's disease is a genetic dominant autosomal disorder due to fibrillin-1 gene dysfunction. It is grossly characterized by arachnodactyly and joint hyperlaxity and aortic aneurysm. Collagen coding gene dysfunction corresponds to Ehlers-Danlös syndrome.

5. b. Familial hypercholesterolemia is possibly the most frequent Mendelian disorder. The other choices are less common.

6. a. Turner's syndrome is a cytogenetic disorder involving monosomy of the X chromosome. The karyotype is 45XO. Turner's syndrome is the most common female sex chromosome disorder, affecting approximately 1 in 2000. It is characterized by prepubescent habitus, streak ovaries, a broad chest, coarctation of the aorta, webbed neck, obesity, and insulin resistance.

7. a. Neurofibromatosis (formerly von Recklinghausen disease) is an autosomal dominant disorder characterized by neurofibromas within nerve trunks anywhere in the skin and also internally. Café au lait spots are light brown cutaneous pigmentations. Lisch nodules are pigmented hamartomas in the iris.

Disorders of the Immune System

1. Which disorder is associated with the CREST syndrome?
   a. Sjögren's syndrome
   b. rheumatoid arthritis
   c. systemic lupus erythematosus
   d. scleroderma

2. In type IV delayed hypersensitivity reactions, which cell type is involved in the process?
   a. CD4$^+$ T helper 1 cells
   b. CD4$^+$ helper 2 cells
   c. mast cells and basophils
   d. eosinophils and platelets

3. Antibody-mediated cellular dysfunction is seen in which disorder?
   a. autoimmune hemolytic anemia
   b. hypersensitive allergic reaction
   c. Graves' disease
   d. rheumatoid arthritis

4. The most common leukemia of children is:
   a. acute myelogenous leukemia
   b. acute lymphoblastic leukemia
   c. chronic myelogenous leukemia
   d. chronic lymphoblastic leukemia

5. A triad of symptoms to include xerophthalmia (dry eyes), xerostomia (dry mouth), and the diagnosis of rheumatoid arthritis is known as:
   a. Sjögren's syndrome
   b. Felty's syndrome
   c. Still's disease
   d. Reiter's syndrome

6. Bronchial asthma (atopic form) is an example of what type of hypersensitivity reaction?
    a. type I
    b. type II
    c. type III
    d. type IV

Answers

1. d. CREST is an acronym for calcinosis, Raynaud's phenomenon, esophageal dysmotility, sclerodactyly, and telangiectasia. This disorder is characterized by abnormal fibrosis of the skin and several organs. Although the etiology is unknown, the likely trigger is an abnormal immune response coupled with vascular damage leading to growth factor–induced collagen production.

2. a. In delayed type IV hypersensitivity, the main mediators involved are CD4+ TH1 and monocytes or Langerhans cells, as encountered in the tuberculin reaction. In contrast, all of CD4+ TH2 cells, plasmocytes, and others are type I hypersensitivity specific mediators.

3. c. In Graves' disease, the antibodies directed against cell-surface receptors impair or cause dysfunction without causing cell injury or inflammation. Autoimmune hemolytic anemia is associated with antibody-mediated erythrocyte destruction. Hypersensitive allergic reaction is a rapidly developing immunologic reaction in a previously sensitized patient to an antigen. Rheumatoid arthritis is an autoimmune disorder characterized by antigen-antibody complexes that produce tissue damage by causing inflammation at the site of deposition.

4. b. Leukemias of myelogenous origin and of chronic nature affect an older age group in comparison to acute lymphoblastic leukemia.

5. a. Sjögren's syndrome is an immunologically mediated autoimmune disorder associated with destruction of lacrimal and salivary glands; in conjunction with the presence of rheumatoid arthritis.

6. a. Immediate or type I hypersensitivity reaction is a rapidly developing immunologic reaction occurring within minutes after the combination of antigen and antibody bound to mast cells in individuals previously sensitized to the antigen. Bronchial asthma and allergic rhinitis are type I reactions.

CHAPTER 36

Environmental and Nutritional Diseases

1. Tetany in children is an outcome of:
   a. vitamin A deficiency
   b. vitamin C deficiency
   c. vitamin D deficiency
   d. vitamin E deficiency

2. Which of the following is the MOST common type of elder abuse?
   a. neglect
   b. emotional abuse
   c. financial abuse
   d. sexual abuse

3. Which of the following is NOT an example of emotional or psychological elder abuse?
   a. enforced social isolation
   b. giving an elderly person the "silent treatment"
   c. inappropriate touching
   d. treating an elderly individual like an adolescent

4. Which of the following features is consistent with lead poisoning?
   a. it competes with bone calcium incorporation
   b. it acts as a potent carcinogen in skin carcinoma
   c. it promotes mesothelioma development if inhaled
   d. it causes chronic recurrent lung hypersensitivity

5. Flaky (enamel) paint dermatosis occurs in which condition?
   a. psoriasis
   b. marasmus
   c. niacin deficiency
   d. kwashiorkor

6. Which of the following contaminates fish and, with chronic poisoning, can produce cerebral and cerebellar atrophy, failure of coordination, and visual and auditory disturbances?
    a. lead
    b. arsenic
    c. mercury
    d. iron

7. Which of the following is the most common cause of thiamine deficiency in the United States?
    a. malabsorption syndromes
    b. poor diet
    c. alcoholism
    d. pernicious anemia

Answers

1. c. Vitamin D deficiency results in hypocalcemia, which is accompanied by excessive excitatory muscle action and thus tetanic convulsions. Vitamins A, C, and E are unrelated to tetanic convulsions.

2. a. All of the selections are examples of elder abuse, but neglect is the most common type of elder abuse.

3. c. Inappropriate touching is a type of elder abuse, but it is not an example of emotional or psychological abuse.

4. a. Lead poisoning is responsible for a wide range of disorders. Lead competes with bone calcium incorporation, whereas arsenic accounts for skin carcinoma development. Asbestos inhalation causes mesothelioma, and beryllium induces chronic lung hypersensitivity.

5. d. Children with kwashiorkor have characteristic skin lesions with alternating zones of hyperpigmentation, areas of desquamation, and hypopigmentation, giving a "flaky paint" appearance.

6. c. Environmental exposure to mercury is most often associated with consumption of contaminated food sources (fish, etc.). Symptoms include muscle tremors, dementia, and cerebral palsy.

7. c. As many as one fourth of chronic alcoholics suffer from thiamine deficiency, which is often referred to as Wernicke-Korsakoff syndrome. It is characterized by polyneuropathy, cardiovascular insufficiency, ophthalmoplegia, nystagmus, ataxia, and confusion. Dietary thiamine deficiency (called beriberi) is seen more often in developing countries in which refined rice is the primary food source.

Disorders of the Musculoskeletal System

1. Dystrophin protein levels are minimal to absent in which of the following conditions?
   a. Becker muscular dystrophy
   b. Duchenne muscular dystrophy
   c. Infantile motor neuron disease
   d. Emery-Dreifuss muscular dystrophy

2. Osteogenesis imperfecta is caused by a deficiency in what protein?
   a. elastin
   b. collagenase
   c. type I collagen
   d. type II collagen

3. Which disease is characterized by osteolysis followed by a mixed osteoclastic-osteoblastic stage, then an osteoblastic stage, ending in osteosclerosis?
   a. osteoporosis
   b. hyperparathyroidism
   c. osteogenesis imperfecta
   d. Paget's disease

4. In osteomyelitis, subperiosteal abscesses may form leading to ischemia and necrosis of a piece of bone. Which term is used to describe this dead fragment of bone?
   a. woven bone
   b. sequestrum
   c. limbus bone
   d. involucrum

5. Pain originating in the proximal tendons of the wrist extensors is aggravated by wrist extension against resistance. What overuse injury does this describe?
   a. lateral epicondylitis
   b. carpal tunnel syndrome
   c. de Quervain's tenosynovitis
   d. medial epicondylitis

6. Where is the most common site of fracture in osteoporosis?
   a. metacarpals
   b. skull
   c. proximal radius
   d. vertebral bodies

7. Acute alcoholic myopathy is characterized by which of the following?
   a. fiber atrophy
   b. fatty infiltration of muscle
   c. rhabdomyolysis and myoglobinuria
   d. a, b, and c

8. Osteochondroma commonly arises from what area of a bone?
   a. epiphysis
   b. diaphysis
   c. metaphysis
   d. cartilage

9. The pain in osteoid osteoma is caused by what mechanism?
   a. vasodilation
   b. excess PGE_2 production
   c. pressure on nerves
   d. stretching of surrounding tissues

10. Charcot's joint occurs in all of the following conditions EXCEPT which one?
    a. tabes dorsalis
    b. diabetic neuropathy
    c. tuberculous arthritis
    d. peripheral neuropathy

11. Which one of the following conditions is characterized by reduced osteoclastic bone resorption?
    a. Paget's disease of the bone
    b. osteoporosis
    c. osteopetrosis
    d. osteomalacia

12. Which of the following is a joint disease in which the articular cartilage is the primary tissue involved?
    a. rheumatoid arthritis
    b. Lyme disease
    c. ochronosis
    d. osteoarthritis

13. Periosteal reactive bone formation on the external surface is characteristically seen in:
    a. osteochondroma
    b. enchondroma
    c. osteosarcoma
    d. nonossifying fibroma

14. Which of the following conditions is accompanied by a pathological process known as metaplasia?
    a. nodular fasciitis
    b. myositis ossificans
    c. palmar fibromatoses
    d. neurofibromatosis

15. A patient has a history of oat cell carcinoma of the lung of 1.5 years' duration, has muscle weakness, and has a negative serum test for anti-acetylcholine receptor antibody. What is your clinicopathological diagnosis?
    a. amyloid peripheral neuropathy
    b. Lambert-Eaton syndrome
    c. familial periodic paralysis
    d. myasthenia gravis

16. Which of the following characteristics is associated with Ewing's sarcoma?
    a. neuroectodermal tumor arises in the medullary cavity
    b. well-differentiated tumor, resembling osteosarcoma
    c. anaplastic tumor that mimics lung small cell carcinoma
    d. multicentric IgM-secreting plasma cell tumor in bone

17. Which of the following statements characterizes fibrous dysplasia, also known as progressive myositis ossificans?
    a. it is a T cell–mediated immune and inflammatory disease
    b. it is probably due to a gene encoding osteomorphogenic proteins
    c. it is a rare dominant hereditary pseudoneoplastic disease
    d. it is a recessive X-linked hereditary disease of muscle

18.   Which statement BEST describes trichinosis?
    a. it is due to the ingestion of larvae-contaminated raw pork
    b. it provokes septicemia, shock, and hemodynamic disorders
    c. it induces severe bacterial disease with polynuclear infiltration
    d. it provokes severe granulomatous myositis and meningitis

19.   Which of the following conditions is descriptive of osteoarthritis?
    a. it provokes giant cell pigmented villonodular synovitis
    b. it is associated with decreased type II collagen, cytokines, and chondrolysis
    c. ankylosis and follicular inflammation are predominant
    d. it is associated with increased cartilage matrix synthesis and deposition

20.   Which of the following descriptions is associated with Paget's disease?
    a. there is a decrease in osteocalcin and alkaline phosphatase levels
    b. it typically appears as a mosaic consisting of osteoclastic and osteoblastic activity
    c. it is due to an infection of osteoblastic and osteoclastic bone cells by a paramyxovirus
    d. it is associated with distal metaphysic (Erlenmeyer flask) bone deformity

21.   Which of the following is the benign tumor of striated muscle?
    a. lipoma
    b. leiomyoma
    c. lymphoma
    d. rhabdomyoma

22.   A 6-month-old child is brought to the emergency department with a fractured humerus. On further evaluation, it is discovered that this child has experienced numerous fractures since birth. It is also noted in the patient's chart that the patient may have an inherited disorder. Two older siblings show no similar signs to indicate possible abuse. The physical exam reveals some delayed ability to sit up without assistance, signs of a possible hearing impairment, and blue sclera. Which is the most probable cause of these findings?
    a. severe parental abuse and neglect
    b. osteogenesis imperfecta
    c. multiple myeloma
    d. vitamin C deficiency

23. Which is a primary bone tumor that is characteristically seen in women aged 20 to 40 years and has a "soap-bubble" appearance on radiography?
    a. chondrosarcoma
    b. giant cell tumor
    c. osteosarcoma
    d. Ewing's sarcoma

24. During the course of taking an initial history from a new patient, the individual reports that his hat no longer fits him right and he recently had to switch to a larger size. On radiography, you detect that some of his vertebrae are denser than normal and that his skull also appears denser than normally expected. The most likely explanation is:
    a. multiple myeloma
    b. osteopetrosis
    c. Paget's disease of bone
    d. enchondroma

25. A patient has a malignant tumor that is found within bone but is a tumor of plasma cells. It presents with the presence of high titers of monoclonal antibodies, pathological fractures, and "punched-out" lytic lesions of bone on radiography. Which of the following does this describe?
    a. multiple myeloma
    b. myasthenia gravis
    c. Graves' disease
    d. Bruton's agammaglobulinemia

Answers

1. b. In both Duchenne and Becker muscular dystrophy, there is a decrease in dystrophin levels; however, in Duchenne, muscle biopsy shows very little, if any, dystrophin. In Becker muscular dystrophy, there is some dystrophin in the muscle, but it has an abnormal molecular weight. Dystrophin functions as a link between intracellular contractile proteins and the extracellular matrix proteins, thereby transferring forces through the muscle tissue.

2. c. Osteogenesis imperfecta is group of disorders in which there is a deficiency in type I collagen synthesis. These patients have multiple fractures due to the fragility of their bones and have blue sclera.

3. d. Paget's disease (also known as osteitis deformans) ultimately results in an increase in bone mass; however, the bone is haphazard and structurally weak. The typical pattern starts with an osteolytic phase, followed by a mixed phase, and ending with an osteosclerotic phase.

4. b. The loss of blood supply (ischemia) to a section of infected bone leads to necrosis. This bone is called a sequestrum. Over time, new bone, called an involucrum, may form around the damaged bone.

5. a. In reality, it is not the epicondyle that is inflamed but rather the wrist and hand extensor tendons that originate there. Lateral epicondylitis is also often called "tennis elbow."

6. d. Osteoporosis affects all bones of the body, but most commonly it produces symptoms in the major weight-bearing bones.

7. c. Fiber atrophy and fatty infiltration of muscle occur in thyrotoxic myopathy. Alcoholic myopathy produces rhabdomyolysis and myoglobinuria, which may lead to renal failure.

8. c. Osteochondromas develop only in bones of endochondral origin and arise from the metaphysis near the growth plate of long tubular bones.

9. b. The severe nocturnal pain in osteoid osteoma is caused by excess prostaglandin E_2 production. PGE_2 is produced by the proliferating osteoblasts.

10. c. Charçot's joint is a neuvropathic joint that results from loss of
         sensory innervation to the joint, resulting in lack of pain sensation
         to the joint. In tuberculous arthritis, it is painful.

11. c. Osteopetrosis is a genetic disorder characterized by osteoclast
         dysfunction that leads to excessive osteoid tissue formation.
         Paget's disease is an acquired disease in which the osteoclast
         dysfunction initially causes excessive removal of bone (osteolysis).
         Osteomalacia is the softening of bone due to poor and delayed
         calcification. Osteoporosis is due to more than one etiological
         factor, acquired and genetic, accompanied by reduced amount of
         osteoid tissue.

12. d. In osteoarthritis, there is an initial breakdown of articular cartilage
         followed by other morphological changes. Rheumatoid arthritis is
         an autoimmune inflammatory disease initially involving the
         synovial membrane. Lyme disease arthritis is an infectious,
         inflammatory disorder. Ochronosis is a genetic disease involving
         excessive accumulation of homogentisic acid in connective tissues
         of the body, including joints.

13. c. Osteosarcoma is a bone-forming malignant tumor in which there
         is a periosteum reaction on the surface of bone known as
         Codman's triangle. Enchondroma is an anomaly of cartilaginous
         growth within the metaphysis. Osteochondroma is a tumor on the
         surface of long bones due to a misplaced epiphyseal cartilage that
         grows continuously, but it is not a reactive bone. Nonossifying
         fibroma is also an anomalous growth within the bone.

14. b. Myositis ossificans is a posttraumatic inflammatory disorder of
         muscle in which the muscle tissue changes into bone-forming
         tissue (metaplasia). This bony tissue may develop into
         osteosarcoma. Nodular fasciitis (reactive pseudosarcoma), palmar
         fibromatoses, and neurofibromatosis are genetic disorders.

15. b. Lambert-Eaton syndrome is an autoimmune disease secondary to
         oat cell carcinoma of lung. Autoantibodies block the secretion of
         acetylcholine, leading to muscle weakness. Amyloid neuropathy
         may be seen in patients with multiple myeloma, in which there is
         systemic deposition of amyloid protein (amyloidosis). Myasthenia
         gravis is an autoimmune disorder in which anti-acetylcholine
         receptor antibodies are produced, causing receptor destruction and
         muscle weakness. Familial periodic paralysis is a channelopathy
         associated with low serum potassium levels periodically leading to
         hypotonia and muscle weakness.

16. a. Ewing's sarcoma (EWS) is an anaplastic and highly aggressive tumor that exhibits a neuroectodermal pattern. EWS does not resemble well-differentiated osteosarcoma but is similar to malignant lymphoma. EWS is not an IgM-secreting plasma cell tumor.

17. c. Fibrous dysplasia, also referred to as pseudoneoplastic myositis ossificans, is common in young adults. It is a rare dominant hereditary disease, to be distinguished from other forms, such as immune myositis and X-linked Duchenne myodystrophy.

18. a. Trichinosis is a disease due to a larvae parasite infestation, characterized by eosinophilic myositis and meningitis. *Trichinella spiralis* larvae are transmitted to humans by the ingestion of either smoked or incompletely cooked contaminated pork meat.

19. b. Osteoarthritis is induced by aging, trauma, and genetic factors. Hence, fibrillation, osteophytes, and decreased collagen II synthesis are the main features. In contrast, synovitis and inflammation occur in other forms, such as rheumatoid, and giant villonodular arthritis.

20. b. Paget's disease is of unknown origin. It is characterized by a typical mosaic bone pattern that seems to be pathognomonic for this condition. Distal metaphysic enlargement (Erlenmeyer flask) bone deformity is remarkable in osteopetrosis, not Paget's disease.

21. d. Rhabdomyomas are benign tumors that are often found in the hearts of preschool children. Lipomas are benign adipose tumors. Leiomyomas are benign smooth muscle tumors. Lymphomas are malignant tumors of lymph nodes.

22. b. Also known as brittle bone disease, osteogenesis imperfecta is an autosomal dominant defect in the synthesis of collagen type 1. The disorder results in an osteoporotic bone with cortical thinning and attenuation of trabeculae. Clinically, it presents with multiple fractures after birth, blue sclera, and hearing loss.

23. b. Giant cell tumor is a locally aggressive, potentially malignant tumor characterized by osteoclastic, multinucleated giant cells. It is more common in Asian women aged 20 to 40 years. Ninety percent of the tumors originate at the epiphyseal/metaphyseal junction. Hemorrhagic areas result in the appearance of a sponge filled with blood.

24. c. Also called osteitis deformans, Paget's disease is a chronic condition characterized by lesions of disordered remodeling. Initially, the disorder begins with an osteolytic stage with excessive resorption of bone and is followed by excessive and disorganized osteoblastic bone formation. These solitary painful lesions occur in multiple sites.

25. a. Multiple myeloma is a malignant disorder of terminally differentiated B-lymphocytes (plasma cells). Factors produced by neoplastic plasma cells mediate bone destruction, "punched out" lesions in vertebrae, ribs, and skull, etc. Patients tend to be 50 to 60 years old and exhibit neurological manifestations.

Disorders of the Nervous System

1. The histologic structure known as a "glomeruloid body" is present in which of the following neoplasms of the central nervous system?
    a. fibrillary astrocytoma
    b. ependymoma
    c. glioblastoma
    d. meningioma

2. Which of the following conditions is not accompanied by damage to or degeneration of the nigrostriatal dopaminergic system?
    a. Parkinson's disease
    b. progressive supranuclear palsy
    c. Huntington's disease
    d. Pick's disease

3. Which of the following is NOT characteristic of Wernicke-Korsakoff syndrome?
    a. related to alcohol abuse
    b. involvement of the CNS
    c. tinnitus
    d. nystagmus

4. Which is the LEAST likely cause of dementia in the elderly?
    a. stroke
    b. Alzheimer's disease
    c. depression
    d. cerebrovascular accident

5. Which of the following is the MOST common cause of subarachnoid hemorrhage?
    a. head trauma
    b. saccular (berry) aneurysm
    c. middle cerebral artery rupture
    d. hypertension

6. An expansion of the central canal of the cervical spinal cord with destruction of adjacent gray and white matter BEST describes which of the following disorders?
    a. hydrocephalus
    b. anencephaly
    c. syringomyelia
    d. multiple sclerosis

7. Which statement BEST characterizes Arnold-Chiari syndrome?
    a. it is due to tonsillar herniation through the magnum foramen
    b. it is due to transtentorial herniation and causes Duret hemorrhages
    c. it is due to subfalcine (cingulate) herniation under the falx cerebri
    d. it causes compressive ischemia of the anterior cerebral artery

8. Which of the following is associated with Parkinson's disease?
    a. there is amyloid angiopathy with frontal and temporal cortical atrophy
    b. there is a spongiform vacuolar cortex with putamen degeneration
    c. there are senile plaques and neurofibrillary tangles with astrogliosis
    d. Lewy's bodies are found in the substantia nigra with loss of pigmentation

9. Which of the following is NOT true regarding multiple sclerosis?
    a. it is an autoimmune disease
    b. it is a demyelinating disorder
    c. there are neurofibrillary tangles in the cytoplasm of neurons
    d. it is characterized by relapsing and remitting episodes involving the brain and spinal cord

10. Postinfectious ascending paralysis and radiculoneuropathy are characteristics of what condition?
    a. Guillian-Barré syndrome
    b. myasthenia gravis
    c. amyotrophic lateral sclerosis
    d. multiple sclerosis

11. Which of the following is classified as a prion encephalopathy in which the patient experiences a rapidly progressive dementia, ataxia, weakness, and eventually death within 1 to 2 years?
    a. metachromatic leukodystrophy
    b. amyotrophic lateral sclerosis
    c. progressive multifocal leukoencephalopathy
    d. Creutzfeldt-Jacob disease

12. Which of the following is NOT a microscopic characteristic of Alzheimer's disease?
    a. granulovacuolar degeneration
    b. perivascular cuffing
    c. neuritic plaques
    d. neurofibrillary tangles

Answers

1. c. Glioblastoma is a high-grade malignant astrocytoma accompanied by necrosis, angiogenesis, and the presence of glomeruloid bodies. Fibrillary astrocytoma is a well-differentiated neoplasm that normally does not have vascular proliferations. Ependymomas are associated with perivascular pseudorosettes, and meningiomas are benign neoplasms found on the external surface of the brain.

2. d. Parkinson's disease, progressive supranuclear palsy, and Huntington's disease are all accompanied by degeneration of the nigrostriatal dopaminergic pathway and thus accompanied by Parkinson's-like movement disorders. Pick's disease involves the cerebral frontal and temporal lobes only, and not nigrostriatal dopaminergic pathways.

3. c. Wernicke-Korsakoff syndrome is a finding in alcohol abuse with involvement of the CNS, ataxia, and nystagmus. Tinnitus ("ringing" of the ears) may be seen in other conditions such as salicylism, but it is not seen in Wernicke-Korsakoff syndrome.

4. c. Alzheimer's and stroke (cerebrovascular accident) are the two most common causes of dementia in the elderly. Depression may coincide with dementia but is not a cause.

5. b. Berry aneurysms are saccular outpouchings occurring typically at branch points of the circle of Willis arteries. The cause of berry aneurysms is unknown, but there is evidence of a genetic predisposition to the condition. Rupture most often occurs in women in their 40s, with bleeding into the subarachnoid space. Patients often say they are having the "worst headache of my life." Head trauma is more likely to produce subdural hematomas.

6. c. Syringomyelia presents with a loss of pain and temperature sensation in the upper extremities due to the interruption of crossing sensory fibers in the central cord. Because the nerve fibers carrying fine touch and proprioception do not cross at the cord level, these sensory modalities are intact.

7. a. Arnold-Chiari syndrome results from cerebellar tonsillar herniation through the magnum foramen. This condition may induce compression on the vital respiratory center in the medulla oblongata and can be fatal.

8.   d.   Parkinson's disease is characterized by an alteration of the nigrostriatal dopaminergic system, with a loss of pigmentation and the presence of Lewy's bodies in the substantia nigra. Brain spongiform degeneration is specific to Creutzfeldt-Jacob disease.

9.   c.   Presence of neurofibrillary tangles in the cytoplasm of neurons is found in Alzheimer's disease.

10.   a.   About two thirds of the cases of Guillian-Barré syndrome are preceded by an acute influenza-like illness. It is also characterized by weakness beginning in the distal limb and advancing to affect the proximal muscles and inflammation and demyelination of spinal nerve roots and peripheral nerves.

11.   d.   Creutzfeldt-Jacob disease is a spongiform encephalopathy associated with exposure to an infectious protein, a "prion." It manifests as a rapidly progressive dementia. Metachromatic leukodystrophy is a demyelinating disorder, progressive multifocal leukoencephalopathy is a viral JC polyomavirus, and amyotrophic lateral sclerosis is associated with motor neuron degeneration.

12.   b.   Perivascular cuffing is associated with viral encephalitis.

Diseases of the Organ Systems

1. In males, which of the following is the most common cause of both bilateral hydroureters and hydronephrosis?
   a. acute pyelonephritis
   b. benign prostatic hyperplasia
   c. stones in the renal pelvis
   d. hypospadias

2. Which of the following is the malignant tumor that is the most common cause of death from cancer in females?
   a. carcinoma of the breast
   b. carcinoma of the lung
   c. carcinoma of the ovary
   d. carcinoma of the uterus

3. Which one of the following is characterized by intracytoplasmic negri bodies in neurons?
   a. rabies
   b. herpes simplex encephalitis
   c. progressive multifocal leukoencephalopathy
   d. subacute sclerosing panencephalitis

4. While examining a 25-year-old patient, you notice that the head and neck appear pink and flushed. Radiographic examination shows evidence of "notching" of the ribs. During further examination, you discover that the femoral pulse is weak and delayed compared with the brachial pulse, whereas the femoral blood pressure is lower than that obtained from the brachial artery. Which of the following diseases or conditions is the most likely cause of these findings?
   a. berry aneurysm
   b. Marfan's syndrome
   c. coarctation of the aorta
   d. right ventricular failure

5. Which is the type of bacteria very commonly associated with the development of subacute bacterial endocarditis in a previously damaged, native heart valve?
    a. *Staphylococcus aureus*
    b. *Streptococcus viridans*
    c. *Pseudomonas* species
    d. *Candida* species

6. Which of the following is associated with ulcerative colitis?
    a. transmural inflammation
    b. presence of granulomas
    c. regional ileitis
    d. continuous colonic involvement

7. The most common cause of a sporadic case of acute interstitial pneumonia (pneumonitis) otherwise known as "walking pneumonia" is which of the following?
    a. *Legionella pneumophila*
    b. *Streptococcus pneumoniae*
    c. *Mycoplasma pneumoniae*
    d. varicella pneumonia

8. Analgesic nephropathy, a condition associated with excessive chronic use of aspirin and acetaminophen, usually presents with what microscopic feature?
    a. hyaline arteriolosclerosis
    b. interstitial nephritis/fibrosis
    c. pyelonephritis
    d. glomerulonephritis

9. What is the characteristic pathological feature of malignant mesothelioma?
    a. primarily related to smoking
    b. histologically, it is an adenocarcinoma
    c. a localized focal lesion in pleura
    d. accompanied by pleural effusion

10. Which of the following pulmonary malignancies is predominantly involved with paraneoplastic syndrome?
    a. well-differentiated squamous cell carcinoma
    b. undifferentiated small cell carcinoma
    c. pulmonary carcinoid tumor
    d. well-differentiated adenocarcinoma

11. In malabsorption syndrome, which one of the following conditions is accompanied by both infection and lymphatic obstruction as pathogenetic factors?
    a. Crohn's disease
    b. Whipple's disease
    c. parasitic infection
    d. celiac disease

12. The primary cause of endometrial hyperplasia is a high serum level of which hormone?
    a. progesterone
    b. dihydrotestosterone
    c. estrogen
    d. adrenocorticotrophic hormone

13. Which is the primary cause of central hemorrhagic necrosis of the liver?
    a. severe protein deficiency
    b. right-sided heart failure
    c. alcoholism
    d. viral hepatitis

14. What is the main cause of anemia in chronic renal failure?
    a. deficiency of vitamin B12
    b. deficiency of erythropoietin
    c. deficiency of folic acid
    d. deficiency of hematopoietic stem cells

15. Which one of the following factors is NOT involved in crescent formation in rapidly progressive glomerulonephritis?
    a. fibrin
    b. interleukin 1
    c. amyloid material
    d. tissue necrotic factor

16. Which is the most common cause of nephrotic syndrome in adults in the United States?
    a. minimal change disease
    b. focal segmental glomerulosclerosis
    c. IgA nephropathy
    d. membranoproliferative glomerulonephritis

17. Which of the following is indicative of left heart failure?
    a. pitting pedal edema
    b. neck vein distention
    c. orthopnea
    d. ascites

18. The usual source of pulmonary embolism is thrombus formation in what location?
     a. superficial veins of leg
     b. deep veins of leg
     c. heart
     d. superficial veins of arm

19. Which of the following dietary factors does NOT increase one's risk of colon cancer?
     a. decreased intake of protective micronutrients
     b. increased intake of red meat
     c. high content of nonabsorbable vegetable fiber
     d. high content of refined carbohydrates

20. What is the hallmark of hypocalcemia?
     a. bone pain
     b. nephrolithiasis
     c. tetany
     d. peptic ulcers

21. Skin cancer is caused by which of the following carcinogens?
     a. nitrosamine
     b. vinyl chloride
     c. arsenic
     d. asbestos

22. Which of the following increases the risk of breast carcinoma?
     a. obesity
     b. nulliparity
     c. early menarche and late menopause
     d. a, b, and c

23. The Gleason system is a system of grading for what carcinoma site?
     a. stomach
     b. prostate
     c. colon
     d. thyroid

24. Alpha-1 antitrypsin deficiency may lead to which of the following?
     a. chronic bronchitis
     b. bronchial asthma
     c. emphysema
     d. cystic fibrosis

25. Which of the following descriptions characterizes Barrett's esophagus?
    a. there are dilated submucosal esophageal veins, due to portal hypertension
    b. there is cylindrical muciparous epithelium metaplasia, due to reflux
    c. there is squamous dysplasia in response to sustained peptic acid injury
    d. there is achalasia induced by the destruction of the myenteric plexus by trypanosomes

26. Which of the following characteristics is consistent with hepatic stellate cells or Ito cells?
    a. they are located in portal spaces and are in charge of vitamin B storage
    b. they are endothelial cells that stimulate fibrosis, through TNF-α and IL-1
    c. they store perisinusoidal fat and synthesize collagen
    d cytokines promote collagen synthesis by Kupffer cells

27. Which of the following conditions is associated with acute pancreatitis?
    a. shock, disseminated intravascular coagulation, and peritonitis
    b. pathognomonic diabetes mellitus type 1 onset
    c. decreased serum lipase and amylase levels and loss of surfactant
    d. always results in obstructive jaundice onset

28. Which statement BEST defines "pulmonary microatelectasis"?
    a. lung tissue collapse due to hydrothorax compression
    b. chronic fibrous adherent pleuropneumonia
    c. hyaline membranes owing to lack of surfactant
    d. tissue collapse due to bronchial foreign body aspiration

29. Which of the following pathologies is responsible for left cardiac concentric hypertrophy?
    a. pulmonary emphysema secondary to smoking
    b. thrombus-induced pulmonary artery obstruction
    c. sustained diastolic pressure over 90 mm Hg
    d. myxomatous degeneration of the mitral valve

30. Which of the following conditions is associated with nephrotic syndrome?
    a. abnormal glomerular cell proliferation resulting in massive uremia
    b. glomerular filter alteration causing proteinuria and edema
    c. glomerulopathy responsible for oliguria, hematuria, and hypertension
    d. acute tubular necrosis resulting in ischemia and necrosis

31. Which of the following conditions is MOST involved in the occurrence of cervical carcinoma?
    a. HPV (types 6 and 11) genomes are maintained in a free episomal form
    b. HPV (types 16 and 18) inactivates *p53* and *Rb* tumor-suppressor genes
    c. type 2 herpes simplex virus integrates into host cell genome
    d. increased estrogen levels stimulate cervical squamous epithelium

32. Which of the following descriptions BEST describes Conn's syndrome?
    a. bilateral hyperplasia of the zona fasciculata, resulting in hypercorticism
    b. increased renin levels stimulate aldosterone secretion by the zona glomerulosa
    c. an aldosterone-secreting adenoma, which inhibits renin production
    d. a primary adrenocortical deficiency resulting in hyperpigmentation and hypotension

33. Which of the following is NOT an infant risk factor for SIDS?
    a. brain stem abnormalities
    b. female gender
    c. SIDS in a sibling
    d. low birth weight

34. Which of the following is NOT an environmental risk factor for SIDS?
    a. prone sleep position
    b. hypothermia
    c. passive smoke
    d. sleeping on a soft surface

35. Which is NOT a cause of sudden infant death?
    a. viral meningitis
    b. bronchopneumonia
    c. metabolic defects
    d. genetic defects

36. Which is the MOST common tumor of infancy?
    a. Wilms tumor
    b. leukemia
    c. hemangioma
    d. rhabdomyosarcoma

37. Which of the following is the correct order of frequency of childhood malignancies?
    a. neuroblastoma, Wilms tumor, retinoblastoma, leukemia
    b. neuroblastoma, retinoblastoma, leukemia, Wilms tumor
    c. leukemia, neuroblastoma, retinoblastoma, Wilms tumor
    d. leukemia, retinoblastoma, neuroblastoma, Wilms tumor

38. What is the prognosis (2-year survival with combined nephrectomy and chemotherapy) for Wilms tumor?
    a. <10%
    b. 10% to 20%
    c. 40% to 60%
    d. 90%

39. Which is NOT true of Whipple's disease?
    a. central nervous system may be involved
    b. thinning of the intestinal wall
    c. presence of gram-positive bacteria in the lamina propria of the intestine
    d. blunting of the intestinal villi

40. Certain neoplasms of the intestines may cause increased production of serotonin that will most likely result in what type of diarrhea?
    a. secretory
    b. osmotic
    c. exudative
    d. bloody

41. Lactase deficiency is most likely to result in what type of diarrhea?
    a. secretory
    b. osmotic
    c. exudative
    d. bloody

42. An edema that develops in a hypertensive individual is most likely due to what factor?
    a. osmotic forces
    b. hydrostatic forces
    c. lymphatic obstruction
    d. reduced albumin concentration in the plasma

43. The nephrotic syndrome is most likely to be accompanied by what finding?
    a. hydrostatic edema
    b. osmotic diarrhea
    c. edema due to lymphatic obstruction
    d. bloody diarrhea

44. Which of the following is NOT a type of shock?
    a. nephrogenic
    b. cardiogenic
    c. hypovolemic
    d. septic

45. Which of the following is NOT characteristic of alcoholic hepatitis?
    a. liver tenderness
    b. shrunken liver
    c. fever
    d. risk of progressing to cirrhosis

46. "THC" is the active ingredient in which of the following drugs?
    a. cocaine
    b. marijuana
    c. heroin
    d. barbiturates

47. Which of the following is LEAST likely to be seen in an elderly patient with hypothyroidism?
    a. weight loss
    b. cognitive loss
    c. heart failure
    d. diarrhea

48. Which one the following is the least likely complaint of an elderly patient with a UTI (urinary tract infection)?
    a. dysuria
    b. frequency
    c. anorexia
    d. hematuria

49. For which of the following conditions is hypertension NOT a risk factor?
    a. peripheral vascular disease
    b. stroke
    c. renal disease
    d. diabetes mellitus

50. Which endocrine disorder is characterized by bone fractures secondary to osteopenia, nephrolithiasis, constipation and nausea, depression, lethargy, and eventually seizures?
    a. senile osteoporosis
    b. acromegaly
    c. Graves' disease
    d. hyperparathyroidism

51. Which of the following BEST describes ulcerative colitis?
    a. it is an inflammatory disease of the colon involving a continuous segment of the organ from the rectum proximally
    b. it is an inflammatory disease of the colon involving "skip lesions," where there are several isolated areas of the colon involved
    c. it is a chronic disease of the small intestine due to gluten sensitivity characterized by diarrhea, flatulence, weight loss, and fatigue
    d. it is characterized by multiple polyps in the colon

52. What is the pathophysiology of resorption atelectasis?
    a. it results from accumulation of blood, air, or and exudates into the pleural cavity
    b. it is caused by a complete airway obstruction
    c. it is secondary to fibrosis of the lung tissue
    d. it is most often caused by a pneumonia

53. Which is NOT true of giant cell arteritis?
    a. it is associated with polymyalgia rheumatica
    b. it involves inflammation of the temporal artery
    c. it may lead to vision loss
    d. the condition is unresponsive to anti-inflammatory drugs

54. Longitudinal tears in the distal esophagus may occur in patients with severe retching or vomiting, such as chronic alcoholics. What is this condition called?
    a. esophageal varices
    b. Barrett's esophagus
    c. Mallory-Weiss syndrome
    d. Zenker's diverticulum

55. Which form of hepatitis is transmitted by the fecal-oral route, is an acute illness that is self-limited, and is not associated with hepatocellular carcinoma?
    a. hepatitis A
    b. hepatitis B
    c. hepatitis C
    d. hepatitis D

56. In which of the following conditions is a "bread and butter" pericarditis found?
    a. rheumatic heart disease
    b. Libman-Sacks disease
    c. dilated cardiomyopathy
    d. hypertrophic cardiomyopathy

57. Which of the following is NOT a feature of the tetralogy of Fallot?
    a.   overriding aorta
    b.   interventricular septal defect
    c.   right ventricular hypertrophy
    d.   patent ductus arteriosus

Answers

1. b. Bilateral hydronephrosis and hydroureters would require obstruction below the bladder. Within the bladder, it would involve a tumor at the level of the trigone. Hypospadias is an abnormal opening of the urethral canal on the ventral surface of the penis.

2. b. Carcinoma of the lung is the most common cause of cancer deaths in both males and females.

3. a. Negri bodies are intracytoplasmic eosinophilic inclusion bodies found in pyramidal neurons of the hippocampus and Purkinje cells of the cerebellum in cases of rabies.

4. c. Postductal coarctation of the aorta becomes symptomatic in adults. It is characterized by hypertension in the upper extremities and weak pulses and lower blood pressure in the lower extremities. Patients develop collateral circulation with rib notching.

5. b. The viridans streptococci are associated with subacute endocarditis in high-risk groups (those with previously damaged or otherwise abnormal valves). Patients require prophylactic antimicrobial treatment prior to dental work.

6. d. Ulcerative colitis involves the rectum and extends in a retrograde fashion to involve the entire colon. Continuous superficial lesions with pseudopolyps are characteristic. Crohn's disease has transmural, skip lesions with fissures/ulcerations, and granulomas.

7. c. *Mycoplasma pneumoniae* is also called the Eaton agent. Bacterial colonies appear as "fried eggs" on blood agar plates. They lack a cell wall and cause interstitial pneumonia.

8. b. Interstitial nephritis/fibrosis is associated with chronic combined use of aspirin with acetaminophen over a 3- to 5-year period. The end stage of the disease involves bilateral papillary necrosis and interstitial nephritis and fibrosis. Transplantation is the treatment of choice.

9. d. Pleural effusion is very characteristic of malignant mesothelioma and also of any primary or metastatic pleural malignancies. Smoking does play a role in the etiology of pleural malignancy, but it is secondary. Asbestos plays the primary role. Histologically, it is not an adenocarcinoma but a combination of epitheloid and mesenchymal type tumor. Mesothelioma is a diffuse lesion and not a focal lesion.

10. b. Undifferentiated small cell carcinoma (also known as oat cell carcinoma) is predominantly involved with paraneoplastic syndromes because highly anaplastic undifferentiated cells produce neuroendocrine substances. Well-differentiated squamous cell and adenocarcinomas behave functionally as normal cells. Carcinoid tumor is largely responsible for carcinoid syndrome.

11. b. The most recent understanding of Whipple's disease is that it causes infection and lymphatic obstruction and thus malabsorption. Crohn's disease, parasitic infection, and celiac disease are not accompanied by lymphatic obstruction but cause malabsorption due to other pathogenetic factors.

12. c. Estrogen hormone is normally responsible for proliferative activity of the endometrium, but persistently high levels of estrogen will lead to hyperplasia. Progesterone causes secretory changes in the endometrium. It lacks proliferative and mitotic activity. Dihydrotestosterone is a male hormone that causes benign prostatic hyperplasia, and adrenocorticotrophic hormone stimulates the adrenal cortex.

13. b. The pathogenetic mechanism for central hemorrhagic necrosis is chronic passive congestion caused by right-sided heart failure. Severe protein deficiency and alcoholism lead first to fatty change and eventually to coagulative necrosis followed by cirrhosis of the liver. Viral hepatitis is accompanied by hepatic cellular injury and eventually coagulative necrosis.

14. b. Erythropoietin, necessary to produce RBCs, is produced in the kidneys. In chronic renal failure, normal kidney tissue is replaced by diffuse hyalinization and fibrosis and thus lacks of erythropoietin secretion. Vitamin B12 and folic acid deficiency causes anemia but not related to chronic renal failure. Deficiency of hematopoietic stem cells is not related to chronic renal failure but is related to the suppression of stem cells by other mechanisms.

15. c. Amyloid material is an outcome of many pathological processes that cause deposits in glomerular capillary basement membrane in nephrotic syndrome and does not promote epithelial cell proliferations. Fibrin (procoagulant factor), interleukin 1, and tissue necrotic factor (cytokine) promote glomerular epithelial cell proliferations.

16. b. The most common cause of nephrotic syndrome is focal segmental glomerulosclerosis. Minimal change disease, IgA nephropathy, and MPGN are uncommon causes of nephrotic syndrome.

17. c. Orthopnea, which is dyspnea in the recumbent position, is a typical symptom of chronic left heart failure. All of the other symptoms and signs are due to right heart failure.

18. b. Ninety percent of pulmonary emboli originate from deep leg vein thrombi.

19. c. Low (not high) content of nonabsorbable vegetable fiber is associated with a higher incidence of colon cancer.

20. c. Bone pain, nephrolithiasis, and peptic ulcers are symptomatic presentations of hypercalcemia. Tetany, the neuromuscular irritability resulting from decreased serum ionized calcium concentration, is the hallmark of hypocalcemia.

21. c. Among these chemical carcinogens, arsenic is the major carcinogen for skin cancer. Nitrosamine leads to stomach cancer, vinyl chloride for liver cancer, and asbestos for pleural and lung cancers.

22. d. Statistically, the risk of breast cancer is increased in obese women, nulliparous women, and women with a menstrual history of early menarche and late menopause.

23. b. Several grading systems have been described, of which Gleason system is the best known for prostate cancer.

24. c. Alpha-1 antitrypsin is a major inhibitor of proteases secreted by neutrophils during inflammation. Its deficiency causes alveolar wall destruction in emphysema.

25. b. Barrett's esophagus occurs as a consequence of gastroesophageal reflux disease (GERD), in which stomach acid juices irritate the mucosal lining of the organ. Normal squamous epithelium undergoes a cylindrical muciparous metaplasia (it becomes a columnar epithelium with intestinal goblet cells).

26. c. Ito cells, also referred to as stellate cells, are located in Disse's spaces but are not located in portal spaces. Under normal conditions, Ito cells are involved in fat and vitamin A storage. Ito cells activated by cytokines may secrete excessive collagen, responsible for cirrhosis.

27. a. Acute pancreatitis is a serious necrotic condition mainly resulting from pancreas auto digestion. It is characterized by increased serum lipase and amylase levels, peritonitis, shock, and disseminated intravascular coagulation. Jaundice is seen in bile duct obstruction.

28. c. Hyaline membrane deposits lining alveoli walls, as observed in neonate and adult respiratory distress syndrome, is a condition in which microatelectasis onset occurs, owing to loss of surfactant.

29. c. Left ventricle concentric hypertrophy results from hypertension-induced pressure overload or occurs in aortic stenosis. Mitral valve degeneration and other conditions result in hypertrophic right ventricle dilatation or right heart failure.

30. b. Nephrotic syndrome is grossly characterized by glomerular selective permeability impairment, which results in protein leakage into the urine, albuminuria, and severe edema.

31. b. Types 16 and 18 human papilloma viruses are most involved in cervix carcinoma. The viral genome is integrated into the host genome, resulting in *p53* and *Rb* gene inactivation. In contrast, HPV (6 and 11), HSV, and elevated estrogen levels are not involved.

32. c. Conn's syndrome, or primary hyperaldosteronism, is a disorder caused by excess production of mineralocorticoids, due to an aldosterone-secreting adenoma, or zona glomerulosa hyperplasia. This results in the inhibition of renin production.

33. b. SIDS is idiopathic, but there are some identified risk factors. Brain stem abnormalities, being one of a multiple birth, previous history of SIDS in a sibling, and low birth weight are all infant risk factors for SIDS. Female gender is not a risk factor for SIDS.

34. b. SIDS is idiopathic, but there are some identified risk factors. All of the selections are risk factors for SIDS except hypothermia. Hyperthermia, however, is a risk factor for SIDS.

35. a. Viral meningitis is self-limiting, but the others, including child abuse, are documented causes of sudden infant death. These causes, however, are not causes of SIDS.

36. c. Although Wilms tumor, leukemia, and rhabdomyosarcoma are some of the more common malignancies of childhood, the most common tumor of childhood is hemangioma (a benign neoplasm).

37. d. Leukemia is the most common malignancy of childhood followed by retinoblastoma, neuroblastoma, and Wilms tumor.

38. d. Although at one time the prognosis for Wilms tumor was not very good, improved therapies have increased the 2-year survival to 90% when chemotherapy is combined with nephrectomy.

39. b. Actually, there is thickening of the intestinal wall. The other choices are also true of Whipple's disease, which is probably caused by the gram-positive bacteria *Tropheryma whippelii.*

40. a. Serotonin is a secretory product occurring in some carcinoid neoplasms that can result in a secretory diarrhea.

41. b. A deficiency of lactase will result in malabsorption of lactose, which results in an osmotic diarrhea.

42. b. An increase in blood pressure (hypertension) will increase the hydrostatic pressure within the blood vessels, resulting in edema.

43. b. In the nephrotic syndrome (nephrosis), there is proteinuria that results in an osmotic diarrhea.

44. a. All of the selections except "nephrogenic" are causes of shock. In addition, anaphylaxis may also cause shock.

45. b. The liver will actually be enlarged with hepatitis and is likely to be shrunken with cirrhosis. The other choices are also true of alcoholic hepatitis.

46. b. THC (tetrahydrocannabinol) is the active ingredient in marijuana.

47. d. The elderly often present with symptoms different from those of the nonelderly. Diarrhea is not a common finding in hypothyroidism in the elderly.

48. d. The first three selections are possible complaints of a UTI in an elderly person. Hematuria (especially painless hematuria) is more likely to portend a more serious situation such as bladder cancer.

49. d. Hypertension may increase the risk of peripheral vascular disease, stroke, and renal disease. On the other hand, diabetes mellitus may accelerate atherosclerosis that can contribute to hypertension.

50. d. Hyperparathyroidism is most commonly due to an adenoma of the parathyroid gland with resulting increased secretion of parathyroid hormone. The resulting hypercalcemia leads to the collection of symptoms described as "painful bones, renal stones, abdominal groans, and psychic moans."

51. a. Ulcerative colitis is an inflammatory bowel disease involving the distal colon. This disorder presents with bloody diarrhea, which is episodic in nature. Crohn's disease is associated with "skip lesions," gluten sensitivity causes celiac disease, and polyps are not found with ulcerative colitis.

52. b. Atelectasis refers to the collapse of part of a lung. There are three types: resorption, compression, and contraction atelectases. Resorption atelectasis is due to an obstruction of an airway, followed by resorption of air from the alveoli distal to the obstruction. Compression atelectasis is due to accumulation of air or fluid in the pleural cavity. Contraction atelectasis is due to fibrotic changes in the lung tissue.

53. d. Giant cell arteritis is also known as temporal arteritis. It occurs in older individuals and is characterized by temporal headaches, and the temporal arteries may be tender to the touch. In some cases, the ophthalmic arteries are involved, which may lead to blindness. This disorder may accompany polymyalgia rheumatica and is effectively treated with anti-inflammatory agents such as prednisone.

54. c. Esophageal lacerations may not need surgical intervention, although hematemesis may occur. Rarely, there may be complete rupture of the esophagus termed Boerhaave's syndrome, which is life threatening. Zenker's diverticulum is an outpouching of the esophagus above the upper esophageal sphincter. Esophageal varices are secondary to portal hypertension. Barrett's esophagus refers to the metaplasia that occurs in the distal esophagus in patients with reflux disease.

55. a. Hepatitis A is generally an acute, self-limited disease. The other types of hepatitis are associated with malignant potential and can become chronic. Hepatitis B and C can lead to hepatocellular carcinoma.

56. a. Rheumatic heart disease is due to a hypersensitivity reaction in which antibodies directed against streptococcal bacteria cross-react with heart antigens. The endocardium, myocardium, and pericardium are all affected, but most significantly, the mitral valve develops vegetations that lead to valve insufficiency. The appearance of the pericardium is that of "bread and butter."

57. d. Classically, tetralogy of Fallot consists of four features: overriding aorta, ventricular septal defect, right ventricular hypertrophy, and pulmonary stenosis.

Section Five Recommended Reading

Chandrasoma P, Taylor C: *Concise pathology*, ed 3, Stamford, Conn, 1998, Appleton & Lange.

Kumar V, Fausto N, Abbas A: *Robbins & Cotran pathologic basis of disease*, ed 7, Philadelphia, 2004, WB Saunders.

Kumar V, Cotran R, Robbins S: *Robbins basic pathology updated edition*, ed 7, Philadelphia, 2005, WB Saunders.

Rubin E, Gorstein F, Schewarting R, Strayer D, Rubin S: *Pathology: clinicopathologic foundations of medicine*, ed 4, Baltimore, 2005, Lippincott Williams & Wilkins.

Microbiology and Public Health

Sameh A. Awad, Samir Ayad, Jill M. Davis,
Martha J. Friesen, Jaya Prakesh, Subramanyam Vemulpad

Microbiology and Public Health

Principles of Microbiology

1. Which of the following is a feature unique to prokaryotic cells?
   a. they have a cell wall
   b. they have circular DNA
   c. they are unicellular organisms
   d. they lack ribosomes

2. What characteristic makes agar a useful culture medium?
   a. it is liquid at room temperature
   b. it is resistant to contamination by fungi
   c. it cannot be digested by most microorganisms
   d. it both melts and solidifies at 100° C

3. Who first used pure cultures to establish the cause of microbial diseases?
   a. Robert Koch
   b. Antonie van Leeuwenhoek
   c. Joseph Lister
   d. Louis Pasteur

4. Which of the following contains LPS (lipopolysaccharides), which forms the basis of endotoxins?
   a. both gram-positive and gram-negative cells
   b. gram-positive cells
   c. gram-negative cells
   d. fungi

5. Bacilli can be described as having what shape?
   a. spherical
   b. spiral
   c. spring
   d. rod

6.   Which two bacteria genera are spore-forming?
    a.   *Bacillus and Clostridium*
    b.   *Staphylococcus and Streptococcus*
    c.   *Neisseria and Mycobacteria*
    d.   *Escherichia and Salmonella*

7.   Which of the following describes a plasmid?
    a.   it is an extrachromosomal DNA for antibiotic resistance
    b.   it is a single-stranded extrachromosomal RNA for toxin resistance
    c.   it is an extrachromosomal DNA for heat resistance
    d.   it is a single-stranded DNA for dehydration resistance

8.   Which of the following bacterial structures is MOST involved in adherence?
    a.   capsule
    b.   lipopolysaccharide
    c.   ordinary pili
    d.   O-specific side-chain

9.   All of the following procedures are useful for the diagnosis of fungal infection EXCEPT which?
    a.   serology test
    b.   gram stain test
    c.   direct microscopic examination
    d.   culture fungi on Sabouraud's agar

10.   Why are gram-negative bacteria more resistant to antimicrobial agents (compared with gram-positive bacteria?
    a.   the peptidoglycan layer in gram-negative bacteria is thicker
    b.   there is an outer membrane
    c.   all medically important gram-negative bacteria form endospores
    d.   a capsule forms a physical barrier in all gram-negative bacteria

11.   Which of the following stains is considered differential?
    a.   capsule stain
    b.   crystal violet
    c.   malachite green
    d.   acid-fast stain

12.   If a process kills 90% of the organisms per minute, how many minutes would it take to kill all organisms when starting with 10,000 organisms?
    a.   5 minutes
    b.   6 minutes
    c.   4 minutes
    d.   3 minutes

13. Koch's postulates are used for which of the following purposes?
   a. to determine if a given organism causes the given disease
   b. to determine if the given organism is a bacterium or a fungus
   c. to determine an organism's growth requirements
   d. to determine if a given organism will produce an immune response

14. Why would a flagellated strain be more virulent than a nonflagellated strain?
   a. flagella can kill the white blood cells
   b. flagella allow the bacteria to negotiate in the mucus layers protecting body surfaces
   c. flagella give metabolic advantage to the bacterium
   d. flagella are major adhesive structures

15. What is the type of virus replication where the virus remains dormant in the host cell called?
   a. lytic cycle
   b. lysogenic cycle
   c. abortive infection
   d. subclinical infection

16. Bacterial cells reproduce by what mechanism?
   a. spore formation
   b. binary fission
   c. sexual reproduction
   d. fusion

17. Which of the following best describes a capsomer?
   a. a viral inclusion body
   b. the lipid envelope
   c. a protein spike
   d. part of a viral capsid

18. Which of the following is characterized by possessing a thick layer of peptidoglycan?
   a. all bacteria
   b. all viruses
   c. gram-positive bacteria
   d. gram-negative bacteria

Answers

1. b. Prokaryotic organisms, such as bacteria, contain circular DNA in their cytoplasm and lack nuclei. Although prokaryotes have cell walls and are unicellular, these are not unique to prokaryotes. For example, plants are eukaryotes with cell walls, and yeasts and protozoa are unicellular eukaryotes. Both prokaryotes and eukaryotes have ribosomes for protein synthesis.

2. c. Agar is a complex polysaccharide obtained from red algae. Although nutrients added to agar are digested by microorganisms, the agar itself is not. It melts at 100° C and solidifies at 42° C and is solid at room temperature.

3. a. Robert Koch developed pure culture methods to prove that certain microbes cause infectious disease. These came to be known as "Koch's postulates." van Leeuwenhoek used a simple microscope to describe microorganisms. Pasteur, the "father of microbiology," developed pasteurization and studied fermentation. Lister developed antiseptic surgical techniques.

4. c. Endotoxin is an intracellular toxin released from disrupted gram-negative bacteria that can cause severe shock and fever. It is derived from lipopolysaccharides (LPS).

5. d. Bacilli are rod-shaped bacteria. Cocci are spherical, spirochetes are spiral shaped, and spirilla are spring shaped.

6. a. *Bacillus* and *Clostridium* form endospores that are capable of withstanding extremes of temperature, desiccation, radiation, and chemicals that would ordinarily destroy vegetative cells.

7. a. Plasmids are small genetic elements (extrachromosomal DNA) that are capable of replication within one prokaryotic (bacteria) cell and may be transferred to another cell, which confers a resistance to antibiotic treatment.

8. c. Pili are hairlike filaments that extend from cell surface, are shorter than flagella, and are found mainly on gram-negative bacteria. They mediate the adherence of bacteria to specific receptors on human cell surfaces to initiate infection.

9. b. The gram stain test is useful for prokaryotic cells (bacteria) and not for eukaryotic cells such as fungi. Most of the cell walls of the bacteria have peptidoglycan and lipopolysaccharides that are sensitive to the staining procedures.

10. b. The outer membrane, made up of lipopolysaccharides, is present only in gram-negative bacteria and acts as a protective barrier to the passage of many molecules, including certain antimicrobial agents. Peptidoglycan is thicker in gram-positive bacteria, and neither capsules nor endospores are present in all gram-negative bacteria.

11. d. Gram stain and acid-fast stain are two important differential stains, both based on the cell wall constituents of bacteria. Gram stain differentiates between gram-positive and gram-negative bacteria, and acid-fast stain differentiates between acid-fast and non–acid-fast bacteria.

12. a. At the rate of 90% killing per minute, there will be 1000 (10%) organisms left at the end of 1 minute, 100 at the end of 2 minutes, 10 at the end of 3 minutes, 1 at the end of 4 minutes, and none at the end of 5 minutes.

13. a. Robert Koch, in order to bring a scientific basis for causation of the disease by microorganisms, adopted the principles put forth by Henle. Koch's postulates state that a given organism must be consistently associated with the disease, be able to isolated from the infected host, and then upon introduction into a suitable animal species should give rise to the same disease and then be reisolated.

14. b. Flagella are the major locomotor organ of microorganisms. They do not have the capacity to kill phagocytes or have any function in metabolism. Fimbriae are the major adhesive structures, and not flagella.

15. b. In lysogeny, the viral DNA or pro-DNA (for RNA viruses) will remain the cell without expressing the full viral replication cycle. It may, however, express some of its genes. In lytic cycle, the cell will be lysed or be destroyed. In abortive infection, which may result in subclinical infection, there is no persistence of the virus.

16. b. Bacteria replicate by asexual binary fission, meaning they grow to a certain size, replicate their DNA, and split into two cells. There is no such thing as sexual reproduction in bacteria. Spores are survival structures that protect bacteria against harsh environmental conditions and are not used for reproduction. Fusion typically does not indicate replication.

17.   d.   Most viruses are composed of a piece of nucleic acid inside a protein shell. The protein shell (called a capsid) is made up of individual proteins called capsomers. An inclusion body is an area of active viral replication inside a host cell. The lipid envelope is picked up from the host cell membrane and is phospholipid in composition. Protein spikes are on the capsid and are part of the capsomers when present.

18.   c.   Both gram-positive and gram-negative cells possess peptidoglycan, a substance unique to bacterial cell walls. The gram-positive bacteria possess a very thick layer. The gram-negative bacteria peptidoglycan is thinner and is covered by an outer layer of lipopolysaccharide. Viruses do not possess any peptidoglycan.

Communicable and Infectious Diseases

1. A 27-year-old man went to the hospital for a deep laceration on his foot that he received during his construction job. He received a shot for a specific type of organism. This organism is classified as which of the following?
   a. gram-positive cocci, ferments lactose
   b. gram-positive rod, anaerobic, and spore forming
   c. gram-negative bacilli, aerobic, and spore forming
   d. it is difficult to stain with gram stain

2. Acute rheumatic fever is a nonsuppurative complication that follows infection by which of the following organisms?
   a. *Streptococcus pneumoniae*
   b. *Streptococcus pyogenes*
   c. *Enterococcus faecalis*
   d. *Salmonella typhi*

3. Following a barbecue hosted by a hunter who served "pork hamburgers," several guests developed abdominal pain and diarrhea. Their condition progresses about a week later to fever, myalgia, and periorbital edema. Blood analysis shows an increased eosinophil count. Which of the following is the most likely cause of these symptoms?
   a. anthrax
   b. botulism
   c. *Escherichia coli* gastroenteritis
   d. trichinosis

4. All of the following agents cause opportunistic infection in AIDS patients except for:
   a. *Candida*
   b. cytomegalovirus
   c. *Plasmodium*
   d. *Mycobacterium avium-intercellular*

5. Negri bodies are the major pathological changes seen in which disease?
   a. rabies
   b. bronchiolitis
   c. croup
   d. AIDS

6. A "slapped-cheek" rash in children is characteristic of which disease?
   a. papillomavirus
   b. measles virus
   c. chickenpox
   d. parvovirus B19

7. A 31-year-old woman with systemic lupus erythematosus (SLE) is found to have a positive serologic test for syphilis (VDRL test). She denies having had sexual contact with a partner who had symptoms of a venereal disease. What would be the next best step to confirm a venereal syphilitic disease?
   a. reassure her that the test is a false-positive reaction for autoimmune disease
   b. trace her sexual contact for serological testing
   c. refer her to a physician to prescribe tetracycline as an antibiotic
   d. perform a fluorescent treponemal antibody-absorbed (FTA-ABS) test

8. Which is NOT an organism that is transmitted by larva or cercaria that penetrates the skin?
   a. *Ancylostoma duodenale*
   b. *Strongyloides stercoralis*
   c. *Wuchereria bancrofti*
   d. *Schistosoma haematobium*

9. Poliovirus replicates in and causes damage to which of the following structures?
   a. sensory neuron (dorsal horn of the spinal cord)
   b. motor neuron (anterior or ventral horn of the spinal cord)
   c. skeletal muscle fibers
   d. cardiac muscle fibers

10. Which of the following organisms does NOT cross the placental barrier and cause congenital defects in humans?
    a. cytomegalovirus
    b. *Toxoplasma gondii*
    c. rubella virus
    d. herpes simplex virus, type 2

11. What is the most commonly reported tick-borne disease seen in the United States?
    a. AIDS
    b. Lyme disease
    c. Rocky Mountain spotted fever
    d. syphilis

12. *Neisseria meningitidis* uses which of the following virulence factors to survive its passage from the blood to the meninges?
    a. flagellum
    b. pilus
    c. pyrogenic exotoxin
    d. polysaccharide capsule

13. Which of the following has been implicated in hemolytic uremic syndrome (HUS)?
    a. *Salmonella typhi*
    b. *Escherichia coli*
    c. *Salmonella enteritidis*
    d. *Vibrio cholerae*

14. The acid-fast stain is used to identify which of the following types of microorganism?
    a. genus *Treponema*
    b. genus *Mycoplasma*
    c. genus *Mycobacterium*
    d. genus *Corynebacterium*

15. Which of the following has been implicated in peptic ulcer disease?
    a. *Mycobacterium*
    b. *Listeria*
    c. *Helicobacter*
    d. *Corynebacterium*

16. Which virus is most characterized by a bullet-shaped capsid?
    a. Ebola
    b. influenza
    c. rabies
    d. measles

17. Which of the following is the causative agent of genital herpes?
    a. bacterium
    b. fungus
    c. virus
    d. parasitic worm

18. In cases of meningitis, in which age group is *Neisseria meningitidis* most often implicated?
    a. newborns
    b. 3 years to 6 years
    c. young adults, college aged
    d. older adults, elderly

19. The most common cause of skin lesions such as boils or abscesses is which of the following bacteria?
    a. *Streptococcus pneumoniae*
    b. *Staphylococcus aureus*
    c. *Bacillus cereus*
    d. *Listeria monocytogenes*

20. Which of the following water-borne enteric diseases is characterized by massive amounts of fluids passed in the feces?
    a. salmonellosis
    b. cholera
    c. hepatitis A
    d. *E. coli* enteritis

21. Which of the following describes the typical appearance of sputum in the patients with pneumonia due to *Klebsiella pneumoniae*?
    a. sputum is purulent and rusty color
    b. sputum is thin and watery
    c. sputum is bloody and gelatinous
    d. scant amount of sputum

22. If a patient is complaining of chest pain, fever, dry cough, and some confusion and has diarrhea and abdominal pain, which of the following organisms is most likely to be the pathogen?
    a. *Bordetella pertussis*
    b. *Legionella pneumophila*
    c. *Mycobacterium tuberculosis*
    d. *Streptococcus pneumoniae*

23. Antigenic drift seen in influenza is responsible for which of the following epidemiologic phenomenon?
    a. a patient who had suffered from influenza previously has partial immunity to the new influenza virus
    b. a patient who had suffered from influenza previously has no immunity against the new influenza virus
    c. a patient who had suffered from influenza previously has a booster effect to his or her immunity
    d. there is no effect on the immunity of a previously infected patient

24. Which of the following fungi cause granulomas in the lung that are mistaken for tuberculosis?
    a. *Histoplasma capsulatum*
    b. *Blastomyces dermatitidis*
    c. *Coccidioides immitis*
    d. *Pneumocystis carinii*

25. Which of the following could cause hemolytic uremic syndrome?
    a. enterohemorrhagic *E. coli*
    b. enteroaggregative *E. coli*
    c. enteropathogenic *E. coli*
    d. enterotoxigenic *E. coli*

26. Which of the following is one of the characteristics of food intoxication due to preformed toxins?
    a. very long incubation period
    b. very short incubation period
    c. live bacteria must be ingested in the food
    d. only cold foods are involved in transmitting this disease

27. In which of the following tissues would the larvae of *Trichinella spiralis* be commonly found?
    a. striated muscle
    b. brain
    c. bones
    d. lungs

28. In which of the parasitic infections does the filariform larvae directly penetrate through the skin to infect a new host?
    a. common round worm
    b. whipworm
    c. hookworm
    d. thread worm

29. Which of the following causes Whitlow, a lesion commonly seen on the fingers of nurses?
    a. papillomavirus
    b. adenovirus
    c. herpes simplex
    d. rubella

30. Which of the following causes erythema infectiosum?
    a. measles virus
    b. varicella zoster virus
    c. parvovirus B19
    d. herpes virus type 6

31. What is the etiologic agent that causes a patient to have high fever, malaise, and either pneumonia or painful swollen lymph nodes called "bubos"?
    a. *Yersinia pestis*
    b. *Shigella sonneri*
    c. *Yersinia enterocolitica*
    d. *Vibrio cholerae*

32. Which of the following diseases is NOT one of the childhood exanthems?
    a. measles
    b. mumps
    c. rubella
    d. rubeola

33. Pertussis can be a serious life-threatening disease due to what bacterial effect on the respiratory system?
    a. swelling of the epiglottis
    b. formation of a pseudomembrane
    c. destruction of the mucociliary action of the respiratory epithelium
    d. pneumonia

34. Which type of virus possesses a double-stranded RNA and a double capsid?
    a. reovirus
    b. flavivirus
    c. retrovirus
    d. alphavirus

35. *Trypanosoma cruzi* causes which of the following diseases?
    a. African sleeping sickness
    b. toxoplasmosis
    c. Chagas disease
    d. leishmania

36. *Tinea unguium* is a fungal infection of what part of the body?
    a. scalp
    b. between the toes
    c. nails
    d. groin

37. Which of the following is a gram-negative, oxidase-positive, facultative anaerobe?
    a. *Escherichia coli*
    b. *Klebsiella pneumoniae*
    c. *Pseudomonas aeruginosa*
    d. *Haemophilus influenzae*

38. A patient complains of diarrhea, abdominal pain, and flatulence shortly after returning from a rafting trip in Canada. He admits drinking water from the streams. With what flagellate protozoan is he most likely infected?
   a. *Giardia lamblia*
   b. *Toxoplasmosis gondii*
   c. *Entamoeba histolytica*
   d. *Leishmania donovani*

39. Which term refers to an "infection that is acquired in a hospital"?
   a. zoonosis
   b. fomite
   c. nosocomial
   d. septicemia

40. Filaria parasites are transmitted by what means?
   a. ingestion
   b. arthropod bite
   c. sexual contact
   d. penetration through the skin

41. A patient presents with a high fever, pharyngitis, lymphadenopathy, and lymphocytosis with atypical lymphocytes. Which infectious disease do the signs and symptoms BEST characterize?
   a. fifth disease
   b. shingles
   c. parainfluenza
   d. infectious mononucleosis

42. Which virus is currently the only poxvirus that causes disease in humans, which appears as papules and nodules on the skin?
   a. variola major
   b. vaccinia
   c. poxvirus of molluscum contagiosum
   d. varicella zoster

43. Which of the following is NOT a causative agent of the common cold?
   a. adenovirus
   b. rhinovirus
   c. coronavirus
   d. hantavirus

44. Pharyngitis with a diffuse erythematous rash appearing on the head and extremities and the appearance of a "strawberry tongue" is descriptive of what disease?
    a. scarlet fever
    b. rheumatic fever
    c. pyoderma
    d. toxic shock syndrome

45. Which correctly describes the appearance of *Staphylococcus* under the microscope?
    a. gram-negative cocci in clusters
    b. gram-positive cocci in clusters
    c. gram-negative cocci in short chains
    d. gram-positive cocci in short chains

46. Bacteria are often cultured on blood agar to detect the presence of hemolytic cytotoxins. What type of hemolysis is β-hemolysis?
    a. no hemolysis is detected
    b. incomplete hemolysis on blood agar
    c. complete hemolysis
    d. irregular hemolysis

47. When *Staphylococcus aureus* enters the blood and it is carried to the bone, it causes an infection given what name?
    a. osteonecrosis
    b. osteopenia
    c. osteolysis
    d. osteomyelitis

48. Which food-borne disease is MOST associated with home canning?
    a. botulism
    b. cholera
    c. listerosis
    d. typhoid fever

49. The Mantoux test is used to detect prior infection by which agent?
    a. *Clostridium difficile*
    b. *Mycobacterium tuberculosis*
    c. *Mycobacterium leprae*
    d. *Cornybacterium diphtheriae*

50. Select the TRUE statement concerning rabies.
    a. the incubation phase is very short; approximately 2 to 10 days
    b. it is caused by a coronavirus
    c. it is an encephalitis with neuron degeneration
    d. it is a spongiform encephalitis caused by a prion

51. A finding of gram-positive encapsulated diplococci in sputum is
     indicative of what organism?
     a. *Escherichia coli*
     b. *Pseudomonas aeruginosa*
     c. *Streptococcus pneumoniae*
     d. *Neisseria gonorrhoeae*

52. What term is defined as a "symbiotic relationship in which one partner
     benefits and the other is unaffected"?
     a. commensalism
     b. parasitism
     c. mutualism
     d. antagonism

53. In human beings, the most common habitat of *Staphylococcus aureus*
     is the:
     a. throat
     b. urethra
     c. skin
     d. nasal chamber

54. What clinical sign can usually diagnose many childhood diseases
     caused by viral infections of the upper respiratory tract?
     a. type of rash
     b. type of cough
     c. type of fever
     d. incubation period

55. Otitis media and sinusitis are usually preceded by what infection?
     a. middle ear infection
     b. infection with *Pseudomonas*
     c. nasopharyngeal infection
     d. lower respiratory tract infection

56. In adults, about 60% of the bacterial pneumonias that require
     hospitalization are caused by what organism?
     a. *Mycoplasma pneumoniae*
     b. *Streptococcus pneumoniae*
     c. *Staphylococcus aureus*
     d. *Klebsiella pneumonia*

57. During which stage of syphilis is the patient noninfectious?
     a. first stage (primary syphilis)
     b. second stage (secondary syphilis)
     c. third stage (tertiary syphilis)
     d. fourth stage (quaternary syphilis)

58. When epidemics of bacterial meningitis occur, they usually involve which organism?
    a. *Neisseria meningitidis*
    b. *Streptococcus pneumoniae*
    c. *Haemophilus influenzae*
    d. *Streptococcus pyogenes*

59. What is the most common etiological agent(s) causing subacute bacterial endocarditis?
    a. *Streptococcus pyogenes*
    b. *Pseudomonas aeruginosa*
    c. normal skin or mouth flora
    d. *Escherichia coli*

60. Symptoms of AIDS appear when:
    a. CD4 counts are <300/µl of blood
    b. CD4 counts are >900/µl of blood
    c. CD8 counts are >1000/µl of blood
    d. CD8 counts are <700/µl of blood

Answers

1. b. The organism is *Clostridium tetani,* a gram-positive rod. Their spores are widespread in soil, enter through a deep laceration (wound) of the skin, and cause a rigid contraction of the muscle by the organism's toxin (tetanospasmin).

2. b. Approximately 2 weeks after group A streptococcal infection (*Streptococcus pyogenes*), there is usually pharyngitis, and rheumatic fever may develop. Rheumatic fever is due to an autoimmune reaction between cross-reacting antibodies to certain streptococcal M-proteins and antigens of joints and heart tissue.

3. d. These clinical manifestations are characteristic of trichinosis disease, which is caused by *Trichinella spiralis* (an intestinal nematode). Humans are infected by eating raw or undercooked pork meat containing larvae that are then encysted in the muscle.

4. c. *Plasmodium* is a blood protozoan that causes malaria disease. Humans are infected after being bitten by a female Anopheles mosquito. This is most likely to occur in tropical areas such as Asia, Africa, and Central and South America. This disease is not dependent upon immune-suppressed conditions.

5. a. Negri bodies are eosinophilic cytoplasmic inclusion of infected neurons of the central nervous system (CNS) by rabies virus (an enveloped-RNA virus). Transmission is usually from the bite of wild animals. The virus infects the sensory neurons and then is transported to the CNS. Negri bodies then develop within these neurons and are diagnosed by fluorescent-antibody staining of a biopsy specimen.

6. d. Parvovirus B19 causes erythema infectiosum ("slapped cheeks" syndrome, fifth disease). This DNA virus is nonenveloped.

7. d. Syphilis is caused by *Treponema pallidum.* The VDRL test is a nonspecific test for syphilis because it may have a false-positive reaction with other infections such as leprosy, hepatitis, or SLE. This test result becomes negative after treatment, but FTA-ABS is a specific test for syphilis and remains positive for life.

8. c. Humans are infected by *Wuchereia bancrofti* when the female mosquito (*Anopheles* or *Culex* species) deposits infective larvae in the skin. The larva by itself lacks the capability to enter the skin without the mosquito bite, as can the other organisms on the list.

9. b. In the central nervous system, poliovirus preferentially replicates in the motor neurons located in the anterior horn of the spinal canal. Death of these cells results in paralysis of the muscles innervated by those neurons (poliomyelitis disease).

10. d. Herpes simplex virus type 2 (HSV-2) causes neonatal herpes, which originates from contact with active vesicular lesions within the birth canal. Despite their association with neonatal infections, neither HSV-1 nor HSV-2 can cross the placenta and cause congenital diseases.

11. b. Lyme disease is spread by the deer tick (the nymph phase). It is considered the most commonly reported tick-borne disease in the United States. Of the other choices, the only other tick-borne condition is Rocky Mountain spotted fever, which is not reported as often as is Lyme disease. Syphilis and AIDS are sexually transmitted conditions.

12. d. *Neisseria meningitidis* is an encapsulated gram-negative coccus that causes meningitis. It is able to survive in the bloodstream to reach the meninges due to its polysaccharide capsule.

13. b. HUS has emerged as an important food/water-borne disease since it was first identified in the 1980s. The causative agent is *E. coli* O157:H7.

14. c. The acid-fast stain is classically used to identify members of the genus *Mycobacterium*. These bacteria have complex waxes and lipids in their cell wall that allow differentiation from other medically important bacteria. Although there are other acid-fast–positive bacteria, the most important medically important ones are in genus *Mycobacterium*. Members include the causative agents of tuberculosis, leprosy, and a variety of AIDS-associated opportunistic infections.

15. c. *Helicobacter* emerged as a major pathogen in the 1980s and has been linked to peptic ulcer disease. Once thought to be a result of lifestyle, and treated as such, the majority of ulcers can now be treated and cured by getting rid of the organism. *Helicobacter* resides in the stomach, protecting itself from the low pH by producing a powerful urease. It is thought to be part of the normal flora in a large percentage of the world's population.

16. c. Rabies is a viral disease caused by the rabies virus. If you examine an electron micrograph of rabies virus particles, you will see a characteristic bullet shape to the capsid. It will be rounded on one end and blunt on the other. Ebola (a filovirus) is more filamentous. Influenza (an orthomyxovirus) and measles (a paramyxovirus) are more helically shaped.

17. c. Genital herpes is caused by herpes simplex 2, a member of the herpes virus family.

18. c. Many microbes cause meningitis, and sometimes knowing the age of the patient can give a hint as to what might be the cause. Although *Neisseria meningitidis* may cause disease in all age groups, it is most often the culprit when the patient is a young adult, of college age, or a military recruit. In newborns, the common first choices are *E. coli, Listeria*, and *Streptococcus agalactiae* (group B streptococci). In those who are 3 to 6 years old, consider *Haemophilus influenzae*. Older adults are often affected by *Streptococcus pneumoniae*.

19. b. When presented with a case history involving boils or inflamed skin lesions, the first choice should be to rule out *Staphylococcus aureus*. *S. aureus* is common on the skin and has many enzymes and virulence factors that cause inflammation. *Streptococcus pyogenes* may also cause these lesions, however, this option was not given. *Streptococcus pneumoniae* is not associated with skin infections.

20. b. Many organisms may cause diarrheal disease from drinking of contaminated water. The key in the symptomatology presented is "massive amounts of fluids." This points directly to cholera. The other choices cause a much less severe diarrhea, which is usually not life threatening. Without treatment, patients with cholera can dehydrate within 24 to 48 hours.

21. c. *Klebsiella pneumoniae* produces a large amount of capsular material and slime, giving a gelatinous quality to the sputum. It also produces a lot of necrosis in the lung, causing bleeding in the lung. Rusty or purulent sputum is seen in *Streptococcus pneumoniae* infection.

22. b. *Legionella pneumophila* will cause dry cough, fever, and chest pain due to lung infection resulting in microabscesses and pleurisy. It can cause diarrhea and abdominal pain due release of inflammatory mediators during bacteremia in about one fourth of the patients. The confusion is caused by an unknown mechanism, probably due to impending respiratory failure and hypoxia.

23. a. In antigenic drift of the influenza virus, a segmented RNA virus, small mutations occur resulting in minor antigenic changes. The antibodies against the original strain may still be able to attach and neutralize the virus but may not be completely effective.

24. a. *Histoplasma capsulatum* gives rise to chronic granulomatous lesions that resemble tuberculosis due to the presence of central necrosis that appears like caseating necrosis. *Pneumocystis carinii* remains in the alveoli and does not cause granulomas; *Blastomyces* and *Coccidiodes* would more commonly cause a noncaseating or suppurative type of granulomas.

25. a. Enterohemorrhagic *E. coli* possesses a plasmid DNA that allows it to produce the Shiga toxin, which causes hemolytic uremic syndrome. Other strains of *E. coli* do not have this toxin-encoding plasmid.

26. b. Because the toxin responsible for the clinical symptoms is already present in the food being ingested, such food poisoning is also called food intoxication. The toxin just needs to reach the gastrointestinal tract and exert its action, so typically the incubation period is in hours. It does not involve multiplication of microorganisms in the body and establishment of infection.

27. a. *Trichinella spiralis* larvae in humans tend to become encysted in the muscles, including striated muscles, heart muscle, and subcutaneous tissue. It is a dead-end infection in humans.

28. c. In hookworms, *Ancylostoma duodenale* and *Necator americanus*, the filariform larvae developing in the soil and in intermediate hosts are able to penetrate the intact skin, especially in people walking barefoot. In the other three organisms, the eggs containing rhabditiform larvae are ingested, resulting in human infection.

29. c. Herpes simplex can cause vesicular lesions called Whitlow, which is sometimes seen on the hands of nurses who take care of patients with active herpes lesions. The patient's lesions are found around the mucocutaneous junctions, or the virus is shed in the patient's saliva.

30. c. *Erythema infectiosum*, or fifth disease, is an infection characterized by fever, "slapped cheeks" appearance (due to the characteristic rash), and sometimes aplastic anemia because parvovirus B19 preferentially multiplies in the bone marrow, especially in erythroid cells.

31. a. *Yersinia pestis* is the causative agent of bubonic plaque. The plague bacillus reservoir is generally in rodents and is transmitted to humans via flea bites.

32. b. The five childhood exanthems are chickenpox (varicella zoster), measles (a paramyxovirus), rubella or German measles (a togavirus), roseola (human herpes virus 6 or 7), and fifth disease (parvovirus B16). Exanthems are characteristic rashes that appear on affected individuals and are accompanied by a fever. Mumps is not associated with a rash.

33. c. Pertussis, or whooping cough, is caused by *Bordetella pertussis.* It is characterized by paroxysmal coughing due to the buildup of mucus and blockage of respiratory passageways.

34. a. The reoviruses have a double capsid in which the outer capsid consists of structural proteins and the inner capsid contains the enzymes needed to transcribe and replicate the double-stranded RNA.

35. c. The protozoan *Trypanosoma cruzi* is transmitted to humans by triatomine bugs indigenous to North, Central, and South America. The disease is characterized by chronic cardiomyopathy, megaesophagus, or megacolon.

36. c. Fungal infections that are confined to the nonliving layers of the epidermis are referred to as the dermatophytoses, or ringworm. They are caused by a large number of different species of fungus and are classified by the area of the body they infect. Ringworm of the nails is called *Tinea unguium.* Ringworm of the scalp is called *Tinea capitis.* Ringworm of the groin is termed *Tinea cruris.* Generalized ringworm on any smooth area of the skin is termed *Tinea corporis.*

37. d. The only gram-negative oxidase-positive facultative anaerobe in the group is *Haemophilus influenzae,* which causes acute bacterial meningitis. *E. coli* and *Klebsiella* are oxidase negative. *Pseudomonas* is oxidase positive, but it is an aerobe.

38. a. The intestinal symptoms described are due to a *Giardia lamblia* infection. Giardia cysts are very hardy and can be ingested in contaminated water or food. *Toxoplasma* is a sporozoan protozoan that is transmitted to humans by eating undercooked meat or by exposure to oocysts in the cat litterbox. Entamoeba infection can be due to eating or drinking contaminated water but is not a flagellate. *Leishmania* is transmitted via a sand fly vector, causes Kala-Azar (Dumdum fever), and occurs in Asia, Africa, and South America.

39. c. Infectious diseases that are obtained in a hospital or clinic are called nosocomial infections. A zoonosis is an infection in which an animal is the natural host for the disease and the disease is transmitted to humans. Fomites are nonliving objects that can be contaminated with a pathogen. Septicemia refers to an infection in the blood.

40. b. Filaria are nematodes that are transmitted via arthropod bites. Examples include *Wuchereria bancrofti*, which causes elephantiasis, and *Onchocera volvulus*, which causes river blindness.

41. d. Infectious mononucleosis (or "mono") is caused by the Epstein-Barr virus, which is a herpesvirus. The disease is most commonly spread by direct oral contact or by saliva-contaminated fomites. Mono is therefore also termed the "kissing disease."

42. c. The variola viruses cause smallpox, which is a disease that was eradicated in the 1970s. The last reported case was in Somalia in 1977. Vaccinia causes cowpox, and varicella is not classified as a poxvirus.

43. d. The four viruses associated with the common cold are adenovirus, rhinovirus, coronavirus, and coxsackievirus. Hantavirus causes the hantavirus pulmonary syndrome of the lung epithelia obtained by inhalation of airborne particles of dried rodent feces.

44. a. All of the listed diseases are caused by *Streptococcus pyogenes*, group A streptococci, but the symptoms are characteristic of scarlet fever.

45. b. Staphylococci are gram positive, and they divide in more than one plane, forming clusters.

46. c. α-Hemolysis is incomplete hemolysis, β-hemolysis is complete hemolysis, and γ-hemolysis is where no hemolysis is detected. β-Hemolysis is the type produced by *Streptococcus pyogenes*, whereas *Streptococcus pneumoniae* demonstrates α-hemolysis.

47. d. Besides *S. aureus*, other organisms can cause osteomyelitis, including various aerobic and anaerobic bacteria, mycobacteria, and fungi.

48. a. The etiologic agent of botulism is *Clostridium botulinum*. The disease is due to the presence of spores in poorly sterilized food, such as in home canning. The spores germinate and produce botulinum toxin within the can. Ingestion of the toxin leads to flaccid paralysis of skeletal muscle.

49. b. The Mantoux test is a screening test for tuberculin sensitivity. A small amount of tuberculin is injected under the skin. If there is a 10-mm red patch of skin produced within 48 hours at the site of injection, prior exposure to TB is indicated.

50. c. Rabies is caused by a rhabdovirus that is transmitted to humans via the bite of an infected animal. The disease has a long incubation phase of 60 days to 1 year, followed by a short prodrome phase consisting of flu-like symptoms, and then neurologic symptoms follow due to encephalitis. Coma and death are the ultimate outcomes.

51. c. *Streptococcus pneumoniae* is a gram-positive organism, occurring in pairs, and is a common pathogen of the respiratory tract; the other bacteria listed are all gram negative.

52. a. Symbiosis is the living together of two organisms in a more or less permanent relationship. Mutualism is where both the partners benefit; parasitism is where one benefits at the expense of the other; and commensalism is when one partner benefits and the other is unaffected.

53. d. The nose is the most common site of carriage of *Staphylococcus aureus*. The skin usually has *Staphylococcus epidermidis*.

54. a. Most upper respiratory viral infections of childhood manifest as exanthems (rashes). The distribution and appearance of the rash are quite distinctive for different virus infections (for example, measles, chickenpox, rubella, erythema infectiosum, and roseola). The rash, in combination with other clinical findings, is useful diagnostically.

55. c. Otitis media and sinusitis are usually preceded by nasopharyngeal infection with organisms such as *Haemophilus influenzae* and *Streptococcus pneumoniae*.

56. b. *Pneumococcus* is the most common cause of bacterial pneumonia in adults that would require hospitalization. Gram-negative bacteria such as *Klebsiella* cause pneumonia in immunocompromised individuals. Pneumonia due to *Mycoplasma* is very mild (hence called "walking pneumonia"). *Staphylococcus* is not a frequent cause of bacterial pneumonia in adults.

57. c. Of the three stages of syphilis, the first two stages are infectious. Tertiary syphilis represents a hypersensitivity reaction to small numbers of *Treponema pallidum* that persist in the tissues; gummas (granulomatous necrotizing masses) can be seen at this stage. At this stage, the patient is not infectious. There is no fourth stage.

58. a. While *Neisseria meningitidis, Streptococcus pneumoniae,* and *Haemophilus influenzae* can all cause bacterial meningitis, for reasons not well understood, only *Neisseria meningitidis* has the propensity to cause epidemics in crowded and stressed populations.

59. c. Virulent bacterial species such as *Staphylococcus aureus* and *Streptococcus pyogenes* are usually responsible for acute bacterial endocarditis. However, opportunistic pathogens such as members of the normal flora of skin (*Staphylococcus epidermidis*) or mouth (α-hemolytic viridans streptococci) are mostly responsible for subacute bacterial endocarditis. This is usually associated with heart valves that are deformed due to a birth defect or rheumatic fever, etc.

60. a. The normal CD4 (Th cells) count is 1000/μl of blood. These cells are the major targets for viral invasion and replication in HIV infection. These cells diminish in numbers as HIV disease progresses. When the CD4 cell counts fall below 300/μl of blood, symptoms of AIDS start appearing (malignancies and opportunistic infections).

Epidemiology and Disease Management

1. Which of the following is the most effective way to sterilize heat-sensitive liquids?
   a. autoclave
   b. filtration
   c. iodine
   d. freezing

2. Which term is defined as the "spread of disease from parent to offspring"?
   a. nosocomial transmission
   b. horizontal transmission
   c. vertical transmission
   d. vector transmission

3. Which of the following is NOT a communicable infectious disease?
   a. chickenpox
   b. tetanus
   c. hepatitis B
   d. influenza

4. Which precautions would be appropriate to prevent the spread of tuberculosis from an infected patient?
   a. gowns and gloves are necessary
   b. proper disposal of urine- or feces-contaminated items
   c. wear masks and disinfect items contaminated with saliva
   d. no special precautions are warranted

5. Which of the following epidemiologic terms is defined as the "ratio between the number of new cases of a disease divided by the number of healthy individuals in a population"?
   a. incidence
   b. prevalence
   c. morbidity rate
   d. mortality rate

6. A disease that occurs with relative regularity only in the southwestern United States would be described as having what type of disease occurrence?
    a. pandemic
    b. epidemic
    c. sporadic
    d. endemic

7. In 2003, the first cases of severe acute respiratory syndrome (SARS) were reported in Asia. Soon, many cases were reported from four continents. How would this spread of SARS be classified?
    a. an outbreak
    b. an epidemic
    c. sporadic cases
    d. a pandemic

8. Which is a term that refers to a disease that is primarily an infection of animals and is accidentally transmitted to humans?
    a. sporadic
    b. secondary infection
    c. zoonosis
    d. reservoir

9. A patient you treated in the morning has influenza, a viral illness caused by an enveloped RNA virus. Which of the following methods of infection control should you use for your adjusting table?
    a. sterilization
    b. pasteurization
    c. high-level disinfectant
    d. intermediate-level disinfectant

10. Which of the following terms describes an epidemiological study where exposed and non-exposed populations are identified and followed over time?
    a. cohort study
    b. case-control study
    c. descriptive study
    d. cross-sectional study

11. Which of the following rates is calculated by dividing all current cases of a disease (old and new) by the total population?
    a. incidence rate
    b. prevalence rate
    c. attack rate
    d. case-fatality rate

12. The term used to describe the occurrence of a disease in a geographic area all the time is:
    a. epidemic
    b. pandemic
    c. epizoodemic
    d. endemic

13. The number of new cases of a specific disease within a specific time period in a given population is called the:
    a. prevalence
    b. epidemic
    c. mortality rate
    d. incidence

14. The single most important measure to prevent the spread of infectious diseases is:
    a. handwashing
    b. proper cooking
    c. canning
    d. pasteurization

15. The period of time between exposure to an infectious agent and the onset of disease signs and symptoms is called the:
    a. prodromal period
    b. incubation period
    c. acute phase
    d. chronic phase

16. Eating undercooked pork is associated with an increased risk of infection with which of the following?
    a. *Trichinella*
    b. *Escherichia*
    c. *Salmonella*
    d. *Staphylococcus*

17. Which of the following is TRUE of botulism?
    a. it is a viral infection
    b. it is spread by mosquitoes
    c. it is sexually transmitted
    d. it is caused by a toxin

18. What is the major cause of death in the United States?
    a. respiratory infections
    b. enteric disease
    c. lifestyle conditions
    d. lack of prenatal care

Answers

1. b. Filtration removes infectious agents from liquids rather than destroys them. Autoclaving is steam sterilization under pressure (heat), iodine is used as a topical antiseptic, and freezing slows the growth of microbes but does not sterilize.

2. c. Vertical transmission is the spread of a disease from parent to offspring via the gametes, placenta, or milk. Nosocomial infections are those that are obtained at a hospital or clinic. Horizontal transmission of a disease is from one individual to another, not parent to child. Vectors are associated with diseases transmitted from animals to humans.

3. b. Communicable infectious diseases are those in which the pathogen is spread from human to human directly or indirectly. Noncommunicable diseases are acquired from one's own microflora or from the nonliving environment such as soil.

4. c. Because tuberculosis is spread via the respiratory route, masks may prevent infection. Tuberculosis is not an enteric disease, so urine and feces are not a concern. Gowns and gloves are not required.

5. a. The incidence is the number of new cases of a disease found within a population over a specified time. Prevalence is the percent of all affected individuals in a population, not just new cases.

6. d. Endemic diseases are those that occur regularly within a geographical area. Sporadic diseases are randomly distributed cases. Epidemics are sudden outbreaks of a disease within a population, and pandemics are worldwide epidemics.

7. d. A pandemic involves a spread of a communicable disease across more than one continent. An outbreak and an epidemic are geographically limited. Sporadic cases are isolated cases of the communicable disease.

8. c. Zoonoses are primarily maintained in nature by circulation of these pathogens in animals. These animals and their vectors can accidentally transmit the infection to humans who come in contact with animals. These animals serve as a reservoir for these pathogens as in the plague (brucellosis).

9. d. Enveloped viruses such as influenza are easily destroyed by intermediate-level disinfectants such as alcohol-based sprays or Lysol.

10. a. Analytical studies test the relationship between a health condition and possible risk factors that may increase the risk of that condition. Cohort study is one type of analytical studies where a group of healthy people who vary in the degree of their exposure are followed over time.

11. b. Prevalence rate refers to the number of cases that exist at one point in time. It measures the extent of the disease in the community by counting all cases (old and new). It is affected by the duration of the disease.

12. d. "Endemic" is a term used to describe a disease that exists in a geographic area at all times. For example, heart disease is endemic in Northern America.

13. d. Incidence is the number of new cases of a disease occurring within a specified period in a given population; prevalence is the total number of cases (both old and new) in a given population at risk at a point in time; mortality rate is the measure of death due to a particular cause in a given population; and epidemic is the occurrence of a disease at higher-than-expected incidence with in a population.

14. a. While cooking, canning, and pasteurization can reduce the chances of food-borne infections, handwashing is acknowledged as the single most important measure to prevent spread of infectious diseases. Handwashing with plain soap aids in the mechanical removal of dirt and microbes present on the hands, including potential pathogens, thus preventing the spread of many infectious diseases.

15. b. The interval between the exposure of a host to an infectious agent and the onset of illness is the incubation period. This is the time taken for the microbe to colonize the host and elaborate the metabolites that would elicit the signs and symptoms of the disease.

16. a. *Trichinosis* is common in pigs, and if one consumes undercooked infected pork, this roundworm may be transmitted with ingestion. The larvae will hatch in the intestinal tract, move to the skeletal muscles, and encyst. The cysts will eventually calcify, leading to loss of function and pain. *Clostridium perfringens* is most often found in contaminated beef, *Salmonella* in contaminated chicken or eggs, and *E. coli* in contaminated water or hamburger.

17.   d.   Botulism is caused by the toxin produced by *Clostridium botulinum*. The toxin is a neurotoxin, affecting the neuromuscular junction. Nerve impulses are prevented from crossing the synapse; thus, muscles do not contract. Without treatment, death occurs due to respiratory failure.

18.   c.   Lifestyle is the prominent factor for cause of death of U.S. citizens. Heart disease, obesity, alcohol abuse, substance abuse, tobacco abuse, and diabetes all play roles. With the advent of medical care and immunizations, microbial disease is low on the list of killers in the United States. Respiratory and enteric diseases, however, are the top causes of death worldwide.

Environmental Health

1. Indicator organisms are used in water testing for the purpose of detecting which of the following?
    a. fecal contamination
    b. turbidity levels
    c. presence or absence of chemicals
    d. offensive odors

2. Which of the following does NOT describe ground-level ozone?
    a. contributes to smog formation
    b. protects the earth from UV radiation
    c. involves sulfur dioxide reactions
    d. involves nitrogen oxide reactions

3. Which of the following causes anthracosis?
    a. *Anthrax*
    b. asbestos
    c. silica
    d. coal dust

4. Water that contains harmful chemicals is called:
    a. contaminated water
    b. polluted water
    c. potable water
    d. deionized water

5. If a patient has ingested a poison, which is a contraindication to inducing vomiting?
    a. if the patient has ingested a corrosive substance
    b. if the dose is moderate to low
    c. if the patient is agitated
    d. if the patient is obese

6. Which of the following is NOT one of the leading health indicators according to *Healthy People 2010*?
   a. physical activity
   b. obesity and overweight
   c. household income
   d. injury and violence

7. Which source of community water requires the LEAST extensive treatment?
   a. ground water
   b. lakes
   c. reservoirs
   d. rivers

8. Which water safety law protects the bodies of water and regulates sewage treatment in the United States?
   a. Safe Drinking Water Act
   b. Clean Water Act
   c. Wastewater Treatment Act
   d. Wetlands Act

9. On which of the following foods can *Staphylococcus aureus* multiply with little competition?
   a. confectionery
   b. salty ham
   c. egg products
   d. milk

10. Plain soap is very effective in controlling spread of microorganisms for what reason?
    a. it is bacteriostatic
    b. it is microbicidal
    c. it is effective at the mechanical removal of microorganisms
    d. it is bactericidal

11. Which of the following prevents dental caries when added to the public water supply?
    a. nitrate
    b. copper
    c. fluoride
    d. iron

12. What is the primary cause of the depletion of the ozone layer?
    a. global warming
    b. chlorofluorocarbons
    c. acid rain
    d. sulfur coal

Answers

1. a. Fecal contamination of water is assessed by examining for the presence of indicator organisms such as *E. coli* or *Enterococcus*. If these normal enteric organisms are found, the chance the water has been contaminated with fecal matter is increased.

2. b. Ground-level ozone is a primary air pollutant produced from photochemical reactions with heat. It contributes to smog formation and can involve chemical reactions with sulfur and nitrogen oxides. Ground-level ozone, although chemically identical to stratospheric ozone, does not protect the Earth from the sun's incoming UV light. Ozone in the stratosphere is "good" ozone. Ozone at ground level is dangerous.

3. d. Prolonged exposure to coal dust will cause damage to lungs, resulting in fibrosis, which can become progressive. This condition is called anthracosis and is named after the common type of coal called anthracite coal. This was a common condition among coal miners, who referred to it as black lung.

4. b. Polluted water is the water that contains harmful chemicals. Contaminated water contains harmful microorganisms, and potable water is neither contaminated nor polluted. Deionized water is water in which ions have been removed and is free of minerals.

5. a. A corrosive substance burns as it descends through the esophagus; it would burn again as it is vomited. Therefore, it is unwise to induce vomiting. Activated charcoal or dilution with water or milk is preferred for many corrosive materials. Other contraindications for emesis are a comatose patient or one who is prone to seizures.

6. c. The leading health indicators as set by *Healthy People 2010* are physical activity, overweight and obesity, tobacco use, substance abuse, responsible sexual behavior, mental health, injury and violence, environmental quality, immunization, and access to health care. Although household income may affect access to health care, it is not a leading health indicator.

7. a. Ground water, which is obtained from wells, is least likely to be contaminated with wildlife droppings, agricultural run off, and trash.

8. b. The Environmental Protection Agency (EPA) governs two water safety laws. The first is the Safe Drinking Water Act, which sets standards for acceptable levels of various pollutants in drinking water. The second is the Clean Water Act, which regulates the amount of pollutants discharged into rivers, lakes, and costal areas and sets standards for sewage treatment.

9. b. Salt is used as a preservative because it inhibits the growth of a variety of microbes. However, *Staphylococcus aureus* can grow in the presence of high concentrations of salt. In fact, high salt concentrations are used in some microbiologic media to make them selective for *S. aureus*.

10. c. Plain soap has minimal or no microbicidal or static activity; but it aids in the mechanical removal of dirt and microbes present on the hands, including potential pathogens, thus preventing the spread of many infectious diseases.

11. c. The most effective, inexpensive, and simple method of preventing dental caries is the fluoridation of the public water supply. Areas with low incidence of dental caries were found to have a water supply that naturally contains high amount of fluoride. The dental caries increased in areas with lower fluoride content.

12. b. Chlorofluorocarbons drift slowly into the upper regions of the stratosphere and release chlorine after being subjected to ultraviolet rays. The released chlorine atoms react with ozone molecules to produce chlorine oxide and oxygen, decreasing the amount of ozone.

Immunology

1. Which class of antibody binds its Fc portion to mast cells?
   a. IgG
   b. IgA
   c. IgD
   d. IgE

2. MHC class II is principally found on what type of cells?
   a. antigen-presenting cells
   b. gut epithelial cells
   c. cytotoxic T cells
   d. T helper cells

3. What effector T-cell type promotes antibody-mediated immune responses?
   a. cytotoxic T cells
   b. T helper 1 cells
   c. T helper 2 cells
   d. $CD8^+$ T cells

4. What is the *V, D,* and *J* gene rearrangement of antibody heavy chains called?
   a. somatic recombination
   b. somatic hypermutation
   c. clonal anergy
   d. affinity maturation

5. Select the TRUE statement concerning the adaptive (acquired) immune system.
   a. the immune response improves during an immune response, and subsequent immune responses for a given antigen
   b. adaptive immune responses occur within 24 hours after contact with a new infection
   c. it is not associated with immunologic memory
   d. the effector cells of the adaptive immune system include dendritic cells and macrophages

6. Which cell type is a professional phagocyte?
    a. cytotoxic T cell
    b. neutrophil
    c. mast cell
    d. B cell

7. Which type of hypersensitivity reaction is associated with immune complex deposition?
    a. type I
    b. type II
    c. type III
    d. type IV

8. Which of the following is a primary lymphoid tissue or organ?
    a. thyroid gland
    b. thymus gland
    c. Peyer's patches
    d. GALT

9. What occurs in a primary lymphoid tissue?
    a. lymphocytes respond to antigens
    b. lymphocytes process antigens
    c. lymphocytes produce antibodies
    d. lymphocytes mature into T and B cells

10. Which of the following classes of antibodies exists as a pentamer?
    a. IgG
    b. IgA
    c. IgM
    d. IgE

11. Cytotoxic T cells kill foreign cells via what mechanism?
    a. activation of complement
    b. opsonization
    c. producing antibodies
    d. producing lymphokines

12. Cell-associated cytotoxicity occurs in which of the following hypersensitivity reactions?
    a. type 1
    b. type 2
    c. type 3
    d. type 4

13. Which of the following is a characteristic of adaptive immunity?
     a. it is nonspecific
     b. it requires prior exposure
     c. it is present from birth
     d. it is not very protective

14. Which of the following is the most abundant and protective antibody in secretions?
     a. IgG
     b. IgA
     c. IgM
     d. IgD

15. Which of the following receptors is present on a typical T helper cell?
     a. MHC class II
     b. CD4
     c. CD8
     d. CD1

16. Deficiencies of proteins of the lytic complex of complement (C5-9) are associated with increased susceptibility to which organisms?
     a. infections with capsulated organisms
     b. infections with opportunistic pathogens
     c. infections with intracellular bacteria
     d. chronic infections with fungal pathogens

17. A primary immune response in an adult human requires approximately how much time to produce antibody in the blood?
     a. 12 hours
     b. 3 days
     c. 1 week
     d. 4 weeks

18. IgG and IgM antibodies activate the complement system via which mechanism?
     a. activating the alternative pathway
     b. activating the classic pathway
     c. inhibiting C1 synthesis
     d. inhibiting C3 convertase

19. Which one of the following types of cells both phagocytize and present antigen during the immune response?
     a. B cells
     b. T cells
     c. macrophages
     d. mast cells

20. Which of the following immunodeficiency diseases causes tetany?
    a. DiGeorge's syndrome
    b. Bruton's agammaglobulinemia
    c. Wiskott-Aldrich syndrome
    d. Chediak-Higashi syndrome

21. Which leukocyte contains histamine within its granules?
    a. lymphocyte
    b. monocyte
    c. macrophage
    d. basophil

22. Which of the following statements about interferon is INCORRECT?
    a. it only works on a few specific types of virus
    b. it makes cells resistant to viral infection
    c. it is a species-specific molecule
    d. it does not directly inactivate viruses

23. Which of the following is the most abundant immunologic class produced?
    a. IgD
    b. IgA
    c. IgG
    d. IgE

24. Which of the following is NOT an immunologically privileged site?
    a. brain
    b. eyes
    c. testes
    d. kidney

Answers

1.   d.   Following sensitization to a particular allergen, IgE binds to the surface of mast cells resident in body tissues. Upon further exposure to the allergen, the allergen binds to IgE, which then triggers mast cell degranulation. Release of inflammatory mediators from mast cells such as histamine leads to the characteristic symptoms of type 1 hypersensitivity reactions (allergies). It is believed that the beneficial purpose of IgE/mast cell reactions is to fight parasitic infections and that allergies are an unfortunate side effect of this system in many individuals.

2.   a.   Specific molecular interactions occur between MHC (major histocompatability complex) molecules and T cells. T helper cells with their antigen receptor and CD4 co-receptor interact with antigens presented on MHC class II occurring on antigen presenting cells such as dendritic cells, macrophages, and sometimes B cells. The effect is to stimulate proliferation and differentiation of the antigen-specific T cell into effector T cells, which release cytokines. MHC class I is present on most nucleated cells of the body and present antigen to CD8$^+$ cytotoxic T cells. This interaction leads to the destruction of the cell presenting the antigen. In this case, the cell to be destroyed is usually virally infected.

3.   c.   There are two subclasses of CD4$^+$ T helper cells. Type 2 effector T cells release cytokines that promote antibody-mediated immune responses, whereas type 1 effector T cells promote cell-mediated immune responses.

4.   a.   In order to create the enormous repertoire of antigen-specific antibodies, three sets of genes are rearranged at the level of DNA to create unique variable regions (antigen-binding domains). For the heavy chain, the genes are called *V* (variable), *D* (diversity), and *J* (joining) regions. This is referred to as somatic recombination. This process occurs during B-cell development prior to antigen encounter.

5.   a.   Over the course of an immune response, and subsequent responses to the same antigen, the adaptive immune system improves. One reason is that activated B cells undergo somatic hypermutation and affinity maturation to produce higher-affinity antibodies. Another reason is the quicker and larger responses of memory B and T cells in secondary immune responses.

6. b. Neutrophils and macrophages are professional phagocytes and are part of the innate immune system. Neutrophils are shorter lived and are involved with pus formation, whereas macrophages are longer lived.

7. c. Type I hypersensitivity reactions are associated with anaphylaxis, asthma, and hay fever. Type I reactions are IgE mediated. Type II hypersensitivity reactions are ones that lyse cells by activating complement. Type III hypersensitivity reactions are associated with immune complex disease. Type IV reactions are delayed-type reactions that are T-cell mediated.

8. b. Primary lymphoid organs are those sites where B or T cells develop and mature. Both B and T cells are generated in the bone marrow, which is also the site where B cells mature in mammals. In birds, they mature in the bursa of Fabricius. Immature T cells leave the bone marrow to mature in the thymus. Peyer's patches and GALT (gut-associated lymphoid tissue) are secondary lymphoid tissues where mature B and T cells encounter antigen. The thyroid gland is not a lymphoid tissue.

9. d. The primary lymphoid tissues are where undifferentiated lymphocytes develop into mature T and B cells. T cells mature in the thymus. B cells mature in the bone marrow in mammals. Lymphocytes respond to antigens in the secondary lymphoid tissues (such as the spleen or lymph nodes). Lymphocytes do not process antigens; macrophages and dendritic cells do. B-lymphocytes produce antibodies after differentiating into plasma cells in secondary lymphoid tissues.

10. c. All antibody molecules are based on the same structural unit; four polypeptide chains (two heavy and two light) attached to each other by disulfide bonds. IgG, IgD, and IgE are monomers, composed of a single unit. IgA is a dimer composed of two units, and IgM is a pentamer composed of five units.

11. d. Cytotoxic T cells are able to kill foreign cells. They do so by producing chemicals called lymphokines, which damage the target cell's membrane. B cells produce the plasma cells that will produce antibodies; complement is activated by IgG, IgM, or other proteins but not T cells. Opsonization is the coating of foreign material to increase phagocytosis. Opsonization is a function of antibody, complement, and other proteins.

12. b. The hypersensitivity reactions are allergic reactions to certain antigens. The type 2 reactions are IgG- and complement-mediated reactions against antigens that are cell associated. Transfusion reactions are a primary example. Type 1 reactions are the immediate IgE-mediated reactions, type 3 reactions are the soluble immune complex reactions, and type 4 reactions are the delayed-type cell-mediated reactions.

13. b. Adaptive or acquired immunity is specific and the most protective immunity, but it requires prior exposure to the antigen (epitope).

14. b. IgA is secreted in the secretions. It is the most abundant and protective antibody in all secretions. It is a dimer and has a protective secretory component added by epithelial cells to protect from digestive enzymes present in secretions.

15. b. CD 4 receptor (antigen) identifies the T-lymphocyte as a helper/inducer cell. This receptor is essential for T cell to interact with antigen-presenting cell. This receptor is the target of HIV.

16. c. The most effective defense against intracellular bacteria such as *Neisseria* is complement-mediated lysis of the bacteria while still in the extracellular fluid. Deficiency of C3 is associated with susceptibility to capsulated bacteria. Opportunistic pathogens are found in T-cell deficiencies such as AIDS. Fungal infections are generally found in phagocyte deficiencies.

17. c. When an antigen is first encountered, antibodies are detectable in the serum after a longer lag period than occurs in the secondary response. The lag period is typically 7 to 10 days.

18. b. The classic pathway of the complement system is initiated by antigen-antibody complexes. The pathway begins with the activation of C1 to form protease, which then activates and cleaves the other types of complements. The alternative pathway is activated by microbial surfaces.

19. c. Macrophages are the only types of cells listed that phagocytize and kill pathogens and also present antigen to a helper T-lymphocytes (CD4$^+$ T cells).

20. a. DiGeorge's syndrome is called thymic aplasia, which is due to the congenital failure of development of the thymus and parathyroid gland from the third and fourth pharyngeal pouches. This disorder is characterized by immunodeficiency and tetany (hypocalcemia) caused by hypoparathyroidism.

21.   d.   Basophils are a variety of granulocytes derived from myeloblasts. They have a lobed nucleus, and their cytoplasmic granules contain histamine and other vasoactive substances. They are important in causing inflammatory reactions. Mast cells are similar to basophils except that the former are found in tissues rather than in circulating blood. Monocytes are derived from monoblasts, are larger in size, and circulate in blood. When they migrate into tissues, they develop into either macrophages or dendritic cells—both are mononuclear phagocytes. Lymphocytes are derived from lymphoblasts and contain a single nucleus with little cytoplasm, and they are important in adaptive immune responses.

22.   a.   Interferons are glycoproteins with antiviral properties and are active against a variety of viruses. Interferon does not directly inactivate the viruses; rather, it prevents the viral replication in infected cells by inducing mRNA degradation and inhibiting protein synthesis. However, they are species specific with reference to the host species (i.e., interferon from other animals is not effective in humans).

23.   b.   IgA is the most abundant immunoglobulin molecule produced in the body. Even though it accounts for only about 10% to 15% of the circulating antibodies in blood, it is also present in various secretions and is important in mucosal immunity. IgG is the most abundant in circulating blood (80% to 85%); IgD and IgE are present in small quantities in circulating blood (<1% and <0.01%, respectively).

24.   d.   Brain, eyes, and testes are immunologically privileged sites. Antigens leaving these sites do not drain through lymphatic vessels and hence do not encounter antigen-presenting cells. The kidney is not an immunologically privileged site.

Section Six Recommended Reading

Brooks G, Butel J, Morse S: *Jawetz, Melnick & Adelberg's medical microbiology,* ed 23, New York, 2004, Appleton & Lange.

Green L, Ottoson J: *Community health,* ed 7, St Louis, 1994, Mosby.

Joklik W, Willett H, Amos D, eds: *Zinsser microbiology,* ed 20, Norwalk, Conn, 1995, Appleton & Lange.

Levinson W: *Medical microbiology & immunology: examination & board review,* ed 8, New York, 2004, McGraw-Hill.

McKenzie J, Pinger R, Kotecki J: *An introduction to community health,* ed 5, Sudbury, Mass, 2005, Jones and Bartlett.

Nester E, Anderson D, Roberts Jr C, Nester M: *Microbiology: a human perspective,* ed 5, New York, 2007, McGraw-Hill.

Ryan K, Ray C: *Sherris medical microbiology: an introduction to infectious diseases,* ed 4, Stamford, Conn, 2003, Appleton & Lange.

Sell S: *Immunology, immunopathology & immunity,* ed 6, Stamford, Conn, 2001, Appleton & Lange.

Stites D, Terr A, Parslow T: *Basic and clinical immunology,* ed 8, Norwalk, Conn, 1994, Appleton & Lange.

Talaro K, Talaro A: *Foundations in microbiology: basic principles,* ed 5, New York, 2004, McGraw-Hill.

US Department of Health and Human Services: *Healthy people 2010: understanding and improving health,* ed 2, Washington, DC, 2001, US Government Printing Office.

Wallace R, ed: *Maxcy-Rosenau-Last public health & preventive medicine,* ed 14, Stamford, Conn, 1998, Appleton & Lange.

PART II

General Diagnosis

*Fiona Jarrett-Thelwell, Curt A. Krause,
Stephan Nicholas Mayer, Brent da Silva Russell,
Keith Wells, Steve Zylich*

CHAPTER 45

Case History

1. The temporal pattern of a disease or condition is more significant for distinguishing which classification of headaches?
   a. postconcussion headaches
   b. chronic headaches
   c. eye strain headaches
   d. sinus and orofacial pain syndromes

2. Many disease processes have premonitory symptoms that help identify the disease by the clinical pattern. Which of the following disease processes often presents with premonitory symptoms?
   a. concussion, cord contusion, disc herniation
   b. migraine, epilepsy, syncope
   c. whiplash, compression fracture, facet syndrome
   d. stroke, vertebrobasilar ischemia, transient ischemic attack

3. A patient states that he recently had a benign mass removed from his upper neck and that a nerve was damaged during the surgery. His formerly deep voice has become very "raspy" and he is having difficulty swallowing. Which nerve was most likely damaged?
   a. facial
   b. trigeminal
   c. hypoglossal
   d. vagus

4. A 41-year-old woman presents with sudden onset of numbness and drooping of the left side of her face and pain directly behind her left ear. Further questioning and a general assessment of the patient revealed asymmetrical facial expression lateralizing to the right side, mild slurring of speech, dysgeusia, hyperacusis, and difficulty drinking noted as the "dribbling" of a beverage. She was recently diagnosed with a viral upper respiratory infection 3 days ago and treatment consisted of rest and fluids. Ms. Ryan denies a traumatic episode, headache, vertigo, lightheadedness, tinnitus, use of oral contraceptives, and smoking of cigarettes. What is the most likely diagnosis?
   a. Guillain-Barré syndrome
   b. Bell's palsy
   c. Lyme disease
   d. stroke

5. A thin, pale, and distraught 53-year-old man presents to the office with a chief complaint of progressive dysphagia to solids and unintentional weight loss of 25 pounds within the past month. Further questioning of the patient revealed recent hoarseness of his voice and fatigue. Lymphadenopathy of the supraclavicular regions was evident on physical examination. Which of the following is the most likely diagnosis?
   a. gastroesophageal reflux disease
   b. adenocarcinoma of esophagus
   c. scleroderma
   d. diffuse esophageal spasm

6. The part of the case history describing the circumstances surrounding the patient's primary reason for the visit is called the:
   a. family history
   b. history of present illness
   c. personal and social history
   d. past medical history

7. When conducting a case history, what is the most risky type of question that the interviewer can ask?
   a. open-ended question
   b. direct question
   c. clarifying question
   d. leading question

8. Which of the following is the preferred way of inquiring about precipitating factors of a patient's chest pain?
   a. "What brings on your chest pain?"
   b. "What types of activities cause your chest pain?"
   c. "Is your chest pain caused by walking rapidly?"
   d. "Does your chest pain occur with activity or when you are upset?"

9. A patient with joint pain tells you that his father was diagnosed with gout 20 years ago. This information is part of what type of information?
   a. history of the present complaint
   b. review of systems
   c. past medical history
   d. family history

10. Which of the following best describes *objectivity* when interviewing a patient?
    a. multiple interviewers would obtain a reasonably similar history
    b. the physician accurately understands and interprets the patient's history
    c. the interviewer sets aside preconceived conclusions about the patient
    d. the physician is able to determine the diagnosis from the history

11. Which of the following is the definition of *respect* during a patient interview?
    a. the physician behaves naturally, that is, "being herself"
    b. the physician accepts the patient as he is without judgment
    c. the physician understands the patient's complaint
    d. the physician feels sorry for the patient's suffering

Answers

1. b. The "temporal pattern" refers to the time course and presentation of signs and symptoms during the development of a condition. It is a significant characteristic in the diagnosis of all diseases, but it becomes more significant in conditions that do not have a clear mechanism of injury or causative aetiology. By definition, the chronic headaches are diagnosed according to International Headache Criteria, which involve excluding other significant options and identifying the temporal pattern of symptoms.

2. b. Antecedent transient visual symptoms before migraine, preepileptic euphoria or depression, and the progressive "gray-out" of a faint are common warning signs of the associated eminent crisis.

3. d. The vagus nerve is the correct answer because it is the motor supply for the muscles of the pharynx (swallowing) and the larynx (voice). Some may become confused because of the similarity of names of "hypoglossal" (cranial nerve XII, control of the tongue) and "glossopharyngeal" (cranial nerve IX, whose functions are paired with those of the vagus nerve). This is an actual patient case.

4. b. Bell's palsy is a disease process affecting the seventh cranial nerve leading to abrupt facial paralysis/weakness as well as the symptoms presented in the case study, which is usually unilateral and self-remitting within a few months to a year. Several possible causes have been linked to the onset or recurrence of the disease process, one of which is a recent viral infection. Obvious physical examination findings involve those structures innervated by the seventh cranial nerve. Other areas of the body are not affected with Bell's palsy, as would be evident with Lyme disease, Guillain-Barré syndrome, and stroke. In stroke, the patient is able to wrinkle the forehead.

5. b. Chronic GERD may lead to hoarseness of the voice due to irritation of the larynx and is the most common predisposing factor for adenocarcinoma of the esophagus. Chronic heartburn and dysphagia to liquids and solids are common symptoms associated with scleroderma. Chest pain and intermittent dysphagia to solids and liquids are common symptoms of diffuse esophageal spasm.

6. b. The history of present illness is the part of the case history where the interviewer follows a step-by-step process detailing the circumstances of the patient's chief complaint that prompted the visit.

7. d. Leading questions are the most risky to ask because by their format they limit the response of the patient to what he or she thinks the interviewer wants to know and does not allow the patient to elaborate, giving more detail.

8. a. Open-ended questions are always preferable to leading questions. Asking about activities, or walking, makes the assumption that these are precipitating factors. Because patients are often eager to please the physician, leading questions may cause a patient to give an answer that is inaccurate.

9. d. The information provided by the patient is about his father. The history of the present illness, review of systems, and past medical history refer to the patient.

10. c. *Objectivity* is the physician's skill at allowing the patient to speak without making hasty value judgments about the patient or to reach preconceived conclusions about what is wrong with the patient; the physician allows the evidence (what the patient says and how the patient behaves) to speak for itself as much as possible. Choice "a" is an example of reliability, and "b" is an example of precision.

11. b. *Respect* is generally defined as accepting people as they are, even if the patient's values and world views differ from those of the physician. Choice "a" is the definition of *genuineness*, "c" is the definition of *empathy*, and "d" defines *sympathy*.

CHAPTER 46

Inspection

1. Which examination procedure can be performed from the first encounter with the patient to the end of the patient's visit?
   a. percussion
   b. auscultation
   c. inspection
   d. palpation

2. A woman exhibits a round, puffy facial appearance with facial hirsutism and what appears to be a fat pad at the base of the neck posteriorly. This appearance has developed only recently, over the past several months. The patient has not altered her life habits in any way. Which of the following would be the most likely cause?
   a. rapid onset of obesity
   b. diabetes mellitus
   c. Hashimoto's thyroiditis
   d. Cushing's syndrome

3. Raynaud's phenomenon would most likely be an associated complication of which of the following conditions?
   a. scleroderma
   b. cholecystitis
   c. osteoporosis
   d. pancreatitis

4. A patient has been previously diagnosed with hypothyroidism. Which inspection finding is LEAST likely?
   a. her hair appears coarse, dry, and brittle
   b. the patient has some difficulty with swallowing
   c. dark blue or purple striae are noted in the abdomen
   d. her fingernails are bent upward toward the tips

5. Which of the following is NOT true when differentiating muscular disuse atrophy from neurogenic atrophy?
    a. disuse atrophy progresses more rapid than neurogenic atrophy
    b. observe for a peripheral limb pattern of involvement
    c. identify a problematic root, nerve, or type of nerve disease
    d. neurogenic atrophy is associated with tender motor points

6. Xanthelasmas are indicative of:
    a. cerebrovascular accident
    b. hypercholesterolemia
    c. angina pectoris
    d. hypertension

Answers

1. c. Inspection of the patient begins with the first encounter with the patient, including what the examiner both observes and smells, and ends when the patient is released from the visit.

2. d. This question assesses the ability to obtain diagnostic clues from inspection of the facial appearance. The patient's "moon face" and facial hair, along with the "buffalo hump," are classic descriptions of what happens to patients with excessive endogenous cortisol production or who are taking exogenous steroidal anti-inflammatory drugs. Choice "a" would not make sense in light of the patient's steady life habits; "c" might explain the facial appearance to some degree but cannot explain the hirsutism (hairy face) and the fat pad at the neck.

3. a. Scleroderma (progressive systemic sclerosis) is a connective tissue disorder that directly affects the vascular system and presents in different forms such as the CREST syndrome. Cholecystitis, osteoporosis, and pancreatitis do not directly affect the vascular system causing Raynaud's phenomenon.

4. c. Choices "a," "b," and "c" *are* associated with hypothyroidism. Dark blue or purple striae are associated with Cushing's disease.

5. a. Disuse atrophy progresses in proportion to the degree of muscular inactivity. Neurogenic atrophy progresses in proportion to neural involvement disease. Flaccid muscular paralysis resulting from a severed nerve (neurotomesis) would progress most rapidly.

6. b. Xanthelasmas are dermal cholesterol deposits typically seen in the familial hypercholesterolemias. While cerebrovascular accident, angina pectoris, and hypertension are often associated with hypercholesterolemia, xanthelasmas are not specifically indicative of these conditions.

CHAPTER 47

Vital Signs

1. Which of the following is the generally accepted correct measurement range for the stated vital function, assuming all measurements are obtained with the patient awake and at rest?
   a. systolic blood pressure: a maximum of 140 mm Hg and a minimum of 60 mm Hg
   b. oral temperature: a maximum of 101°F and a minimum of 94°F
   c. respirations: a maximum of 24 breaths per minute and a minimum of 10 breaths per minute
   d. pulse: a maximum of 100 beats per minute and a minimum of 60 beats per minute

2. The adult patient temperature measure is the least frequent vital sign measured in general office visits, but it is the most frequent measure in the child's examination. Which of the following is the quickest preferred measure for a child's temperature?
   a. oral
   b. anal
   c. axillary
   d. auricular

3. Palpatory systolic blood pressure may be determined:
   a. by comparing the left and right radial pulses
   b. with a sphygmomanometer
   c. while palpating the intercostal spaces over the heart
   d. by palpating the carotid pulse while auscultating the heart

4. The "pulse pressure" is:
   a. normally about 120 mm Hg
   b. best palpated using the brachial artery
   c. usually equal to the palpatory systolic
   d. the numerical difference between systolic and diastolic blood pressures

5. An "auscultatory gap" might be noticed while:
   a. examining tactile fremitus
   b. evaluating blood pressure
   c. auscultating during systole and diastole
   d. listening for friction rubs

6. A patient comes to see you with a complaint of severe back pain. You suspect a leaking aortic aneurysm. Which of the following set of vital signs is consistent with hypovolemic shock?
   a. BP 140/90 mm Hg, pulse 88/min
   b. BP 70/50 mm Hg, pulse 132/min
   c. BP 180/110 mm Hg, pulse 68/min
   d. BP 210/120 mm Hg, pulse 90/min

7. When taking the patient's blood pressure, the auscultatory gap is defined as:
   a. the period of silence from phase I to phase II of Korotkoff's sounds
   b. the difference between the right and left arm systolic blood pressure readings
   c. the period of silence between the first diastolic sound and the second diastolic sound
   d. the difference between systolic blood pressure readings from the seated to the standing position

8. A respiratory rate of _____ would be considered within normal limits for a 28-year-old man.
   a. 8 to 12
   b. 10 to 15
   c. 12 to 20
   d. 18 to 30

Answers

1. d. The range for systolic blood pressure is 140 mm Hg and 90 mm Hg.

2. d. Auricular (ear) measure with electronic instrumentation has become the most convenient and fastest measure (2 seconds), but the technique must be consistent to get a good result. Many pediatricians prefer rectal temperature in infants and toddlers because it is consistent and accurate and much research is based on it, but it is not convenient if the child is very restless. Axillary temperature is convenient but may be up to 2° inaccurate.

3. b. Palpatory systolic is a step in measuring blood pressure that is frequently skipped in an effort to cut corners; as a result, some students forget what it is. However, omitting this step may cause confusion or incorrect readings and may allow for being misled by an auscultatory gap. Additionally, it is possible to become so accustomed to calling the instrument a "blood pressure cuff" as to forget the actual name of the device.

4. d. This is partly a terminology question and partly conceptual. The term "pulse pressure" is not frequently heard. A palpable arterial pulse is created by the wave of blood flow that follows contraction of the ventricles during systole. The increase of pressure accompanying the pulse is the systolic pressure; the pulse pressure is the increase over that of the "passive" blood pressure of diastole.

5. c. Korotkoff's sounds fade prematurely and then return—an auscultatory gap is a phenomenon often experienced during auscultatory measurement of blood pressure. Auscultatory gaps are common occurrences and can cause confusion for the unaware.

6. b. A falling blood volume would lead to a low blood pressure with a compensatory tachycardia. Choices "a," "c," and "d" all present hypertensive blood pressures with pulse rates in the normal range.

7. a. Typically, when taking a blood pressure reading, there will be two consecutive beats indicating the systolic pressure and the start of phase I of Korotkoff's sounds. However, occasionally there will be a period of silence between the first and second beats of 10 to 15 mm Hg. The second beat indicates the beginning of phase II of Korotkoff's sounds, and this period of silence is known as the auscultatory gap. Awareness of this potential gap is important in order not to underestimate the systolic blood pressure and overestimate the diastolic blood pressure.

8.   c.   Normal ranges for respiration rates are as follows (in breaths/minute): adolescents to adults = 12–20; 6 to 10 years old = 15–30; 6 months to 3 years old = 20–30; 0 to 5 months old = 25–40; newborns = 30–50.

Head and Neck Examination

1. A pale optic cup that is greater than one half of the optic disc diameter is characteristic of:
   a. papilledema
   b. proliferative diabetic retinopathy
   c. stage IV hypertensive retinopathy
   d. glaucoma

2. A patient exhibits a large smooth goiter with exophthalmos. Which of the following exam findings would also be expected in this patient?
   a. thick tongue and hoarseness
   b. loss of the outer third of the eyebrows
   c. hyperreflexia
   d. weight gain

3. DeMussette's sign is _____ and is associated with _____.
   a. bruising around the mastoid processes; skull fracture
   b. fine, thin hair and bulging eyes; hyperthyroidism
   c. jerking and bobbing of the head; tremor or aortic insufficiency
   d. masklike rash or pigmentation of the face; pregnancy or SLE

4. When determining whether the trachea is midline, which of the following is evaluated?
   a. the space between the trachea and the trapezius muscle
   b. the space between the trachea and sternocleidomastoid muscle
   c. the space between the trachea and the clavicle
   d. the space between the trachea and the episternal notch

5. Increased fremitus and no tracheal deviation are usually physical exam findings associated with which condition?
   a. atelectasis
   b. pleural effusion
   c. endobronchial tumor
   d. pneumonia

6. Auscultation of the neck region would NOT be helpful to identify which of the following?
    a. carotid body hypersensitivity
    b. arterial dissection disease
    c. areas with arteriosclerotic plaques
    d. vascular bruit and other pulse sounds

1. d. The increased intraocular pressure in glaucoma displaces the optic cup posteriorly, thereby enlarging it and producing atrophy. In stage IV hypertensive retinopathy, papilledema is seen, in which the optic cup disappears and the optic disc is hyperemic and displaced anteriorly. New blood vessel growth is seen in proliferative diabetic retinopathy.

2. c. The patient has findings of Graves' disease, the one form of hyperthyroidism that includes exophthalmos. The key is to search for other findings associated with accelerated thyroid function, that is, increased metabolic rate. The other findings are associated with decreased metabolic rate, expected in manifest hypothyroid function.

3. c. This is largely a terminology question, as it possible to understand the sign without knowing its name. Although tremor might produce a different pattern of movement from aortic insufficiency, the difference might not be apparent without close scrutiny or additional patient history or information about previous diagnoses from other doctors.

4. b. When evaluating if the trachea is midline, the examiner, while standing in front of the patient, gently places his or her thumbs on both sides of the trachea in the lower portion of the neck and compares the space between the trachea and the sternocleidomastoid muscle on both sides of the neck.

5. d. Atelectasis presents as tracheal deviation toward the affected side and decreased fremitus. Pleural effusion presents as tracheal deviation toward the unaffected side and decreased fremitus. Endobronchial tumor presents as tracheal deviation toward the affected side and decreased fremitus. Pneumonia usually has no tracheal deviation but increased fremitus.

6. a. Carotid body hypersensitivity is a significant red flag condition to be ruled out before auscultation or palpation of the carotid artery. In the older patient, ask about past unexplained fainting spells or light-headedness with touching of the anterior neck (shaving, applying make-up) or an aversion to tight neck clothing.

CHAPTER 49

Thorax Examination

CONTENT AREAS

- Auscultation
- Percussion
- Palpation

1. The presence of a slowly developing intraspinal mass of the thoracic spine (neurofibroma) may not produce "red flag" signs until late in the disease. Which of the following clinical patterns would be the least valuable to warn of the development of this type of disease?
   a. bilateral lower limb symptoms (foot drop)
   b. lower motor neuron pattern (areflexia, atrophy, weakness)
   c. unilateral clonus and hyperreflexia
   d. numbness and paresthesia in both feet

2. If this patient developed bladder symptoms, what neurologic bladder pattern would be present?
   a. uninhibited bladder
   b. spastic reflex bladder
   c. peripheral neurogenic bladder
   d. frontal bladder

3. The presentation of a thin patient with a barrel chest, pursed lips, use of accessory respiratory muscles assuming the tripod sitting position and a hyperresonant chest is most likely which condition?
   a. endobronchial tumor
   b. pneumonia
   c. pleural effusion
   d. emphysema

4. What is Kussmaul breathing and with which condition is it most commonly associated?
   a. increased difficulty with expiration; pulmonary obstruction
   b. respiration rate that is less than 12 breaths per minute; electrolyte imbalance
   c. rapid, deep, and labored breathing; metabolic acidosis
   d. respiration rate that is greater than 20 breaths per minute; anxiety

5. Bronchial breath sounds heard over the right lung base is indicative of:
   a. a normal right lower lobe
   b. emphysema
   c. consolidation at the right lung base
   d. bronchial asthma

6. "Flail chest" is most likely to be seen along with which situation?
   a. an enlarged, failing heart
   b. fractured ribs
   c. pulmonary embolism
   d. bronchopneumonia

7. A 10-year-old asymptomatic patient exhibits a systolic murmur during a pre-participation sports physical. The murmur has the following characteristics: localized to the third intercostal space on the left parasternally, grade II/VI, medium pitch, and it diminishes when the patient sits upright compared to lying supine. Which of the following is most likely?
   a. innocent murmur
   b. patent ductus arteriosus
   c. aortic stenosis
   d. aortic regurgitation

Answers

1. b. The lower motor neuron pattern would be typical of a unilateral root or lateral spinal nerve lesion (i.e. disc herniation, lateral entrapment or lateral recess syndrome) and would not warn of a central mass lesion.

2. d. Spastic reflex bladder – This is due to the mass compressing the lower thoracic spinal cord. An upper motor neuron type of lesion results in a spastic reflex bladder. The detrusor muscle becomes over-active which reduces bladder capacity (frequency symptoms) and the patient cannot control external sphincter (incontinence symptoms).

3. d. The presentation is classic for a patient with emphysema. Percussion of the chest reveals hyperresonance. Percussion of the chest in patients with pneumonia, pleural effusion and endobronchial tumor reveals dullness. Normal percussion may be evident with an endobronchial tumor, however.

4. c. Kussmaul breathing is defined as deep and rapid breathing, which is often labored and due to metabolic acidosis.

5. c. The increased lung density caused by the consolidation will transmit the bronchial sounds to the right lung base. Vesicular breath sounds should be heard in normal peripheral lung fields. Emphysema, with hyperinflation of the lungs, would decrease the intensity of breath sounds, while wheezing is common in asthma.

6. b. Flail chest may be seen following thoracic trauma; multiple rib fractures allow a section of the ribcage to expand and contract somewhat independently. It may also be seen in conjunction with paradoxical breathing; the affected area contracts on inspiration and expands on expiration.

7.   a.   One key is the fact that the murmur diminishes when the patient sits upright; another is the patient is asymptomatic. The murmur of patent ductus arteriosus is both systolic and diastolic. The murmur of aortic stenosis is systolic, but is loud and is likely to be heard throughout the precordium, and most likely will radiate to the neck if advanced. It would be unlikely to find this murmur in a child unless there is a congenital defect or unusual disease that afflicts the valves. The murmur of aortic regurgitation is diastolic. By analyzing the name of the murmur and understanding the pathologic anatomy of the valve, a murmur's gross timing can be deduced, which eliminates answer "d" without having to know anything else about aortic regurgitation.

CHAPTER 50

Abdominal Examination

CONTENT AREAS

- Auscultation
- Percussion
- Palpation

1. A 55-year-old man with a long history of uncontrolled hypertension and atherosclerosis exhibits a pulsatile mass just to the left of the midline in his abdomen. Which of the following is MOST likely?
   a. abdominal aortic aneurysm
   b. abdominal intestinal tumor
   c. large-bowel obstruction
   d. inflamed diverticulum

2. Visible peristalsis would probably be accompanied by what other examination finding?
   a. excessive dullness upon percussion over the spleen
   b. prominent pulsations over the abdominal aorta
   c. hyperactivity of bowel sounds
   d. visible signs of diastasis recti

3. The normal vertical span of the liver at the midclavicular line is:
   a. 4 to 8 cm
   b. 6 to 8 cm
   c. 6 to 12 cm
   d. 8 to 15 cm

4. What is Murphy's sign?
   a. rebound tenderness over the right lower quadrant of the abdomen
   b. right lower quadrant pain that is intensified when the left lower quadrant of the abdomen is palpated
   c. pain over the patient's stomach when palpating McBurney's point
   d. pain with inspiration during deep palpation over the area of the gallbladder

5. Inspection of the abdomen in a 53-year-old man during the physical exam revealed tortuous and dilated superficial veins radiating toward the chest from the umbilical region. This appearance of the abdomen is termed:
   a. Kayser-Fleischer rings
   b. caput medusa
   c. chloasma
   d. melasma

6. An infant with an acute abdominal condition who develops periodic colicky pain, vomiting, and rectal bleeding ("red currant jelly" stool) would be suspected of having:
   a. testicular torsion
   b. acute gastroenteritis
   c. intussusception
   d. appendicitis

Answers

1. a. The history and the findings are classic for abdominal aneurysm, and in this case, a visible pulsatile mass is an ominous finding.

2. c. Visible peristalsis implies increased activity within the alimentary canal, which simultaneously causes an increased rate of bowel sounds.

3. c. The vertical span of the liver is commonly measured at the midclavicular line and the midsternal line. At the midsternal line, the normal span is 4 to 8 cm.

4. d. Murphy's sign is indicative of cholecystitis and is present when pain is experienced by the patient upon inspiration while at the same time the examiner is deeply palpating over the area of the gallbladder.

5. b. Kayser-Fleischer rings are associated most commonly with Wilson's disease. Caput medusa is a sign of severe portal hypertension. Chloasma (also known as melasma) is symmetrical irregular hyperpigmented regions of skin of the forehead, cheeks, and upper lip, which may occur during pregnancy, on sun-exposed areas, with oral contraceptive use, with use of certain medications, and in other instances.

6. c. Intussusception is characterized by periodic colicky pain with screaming, vomiting, and tachycardia followed by whimpering, lethargy, and drowsiness. Rectal bleeding ("red currant stool") and abdominal palpation may reveal an elongated intestinal mass.

Rectal and Urogenital Examination

1. Progressive tailbone tenderness after physical activity or after a period of prolonged sitting is associated with a small opening (or sinus tract) at the level of the lower sacrum or coccyx. Examination reveals a small erythematous draining sinus or abscess. When infected it may present a history similar to a gluteal strain. This condition is:
    a. pilonidal cyst
    b. anorectal fistula
    c. anal fissure
    d. hemorrhoid

2. To aid in confirming the diagnosis of renal cysts, which of the following diagnostic imaging examinations should be ordered?
    a. intravenous pyelogram
    b. KUB
    c. plain film of the abdomen
    d. retrograde pyelogram

3. Palpation of a healthy prostate gland should feel:
    a. firm, smooth, and slightly moveable
    b. rubbery and boggy
    c. hard and stony
    d. nodular and nonmoveable

4. Scrotal examination reveals a nontender mass adjacent to the testis that transilluminates. This finding is descriptive of:
    a. a hydrocele
    b. acute orchitis
    c. acute epididymitis
    d. a testicular tumor

5. Which of the following is the MOST likely diagnosis in a man who exhibits lower abdominal pain and unilateral scrotal enlargement when he is upright?
   a. direct hernia
   b. obturator hernia
   c. femoral hernia
   d. indirect hernia

Answers

1   a.   Pilonidal disease is an acquired condition that involves a combination of skin and perineal flora of the midline pits in the natal cleft. These holes or pits are enlarged hair follicles in the skin that develop a small abscess that may expand.

2.   a.   Intravenous pyelogram consists of injecting contrast medium intravenously, which is excreted via the renal system; therefore, an evaluation of renal function and anatomic information can be obtained. Retrograde pyelogram is a nonfunctional test because the contrast medium does not travel through the vascular system. KUB and plain film imaging do not use contrast medium.

3.   a.   On normal palpation, the prostate gland should be nontender, firm, smooth, and slightly moveable. If the prostate feels rubbery or boggy, it indicates benign hypertrophy. A hard, stony, and nodular prostate indicates possible carcinoma.

4.   a.   In a hydrocele, fluid painlessly accumulates in the tunica vaginalis. Because the mass is fluid filled, it transilluminates. Both acute orchitis and epididymitis are painful and tender. Tumor typically produces a nontender, nontransilluminating mass.

5.   d.   The scrotal enlargement is from the descent of a loop of intestine into the inguinal canal and then the scrotum. Direct hernias do not typically make their way through the inguinal canal and exhibit the characteristic bulging scrotum.

Clinical Diagnosis

1. Of the choices below, which of the following makes the diagnosis of myocardial infarction MORE likely in a patient with chest pain?
   a. the pain can be reproduced by palpation
   b. the pain can be reproduced by certain movements
   c. the pain is accompanied by nausea and vomiting
   d. the pain radiates down the left arm

2. Which of the following is the MOST likely diagnosis in a patient with sharp substernal chest pain, worsening of the pain when the patient lays supine or coughs, shortness of breath, rapid pulse, and a history of a recent viral respiratory infection?
   a. acute pericarditis
   b. acute endocarditis
   c. acute costochondritis
   d. acute myocardial infarction

3. A 15-year-old girl is a highly successful soccer player. She has recently been complaining of chest pressure and shortness of breath during practices and games. Which of the following findings should be searched for, directly related to the complaint?
   a. prolonged exhalation phase of respiration
   b. rales and ronchi
   c. harsh systolic murmur
   d. pericardial friction rub

4. A patient complains of chest pain that seems to be localized along a band from the side of his rib cage to the front of his chest at the sternum. The complaint began yesterday. What is MOST likely to appear in the next several days?
   a. a rash
   b. jaundice
   c. cyanosis
   d. ankle swelling

5. A 55-year-old overweight smoker with a 120 pack-year smoking history has dyspnea and cough with abundant sputum. This complaint is 5 years old, and the patient often gets lung infections. There is mild cyanosis. Which of the following is the MOST likely diagnosis?
   a. emphysema
   b. asthma
   c. cystic fibrosis
   d. chronic bronchitis

6. When comparing chronic bronchitis with emphysema, which of the following primarily relates to emphysema?
   a. history of cigarette smoking
   b. dyspnea during exertion
   c. abundant sputum production
   d. development of lung bullae

7. Which of the following is the MOST likely diagnosis in a patient with rapid development of chest pain, cough, sputum, high fever, and dyspnea?
   a. acute myocardial infarction
   b. acute pneumonia
   c. acute bronchitis
   d. chronic bronchitis

8. Which of the following is the MOST likely diagnosis in a patient with unexplained cough and hemoptysis?
   a. emphysema
   b. lung cancer
   c. acute pneumonia
   d. acute bronchitis

9. Which of the following is MOST characteristic of gastroesophageal reflux disease (GERD) compared with other esophageal disorders?
   a. reflux of acid into the mouth
   b. anginalike chest pain
   c. bleeding from the esophagus
   d. pyrrhosis (heartburn)

10. A patient develops jaundice with no other symptoms. Which of the following is the primary suspicion until proved otherwise?
    a. hepatic cirrhosis
    b. pancreatic cancer
    c. acute hepatitis
    d. acute cholecystitis

11. Which of the following is typical of acute cholecystitis but is NOT typical of acute cholelithiasis?
    a. elevated temperature
    b. right upper quadrant pain
    c. nausea and vomiting
    d. pain radiation to the right scapula

12. Korsakoff's syndrome will MOST likely be associated with which of the following conditions?
    a. hyperthyroidism
    b. pancreatitis
    c. Addison's disease
    d. osteomalacia

13. Which of the following is the most common cause of pancreatitis?
    a. cholelithiasis
    b. pancreatic pseudocyst
    c. hepatitis
    d. diabetes mellitus

14. A "bull's-eye lesion" may be a finding in which of the following conditions?
    a. scleroderma
    b. Whipple's disease
    c. Lyme disease
    d. celiac disease

15. Exacerbations and remissions of progressive muscle weakness and fatigue of skeletal muscles, most commonly those innervated by the cranial nerves, with repetitive use and exercise, without alteration in sensation, reflexes, or coordination, would MOST likely be the result of which condition?
    a. amyotrophic lateral sclerosis
    b. myasthenia gravis
    c. hyperthyroidism
    d. Lambert-Eaton myasthenic syndrome (LEMS)

16. Which of the following is NOT considered to be an autoimmune disorder?
    a. acromegaly
    b. systemic lupus erythematosus
    c. type 1 diabetes mellitus
    d. celiac disease

17. Which condition will MOST likely lead to a pulmonary embolism?
     a. prolonged immobilization
     b. cerebrovascular accident
     c. primary hyperparathyroidism
     d. dyspareunia

18. Which of the following is an associated complication of celiac disease, which is manifested in the form of a skin rash?
     a. Battle's sign
     b. café au lait spots
     c. cutis hyperelastica
     d. dermatitis herpetiformis

19. Which of the following would be evident with an upper motor neuron lesion?
     a. hyporeflexia
     b. spasticity
     c. flaccidity
     d. fasciculations

20. Carpal tunnel syndrome is NOT an associated complication of which condition?
     a. pregnancy
     b. acromegaly
     c. hyperthyroidism
     d. rheumatoid arthritis

21. Unintentional weight gain can be a clinical manifestation of which condition?
     a. tuberculosis
     b. hypothyroidism
     c. depression
     d. malignancy

22. Inadequate intake of which vitamin may lead to pellagra?
     a. niacin
     b. thiamine
     c. vitamin C
     d. vitamin D

23. A 35-year-old woman complains of weakness; she is having more difficulty picking up her 3-year-old son. She also states that she has lost 15 pounds over the past month with no change in her diet and that she is always warm. Of the following, which is the MOST likely diagnosis?
    a. hyperthyroidism
    b. hypothyroidism
    c. Cushing's syndrome
    d. Addison's disease

24. A 55-year-old man presents with a sudden onset of facial muscle paralysis over the right side of his face. He has a history of a recent cold. Upon examination the following is noted: loss of the nasolabial fold on the right; patient is unable to smile, frown, or squint his eyes; patient retains the ability to wrinkle his forehead. Of the following, which is the MOST likely diagnosis?
    a. Bell's palsy
    b. trigeminal nerve palsy
    c. oculomotor nerve palsy
    d. stroke

25. A 33-year-old woman complains of being tired and has the inability or desire to perform her normal daily routine. She also states that she has gained 25 pounds over the past 2 months with no change in her diet. Upon examination the following is noted: she has coarse and brittle hair; there is delayed relaxation of her deep tendon reflexes; there is good muscle strength. She also complains of being cold all the time. Of the following, which is the MOST likely diagnosis?
    a. anemia
    b. hypothyroidism
    c. Cushing's syndrome
    d. hyperthyroidism

26. A 10-year-old boy presents to your office with a complaint of pain and itching in his right ear. The history reveals that the patient has just returned from the summer camp 2 days prior and the pain began on the last day of the camp. He reports that there was a lake at the camp, where he swam everyday. The otoscopic exam reveals a red and swollen external auditory canal and the presence of a foul-smelling discharge in the right ear. The right tympanic membrane is normal. Of the following, which is the MOST likely diagnosis?
    a. otitis externa
    b. otitis media
    c. cholesteatoma
    d. otitis media with effusion

27. When examining a patient's tongue, you note left deviation of the tongue when he attempts to stick the tongue straight out. Of the following, where is the MOST likely site of the lesion?
   a. right CN X
   b. right CN XII
   c. left CN IX
   d. left CN XII

28. Upon examining a patient, you note on passive movement the presence of lead-pipe rigidity. This type of rigidity is MOST commonly associated with which of the following conditions?
   a. disorder of the neuromuscular junction
   b. lesion within the anterior horn cells
   c. basal ganglia lesion
   d. peripheral neuropathy

29. A 50-year-old man presents to your office with the following presentation: +2 muscle strength with left shoulder abduction and elbow flexion; +5 muscle strength of left elbow extension and the intrinsic muscles of the hand; bicipital reflex absent on the left and hypotonia of the biceps and deltoid muscles; triceps reflex +2 with normal triceps muscle tone; spasticity and hyperreflexia in the left lower extremity. Based upon the previous presentation, where is the MOST likely site of the lesion?
   a. left side of the spinal cord at C5
   b. left side of the spinal cord at C7
   c. right side of the spinal cord at T1
   d. right side of the spinal cord at C5

30. A 30-year-old woman presents to your office with the following findings: difficulty in writing, typing, or buttoning her clothes with her right hand; complaint of numbness and burning in her right hand. Which of the following is MOST likely?
   a. traumatic myelopathy
   b. cerebellar lesion
   c. cauda equina syndrome
   d. demyelinating myelopathy

31. Upon performing a sensory examination of a patient, you note a loss of pain and temperature sensation on the right side of the body up to the level of the xiphoid process. There is also a loss of vibratory and proprioception in the left lower extremity but not the left upper extremity. Of the following, which is the MOST likely diagnosis?
    a. Brown-Sequard syndrome on the left side of the thoracic spinal cord
    b. syringomyelia in the thoracic spinal cord
    c. central cord lesion in the thoracic spinal cord
    d. Brown-Sequard syndrome on the right side of the thoracic spinal cord

32. With which of the following would you expect the patient to have bilateral and asymmetrical loss of pain and temperature sensations but normal function of all other sensory modalities?
    a. cord hemisection
    b. posterior cord lesion
    c. anterior cord lesion
    d. syringomyelia

33. A 45-year-old male patient presents with a complaint of muscle weakness in his biceps. EMG study demonstrates increased muscle response to repetitive stimuli to the biceps. Of the following, which is the MOST likely diagnosis?
    a. myasthenia gravis
    b. Eaton-Lambert syndrome
    c. cervical disc prolapse
    d. Duchenne muscular dystrophy

34. Chronic nerve root disease may render innervated muscles tender to the touch due to:
    a. tender motor points
    b. phantom pain
    c. disuse atrophy
    d. hysteresis and creep

35. Where is the "autonomous zone" for the axillary nerve?
    a. mid-biceps area
    b. mid-triceps area
    c. lateral shoulder area
    d. superior trapezius area

36. Spinal nerve root compression will reveal the most sensory deficit in what part of the dermatome?
    a. autonomous zone
    b. anesthetized area
    c. all dermatomes of the peripheral nerve
    d. signature area

37. What is the BEST method to test motor strength of the hypoglossal nerve?
    a. protrude the tongue straight out of the mouth
    b. resisting tongue pressure through each cheek
    c. move tongue side-to-side
    d. push tongue into roof of mouth

38. A peripheral mononeuropathy (neuropraxia) would NOT include which one of the following?
    a. glove and stocking presentation
    b. loss of strength and reflex
    c. motor weakness
    d. autonomic deficit

39. Which statement does NOT apply to the "lower crossed postural syndrome"?
    a. altered firing pattern of hamstring-gluteal-erector spinae
    b. abdominal protuberance
    c. gluteal hypertrophy
    d. pelvic extension

40. A neurologic "deficit" and "release" phenomenon may both help localize a motor system lesion. Which of the following is TRUE?
    a. a release phenomena is seen with the subluxation complex
    b. a deficit phenomenon is related to upper motor neuron lesions
    c. both refer to abnormal sensory reflexes
    d. both are associated with a change of muscle tone

41. What would a muscle test feel like where there is POOR recruitment of motor units?
    a. flaccid contraction
    b. weak and feeble contraction
    c. ratchetlike contraction
    e. giving-out weakness with exertion

42.   A 5-year-old child is strapped into a car seat with a three-point seat belt. After a motor vehicle accident, he sustains a "submarining" injury. What mechanism of injury has occurred?
a.   child was projected out of the harness
b.   child slipped down low under the lap belt
c.   belt compression injury to local subcutaneous tissue and fat necrosis
d.   chest belt applied submandibular pressure to cause choking

43.   Which of the following offers a theoretical rationale for chiropractic care of the child with inner ear fluid build-up?
a.   TMJ dysfunction compresses eustachian tube
b.   normalize ciliary function in the ear canal and tragus
c.   C1 dysfunction blocks the eustachian tube
d.   normalize tone of tensor veli palatini

44.   What is the characteristic differentiation between spasmotic torticollis (ST) and wry neck (capsular joint sprain)?
a.   ST is painful and position aggravated
b.   wry neck develops as a painless torticollis
c.   ST is self-limiting pain condition
d.   wry neck is due to a facet-mediated pain

45.   Clonus is an example of:
a.   diminished cortical control of the lower motor neuron
b.   inhibition of the lower motor neuron by cortical controls
c.   repetitive stimulation and inhibition by cortical controls
d.   lower motor neuron lesion

46.   What is the "capsular pattern" of the cervical spine?
a.   flexion and extension restriction
b.   rotation and extension restriction
c.   extension and lateral flexion restriction
d.   lateral flexion, rotation, and extension restriction

47.   What does Sherrington's law of reciprocal inhibition help to explain?
a.   antagonistic muscle relaxation during agonist contraction
b.   inhibition of antagonist if agonist is short and tight
c.   co-contraction of antagonist and agonist
d.   stabilizer muscle inhibition with core muscle stabilization

48.   A 55-year-old smoker presents with left shoulder pain of 8 months' duration. The pain radiates down the medial arm. He has a partial ptosis on the left along with a miotic pupil. You should suspect:
a.   angina pectoris
b.   adhesive capsulitis
c.   superior sulcus tumor
d.   scalenus anticus syndrome

49. A patient who presents with a complaint of rapidly worsening polyuria and excessive thirst, accompanied by weight loss despite an increased appetite, should make you suspect which of the following as the MOST likely diagnosis?
    a. Graves' disease
    b. type 1 diabetes mellitus
    c. type 2 diabetes mellitus
    d. diabetes insipidus

50. A 30-year-old woman presents with tingling and numbness in the first three digits of the right hand. You suspect carpal tunnel syndrome. She also reports dry skin, a recent onset of constipation, and a lack of energy. You note that she has slow speech, is wearing a thick sweater on a warm day, and is modestly overweight. You suspect that her carpal tunnel syndrome is secondary to:
    a. type 2 diabetes mellitus
    b. acromegaly
    c. primary hyperparathyroidism
    d. hypothyroidism

51. A 62-year-old cab driver with a 35 pack-year history of cigarette smoking has right hip and thigh pain of 3 days' duration. He describes the pain as a tightness that is worse in a dependent position. Yesterday, he developed a sudden onset of left subscapular pain and dyspnea. This presentation is MOST likely due to:
    a. pulmonary thromboembolism
    b. spontaneous pneumothorax
    c. congestive heart failure
    d. thromboangitis obliterans

52. A 60-year-old smoker presents with epigastric abdominal pain that radiates to the back. The pain has been present for 3 months. He has also begun to experience weight loss and recently has become jaundiced. The MOST likely cause of his symptoms is:
    a. cholelithiasis
    b. carcinoma of the head of the pancreas
    c. carcinoma of the esophagus
    d. chronic pancreatitis

53. Which of the following MOST reliably increases the probability that a complaint of episodic chest pain is due to myocardial ischemia?
    a. description of the pain as a chest tightness or constriction
    b. presence of several cardiovascular risk factors
    c. duration that patient has been experiencing episodes
    d. severity of the pain

54. A 66-year-old man has orthopnea, exertional dyspnea, and pedal edema. He has distended jugular veins while sitting. Auscultation of the lungs reveals bibasilar crackles. Which of the following is MOST likely to have caused this condition?
    a. hypertension
    b. tuberculosis
    c. endocarditis
    d. ventricular septal defect

55. A 50-year-old smoker is brought in by her husband because of dizziness and lethargy. He also mentions that his wife has been behaving "irrationally" during the past few days. No other symptoms are reported. Which one of the following conditions BEST explains this presentation?
    a. dehydration secondary to diabetes mellitus
    b. upper cervical subluxation
    c. syndrome of inappropriate antidiuretic hormone secretion secondary to lung cancer
    d. pheochromocytoma

56. A patient complains of pharyngitis. Which one of the following DECREASES the probability of "strep" throat?
    a. difficulty swallowing
    b. fever with temperature of 103°F
    c. peritonsillar cellulitis
    d. cough and rhinorrhea

57. A patient has a cough and erythema nodosum in the pretibial regions bilaterally. Chest radiographs reveal bilateral hilar adenopathy. The MOST likely diagnosis is:
    a. lung cancer
    b. *Pneumocystis carinii* pneumonia
    c. sarcoidosis
    d. asbestosis

58. In virtually all cases, a patient with nephrolithiasis will have:
    a. flank or groin pain
    b. hematuria
    c. pyuria
    d. fever

59. When examining persons with very dark skin, it is possible to mistakenly conclude that such patients have heart or lung disease because:
    a. they may normally have a bluish hue to their lips and gums that looks like cyanosis
    b. they naturally tend to have cooler extremities than lighter-skinned people
    c. pallor may only be evident in the palmar and plantar surfaces of the hands and feet
    d. the brown pigmentation of venous stasis is not as easily seen as in most Caucasians and Asians

60. Observation of a "hairy patch" in the low back might indicate the presence of what underlying lumbar spine abnormality?
    a. facet arthrosis
    b. spondylolisthesis
    c. scoliosis
    d. spina bifida

61. What color is icterus?
    a. yellowish
    b. pale or white
    c. red
    d. blue/cyanotic

62. Blue coloration around the umbilicus is evidence of:
    a. metastatic carcinoma
    b. intra-abdominal bleeding
    c. appendicitis
    d. portal hypertension

63. What type of lesion is BEST described as "irregularly-shaped, elevated, progressively enlarging scar; grows beyond boundaries of wound; caused by excessive collagen formation during healing"?
    a. cicatrix
    b. keloid
    c. excoriation
    d. these are usual characteristics of scars

64. Shortness of breath that begins when an individual lies down is:
    a. dyspnea
    b. hyperpnea
    c. bradypnea
    d. orthopnea

65. A patient's breath has an odd musty odor to it. This may be indicative of:
    a. severe liver disease
    b. intestinal obstruction
    c. tonsil or dental infections
    d. diabetes mellitus

66. One sign of infectious disease is the presence of several lymph nodes that are enlarged and close together such that they feel somewhat like a large mass. These nodes are called:
    a. matted
    b. discrete
    c. moveable
    d. connected

67. A patient has been fighting cancer for several years. During an examination, it would be likely to find some enlarged lymph nodes that could be described as:
    a. tender
    b. movable
    c. discrete
    d. matted

68. As a patient pulls his left knee toward his chest, it might be observed that his right thigh rises a few inches from the examining table. This indicates _____ for the right side of his body.
    a. hypertonic hamstring muscles
    b. a positive Gaenslen test
    c. hypertonic iliopsoas muscle
    d. a normal finding

69. Upon squeezing a patient's calf, the ipsilateral foot may be seen to plantarflex. This should be interpreted as a:
    a. positive Gordon's sign
    b. positive Thompson's sign
    c. positive Homan's sign
    d. normal finding

70. For a patient who admits to having had a long-term, undiagnosed infection with syphilis, the fingernails could be expected to appear:
    a. bent upward toward the tips
    b. pitted with small indentations
    c. with a significant convex curvature
    d. very wide and flat

71. "Borborygmi" would MOST likely be detected during:
    a. palpation of cervical lymph nodes
    b. auscultation of the abdomen
    c. evaluation of respiratory excursion
    d. percussion of the lung fields

72. In a patient with a known chronic venous obstruction in a thigh or leg, you would NOT expect to find what in the affected extremity?
    a. normal pulse amplitude
    b. cool skin temperature
    c. rough skin texture
    d. a cyanotic appearance

73. Which of the following examination findings would NOT be a sign of emphysema?
    a. during inspection of the patient, ribs appear nearly horizontal
    b. in percussion of the lung fields, diaphragmatic excursion is decreased
    c. in auscultation of the chest, spoken words sound loud through a stethoscope
    d. tactile fremitus feels diminished during palpation of the thorax

74. The muscles that allow for the ability to "heel walk" are innervated by which nerve?
    a. superficial tibial
    b. anterior tibial
    c. superficial peroneal
    d. deep peroneal

Answers

1. c. In general, chest pain or pressure that is accompanied by some or all of the classic associated symptoms of myocardial infarction is *more likely* to result from myocardial infarction. However, any patient with chest pressure or pain should be suspected of having myocardial infarction until proved otherwise, regardless of whether there are other symptoms. The diagnosis of chest pain is a science and an art and deals strictly with probabilities as opposed to certainties. Choices "a" and "b" are more likely to be associated with chest pain of a mechanical cause based on what reproduces the complaint. Choice "d" might occur with angina pectoris without infarction, whether classic or unstable angina.

2. a. Viral infections can lead to inflammation of the pericardium, which leads to the classic symptoms of pericardial inflammation—sharp chest pain that increases with any movement of the pericardial sac caused by deep breathing, coughing, or sneezing. It is also common for the patient to feel worse lying supine, as the gravitational effects make the discomfort worse. If there is pericardial effusion, cardiac function can be compromised, leading to tachycardia and tachypnea. Pericarditis is a fairly common complication of some rheumatic diseases, especially systemic lupus erythematosus.

3. c. Any young person, and especially a young athlete, who was otherwise healthy and active, should be suspected of the rare but devastating hypertrophic cardiomyopathy (HC) in light of the complaints. The obstructive form of HC is the most common cause of heart-related death in athletes under age 35. In the obstructive form of HC, there might be a harsh systolic murmur that increases with standing upright and decreases with squatting, due to hemodynamic changes that occur with body position change as described. Choices "a" and "b" are more characteristic of asthma and/or respiratory infections, and "d" is characteristic of acute pericarditis, which causes a different clinical picture.

4. a. This clinical picture is typical of an impending outbreak of herpes zoster, or shingles, along a thoracic dermatome. The dermatomal rash is frequently preceded by unexplained pain along the distribution.

5. d. The description is classic for this disease—the long history of smoking, the shortness of breath, the sputum, and the cyanosis are expected findings over time. Emphysema produces little sputum and patients are not typically cyanotic until the end stage of the disease. Asthma is episodic and acyanotic, and cystic fibrosis is a genetic illness that no one survives to the age of 50.

6. d. Development of bullae is characteristic of late emphysema and does not occur in chronic bronchitis. Abundant sputum is characteristic of chronic bronchitis, and the other answers can be found in either disease.

7. b. The description is classic for the explosive onset of acute bacterial pneumonia. The sputum and fever make the lungs the likely source of the problem as opposed to the heart. The rapid onset, the high fever, and the chest pain make pneumonia more likely than the less serious acute bronchitis. Chronic bronchitis is a chronic obstructive pulmonary disease and not an infectious illness.

8. b. Any unexplained cough, especially accompanied by hemoptysis, must be considered lung cancer until proved otherwise. Pneumonia and, in some cases, acute bronchitis can be accompanied by blood-tinged sputum depending on a variety of factors, but these would likely have other symptoms that could be attributed to infectious disease. The key word in the question is "unexplained."

9. a. Reflux of acid is the sine qua non ("without which is not") of GERD. Choice "b" is more likely in diffuse esophageal spasms, choice "c" would occur in esophageal tears or in late hepatic cirrhosis, and heartburn is vague and is associated with many problems.

10. b. Cancer of the head of the pancreas frequently compresses the bile duct, leading to jaundice before any other significant symptoms appear. Choice "a" is incorrect because other symptoms would be expected; the same reasoning applies to "c" and "d."

11. a. All of the other symptoms are characteristic of both illnesses.

12. b. Two of the major courses of pancreatitis are chronic alcoholism and cholelithiasis. Thiamine deficiency is the major cause of Korsakoff's syndrome, which is common in chronic alcoholics. Hyperthyroidism may lead to thiamine deficiency but is not a common complication. Addison's disease and osteomalacia are not associated with the syndrome.

13. a. Chronic alcoholism and cholelithiasis are the most common causes of pancreatitis. Any predisposing factors leading to cholelithiasis (e.g., pregnancy) may therefore result in pancreatitis. Pancreatic pseudocyst may result from chronic inflammation of the pancreas. Hepatitis is a less common cause for pancreatitis. Pancreatitis may lead to diabetes mellitus.

14. c. In the area of tick bite, the patient may develop a painless red papule similar to a target, hence the term "bull's-eye lesion." Morphea skin changes are evident with localized scleroderma, hyperpigmentation with Whipple's disease, and dermatitis herpetiformis with celiac disease.

15. b. Myasthenia gravis is an autoimmune disease process involving an alteration of the transmission of nerve impulses at the neuromuscular junction due to destruction of ACh receptors. Amyotrophic lateral sclerosis is a progressive disease involving progressive degeneration of upper and lower motor neurons. Hyperthyroidism is associated with systemic symptoms such as diaphoresis, diarrhea, tremor, palpitations, nervousness, and weight loss. In LEMS, symptoms are more widespread and reflexes are reduced or absent.

16. a. Acromegaly is a hormonal disorder. Systemic lupus erythematosus, type 1 diabetes mellitus, and celiac disease are all autoimmune disorders.

17. a. Numerous predisposing factors leading to vascular wall damage, hypercoagulability states, and prolonged venous stasis contribute to pulmonary embolism. Some of these include, but are not limited to, prolonged bed rest, history of deep vein thrombosis, pregnancy, medications, trauma, burns, and chemotherapy. A thrombus and an embolism are major causes of a cardiovascular accident. Primary hyperparathyroidism and dyspareunia are not associated with pulmonary embolism.

18. d. Battle's sign is a bruise associated with basilar skull fractures. Café au lait spots are seen with neurofibromatosis and fibrous dysplasia. Cutis hyperelastica is seen in Ehlers-Danlös syndrome.

19. b. Upper MNL signs include spasticity, hyperreflexia, clonus, and pathologic reflexes. Lower MNL signs are flaccidity, hyporeflexia/ areflexia, fasciculations, muscle atrophy, and muscle weakness (paralysis or paresis).

20. c. Hyperthyroidism leads to overactivity of the thyroid gland, thereby increasing metabolism and leading to weight loss. Pregnancy, acromegaly, and rheumatoid arthritis are disease processes, which may lead to an increased pressure on the median nerve and tendons of the wrist through either weight gain or an inflammatory response.

21. b. With tuberculosis, depression, and malignancy, there usually is an unintentional weight loss.

22. a. Deficiency of thiamine leads to beri beri. Deficiency of vitamin C leads to scurvy, and deficiency in vitamin D leads to rickets/osteomalacia.

23. a. Hyperthyroidism typically has a female predilection with common findings of proximal muscle weakness, loss of weight without dieting, fine silky hair, and intolerance to heat.

24. d. Stroke and Bell's palsy can have a similar presentation in facial symptomatology. Bell's palsy is a peripheral lesion affecting all nerve fibers within CN VII; therefore, the entire facial musculature of the side affected will be involved. A stroke is a central lesion; therefore, only the fibers that originate from the cerebral hemisphere where the stroke has occurred will be affected. Fibers originating from the noninvolved hemisphere will be spared. The forehead has dual innervation from both cerebral hemispheres; therefore, a patient who has suffered a stroke will have sparing of the forehead musculature and will not if he or she is has Bell's palsy.

25. b. Hypothyroidism typically has a female predilection and has common findings of weight gain without change in diet, coarse and brittle hair, intolerance to cold, and delayed relaxation phase of deep tendon reflexes with normal muscle strength.

26. a. Otitis externa is also known as swimmer's ear. It is an infection of the external auditory canal, usually bacterial. Therefore, the canal will be red, swollen, and filled with debris. There can be and often is the presence of a foul-smelling discharge coming from the canal.

27. d. A lesion of CN XII will present with deviation of the tongue when the patient attempts to stick it straight out. The tongue will deviate toward the side of the lesion due to the noncontracting musculature on that side.

28. c. Lesions in the basal ganglia will typically present with lead-pipe rigidity with passive movements of the joints.

29. a. Spinal cord lesions usually present with upper motor neuron signs below the level of the lesion; however, if the lesion involves the anterior horn cells, there will also be lower motor neuron signs at the site of the lesion. Therefore, based on the information provided in the question, the lesion must be located at C5 on the left side of the spinal cord and involving the anterior horn cells.

30. d. Useless hand syndrome is a hallmark finding of multiple sclerosis, which is a demyelinating myelopathy. Along with the inability to perform routine functions with the hand involved, there is typically a complaint of numbness and burning. In addition, multiple sclerosis typically has a female predilection.

31. a. Brown-Sequard syndrome is a hemisection of the spinal cord and will present with contralateral loss of pain and temperature sensation due to the fact the spinothalamic tracts cross the cord and ascend up on the contralateral side from where they originate.

32. d. Syringomyelia is a central cord lesion; therefore, the only modalities that will be affected are the ones carried by the spinothalamic tracts because they cross and ascend up on the contralateral side from where they originate.

33. b. Eaton-Lambert syndrome is thought to be due to cross reaction of tumor antigens to voltage-gated calcium channels. As a result, there is impaired release of acetylcholine. However, over time, more and more acetylcholine will be released with repetitive stimulation, causing an increased response that is demonstrable on EMG study.

34. a. A tender motor point occurs because partial muscle denervation causes motor fibers that lose their motor innervation to initiate reinnervation from intact motor neurons. The motor point becomes larger and more sensitive (denervation supersensitivity).

35. c. The "autonomous zone" is the area of a peripheral nerve solely innervated by that nerve. The lateral shoulder area, commonly referred to as the epaulet area of the shoulder, is the autonomous zone for the axillary nerve.

36. d. A dermatome is the area that is innervated by a spinal nerve. There is some dermatomal overlap between adjacent dermatomes. The part of the dermatome that is not innervated by adjacent nerve roots is referred to as the signature area of the dermatome. It is usually the most central or most distal area of the dermatome. Partial root compressions are difficult to test for sensory deficits because of the dermatomal overlap; in chronic radiculopathy, a residual sensory loss may remain in the signature area. This is always confusing to the new clinician.

37. b. Palpating and resisting tongue pressure through each cheek is the easiest method to grade the strength of the tongue. Weakness is felt as the tongue slides forward and cannot apply a constant pressure to the outside finger pressure.

38. a. Glove and stocking presentation is a characteristic pattern for a polyneuropathy presenting with bilateral symptoms.

39. c. In the lower cross-postural syndrome, the gluteal musculature is said to be chronically inhibited due to reciprocal inhibition from overactive hip flexors (psoas muscle). Gluteal disuse atrophy (hypotrophy) is said to occur with weakness and diminished tone.

40. d. Both are associated with a change in muscular tone. A neurologic "deficit" phenomenon occurs when the lower motor neuron is affected by a disease process, giving rise to classic lower motor nerve signs (areflexia, rapid muscular atrophy). A neurologic "release" phenomenon would occur when the lower motor nerve is released from higher cortical controls by a spinal or supraspinal disease process. This would give rise to classic upper motor nerve signs (hyperreflexia, clonus, spasticity).

41. c. Muscles with a poor recruitment pattern will reveal a ratchetlike feel during concentric contraction.

42. a. A "submarining" injury describes a process of the child slipping down low under the lap belt. The belt may then cause significant abdominal visceral, spinal, or rib injury.

43. d. The normalize of the tone of tensor veli palatine has been suggested as a mechanism for cervical manipulation enhancing the drainage of the inner ear for children with acute serious otitis media or chronic otitis media with effusion (noninfectious).

44. d. Wry neck is due to a facet-mediated pain. It is painful with limited neck motions and associated with positions of relief. It often lasts 5 to 10 days. Spasmotic torticollis is a torsional dystonia that is painless and embarrassing and does not respond to physical therapies. It is a permanent disease. The early stages of spasmotic torticollis may be misdiagnosed as a benign cervical torticollis.

45. a. Clonus occurs with diminished cortical control of the lower motor neuron (release phenomenon). The lower motor neuron is restimulated from its own stretch reflex because higher cortical control is not inhibiting the reflex.

46. d. The term "capsular pattern" was first coined by Dr. James Cyriax to describe a characteristic motion loss when a joint capsule tightens due to inflammation or arthritic change. The capsular joint pattern in the cervical spine is diminished lateral flexion and rotation equally limited and extension.

47. b. Sherrington's law of reciprocal inhibition describes how a muscle inhibits muscles that oppose it (antagonists). If a muscle is short and tight, then it is said to continually inhibit its antagonist by way of an inhibitory segmental interneuron.

48. c. Although all of the conditions listed could potentially cause shoulder pain with radiation down the medial arm, only the superior sulcus, or Pancoast's tumor, would affect the stellate ganglion, producing ptosis and miosis.

49. b. The absence of insulin in type 1 diabetes mellitus would produce the polyuria and weight loss with an increased appetite. While hyperthyroidism of any cause will also produce weight loss with an increased appetite, it will not typically cause polyuria. Diabetes insipidus does not affect appetite and weight, and type 2 diabetes does not lead to weight loss until late in the course of the disorder.

50. d. While all of the conditions can lead to carpal tunnel syndrome, only hypothyroidism can explain all of the symptoms. In particular, type 2 diabetes mellitus and hyperparathyroidism do not typically cause dry skin, and both conditions as well as acromegaly would not commonly cause cold intolerance and slow speech.

51. a. Increased age, prolonged sitting, being a cab driver, and smoking are all risk factors for deep vein thrombosis. A patient with risk factors for deep vein thrombosis and sudden onset of chest/thorax pain and dyspnea should be suspected of having pulmonary thromboembolism until proved otherwise.

52. b. Cholelithiasis would have a sudden onset and a duration that would be measured in hours or days. While both esophageal and pancreatic carcinoma are commonly associated with smoking, esophageal carcinoma tends to cause chest pain, dysphagia, and weight loss; jaundice is atypical. Chronic pancreatitis does not cause jaundice.

53. b. Patients with angina may not have the typical pain or may have no pain, while other conditions such as asthma may also cause chest tightness. The severity is largely irrelevant, as is the duration of complaint, because stable angina may be present for years before a catastrophic event occurs. Presence of risk factors, however, such as hypercholesterolemia, smoking, and sedentary lifestyle, should raise one's index of suspicion for cardiovascular disease.

54. a. The patient is exhibiting classic findings of congestive heart failure. The most common causes of this condition in the United States are myocardial infarction and uncontrolled hypertension.

55. c. In a smoker with CNS symptomatology, the possibility of hyponatremia due to syndrome of inappropriate antidiuretic hormone secretion (SIADH) must be considered. Small-cell carcinoma of the lung, which commonly ectopically secretes ADH, often presents with nonpulmonary manifestations.

56. d. While the other symptoms are strongly suggestive of strep throat, cough, rhinorrhea, and generalized myalgias are relatively uncommon and decrease the likelihood that the pharyngitis is due to *S. pyogenes.*

57. c. The combined presence of hilar adenopathy and erythema nodosum suggests sarcoidosis until proved otherwise. Hilar adenopathy indicates sarcoidosis nearly 99% of the time, and the most common cause of erythema nodosum is sarcoidosis.

58. b. While kidney stones commonly cause pain, not all patients report this symptom. Gross or microscopic hematuria, however, is believed to be present in all patients. Pyuria and fever suggest pyelonephritis.

59. a. The question and its answer, "a," are worded very similarly to the source, *Mosby's Guide to Physical Examination.* Distractors "c" and "d" are possible reasons why one might *miss* signs of heart or lung disease. Distractor "b" is simply silly but might be chosen by a student who does not have a grasp of the vascular exam or circulatory system.

60. d. The presence of a patch of hair over the low back implies a congenital problem, which immediately rules out degenerative (facet arthrosis) or traumatic (spondylolisthesis) conditions. And while there may be debate over some types of scoliosis being hereditary, that simply is not the correct answer.

61. a. Icterus is generally considered to be a synonym for "jaundice."

62. b. Blue coloration around the umbilicus is known as Cullen's sign and is a sign of bleeding within the abdomen.

63. b. This is a description of keloid. Keloids tend to occur more often in darker-skinned people and can cause discomfort as clothing (belts, bra straps, waistbands) rub against them.

64. d. Orthopnea is one form of the more general term "dyspnea." Hyperpnea is breathing that is deeper and more rapid than is normal at rest; bradypnea, of course, is abnormal slowness of respiration.

65. a. Intestinal obstructions or diverticulitis tends to cause a fecal odor of the breath; tonsillitis and some dental infections cause a foul, rotten odor; diabetes is well known to generate a sweet, fruity smell.

66. a. It seems to be fairly common knowledge that, in the presence of infection, lymph nodes are tender, moveable, and compressible. *Mosby's Guide to Physical Examination* makes an additional distinction between nodes that are "matted" versus those that are "discrete." This latter seems to be less well known but is almost as important.

67. c. In the presence of malignancy, lymph nodes are nontender, immovable, and hard. *Mosby's Guide to Physical Examination* makes an additional point that nodes tend to be "discrete," meaning that they are well-defined, single nodes, in cancer patients. This seems to be less well known than the other characteristics, but it is also important.

68. c. This describes a positive finding for the Thomas test, a sign of psoas muscle hypertonicity.

69.   d.   Failure of the foot to plantarflex when squeezing the calf muscles is, of course, a positive sign for rupture of the Achilles tendon (Thompson's test). Gordon's sign is a Babinski response upon squeezing the calf. Squeezing the calf is also a secondary maneuver associated with Homan's sign for thrombophlebitis, which will elicit deep pain in the calf upon dorsiflexion of the foot.

70.   d.   Nails that are bent upward toward the tips describes "spoon" nails, which can also be associated with syphilis—as well as iron deficiency anemia, fungal infections, and hypothyroidism. Pitted nails are associated with psoriasis. A significant convex curvature describes "clubbed" nails, which also tend to be enlarged and indicate chronic hypoxia from pulmonary or cardiac conditions.

71.   b.   Borborygmi describes the rumbling or gurgling noises of the alimentary canal (and it is an onomatopoeic word, a vocal imitation of the sounds associated with the word).

72.   b.   Cool skin temperature is a sign of arterial obstruction.

73.   c.   Spoken words usually sound somewhat muffled and indistinct when heard through a stethoscope; when they sound loud and clear, it is a sign of lung consolidation. In emphysema, it would be more difficult than usual to hear the sounds.

74.   d.   The muscles needed to perform this action, including the tibialis anterior, extensor hallicus longus, and extensor digitorum longus, are innervated by the deep peroneal nerve. Inability to perform this action points to a problem with that nerve.

Laboratory Interpretation

1. The clinical use of the laboratory analysis of a hair sample has been highly criticized, but it is still considered an accurate method to assess for:
   a. heavy and toxic metals
   b. water- and lipid-soluble vitamins
   c. calcium and fat-soluble vitamins
   d. protein and manganese

2. Cold water ear irrigation would normally cause:
   a. consensual eye motion to opposite side
   b. nystagmus away from the cold side
   c. optokinetic nystagmus
   d. rotatory nystagmus

3. Nerve conduction velocity/EMG studies of motor nerves are NOT able to differentiate:
   a. peripheral nerve disease from anterior horn cell disease
   b. the specific location—cord, nerve, root, plexus, or peripheral nerve
   c. neuromuscular junction disease from peripheral nerve disease
   d. the specific cause or nature of the neural lesion

4. Hematemesis is usually indicative of bleeding from which structure?
   a. esophagus
   b. jejunum
   c. ascending colon
   d. descending colon

5. The most common causes of megaloblastosis are:
   a. folic acid and cobalamine deficiency
   b. niacin and folic acid deficiency
   c. thiamine and cobalamine deficiency
   d. thiamine and niacin deficiency

6. Which laboratory test aids in confirming the diagnosis of myasthenia gravis?
   a. alanine aminotransferase
   b. CA-125
   c. carcinoembryonic antigen
   d. Tensilon test

7. A patient presents with a complaint of fatigue. The following are the results of a CBC: WBC = 5.0; RBC = 3.9; Hgb = 9.6; Hct = 26.0; MCV = 75.0; MCH = 25.0; MCHC = 33.0. Based upon the lab results, which of the following is MOST likely diagnosis?
   a. no diagnosis, lab work was normal
   b. normocytic hypochromic anemia
   c. microcytic hypochromic anemia
   d. normocytic normochromic anemia

8. A 17-year-old boy presents with generalized malaise and 102° F temperature. The following are the results of a CBC: WBC = 18.7; RBC = 4.5; Hgb = 14.2; Hct = 44.0; MCV = 84; MCH = 29; MCHC = 34; platelets = 190; segs = 86; bands = 5; lymphs = 6; monos = 2; eosins = 1; small toxic granules. Based upon the lab results, which of the following is the MOST likely diagnosis?
   a. viral infection
   b. bacterial infection
   c. anemia
   d. normal labs

9. Upon performing a routine UA for a sports physical exam, you note the following from the results of the UA: color is yellow; character = clear; pH = 5; protein-albumin = negative; sugar = 4+; ketones = negative; bilirubin = negative; occult blood = negative; urobilinogen = 0.2; nitrites = negative; specific gravity = 1.032; WBC/high-power field = 0–1; RBC/high-power field = 0; epithelial cells = 0; bacteria = 0; mucus = negative; crystals = 0; casts = 0. Based upon these results, which of the following is the MOST likely diagnosis?
   a. diabetes
   b. upper urinary tract infection
   c. bladder infection
   d. pyelonephritis

10. In general, the earliest sign of renal parenchymal disease is:
    a. hematuria
    b. elevated BUN and creatinine
    c. proteinuria
    d. hypoalbuminemia

11. A decreased RBC count, decreased hemoglobin concentration, and increased MCV may be caused by:
    a. iron deficiency
    b. thalassemia minor
    c. folate/B12 deficiency
    d. acute blood loss

12. A patient has an elevated lymphocyte count and depressed neutrophil count. Which of the following may cause this pattern?
    a. myocardial infarction
    b. viral pneumonia
    c. pneumococcal pneumonia
    d. corticosteroid therapy

13. Which of the following would be expected in a patient with hemolytic anemia and normally functioning kidneys, intestines, and liver?
    a. decreased urine urobilinogen
    b. normal fecal urobilinogen
    c. increased serum unconjugated bilirubin
    d. increased urine direct bilirubin

14. Which of the following is MOST consistent with cirrhosis of the liver?
    a. increased serum cholesterol
    b. decreased serum albumin
    c. increased serum globulin
    d. decreased prothrombin time

15. Which of the following is the primary diagnostic blood test for acute pancreatitis?
    a. serum aspartate transaminase
    b. serum glucose
    c. serum gastrin
    d. serum amylase

Answers

1. a. Toxic and heavy metals may be seen in hair samples.

2. b. Syringing cold water into a normal ear initiates endolymphatic movement and reflex nystagmus with the fast saccades away from the test ear. Simple mnemonic: COWS: Cold – Other side, Warm – Same side.

3. d. Nerve conduction/EMG studies are useful for identifying the possible injury site along the lower motor nerve reflex but cannot provide a definitive clinical diagnosis.

4. a. Hematemesis is the vomiting of blood from the upper gastrointestinal (GI) tract (esophagus through duodenum). Hematochezia, black or tarry stools, is usually indicative of bleeding from the upper GI tract (stomach through duodenum). Maroon-colored or bright red blood in stools is usually indicative of bleeding from the lower GI tract (colon through rectum).

5. a. Cobalamine (vitamin B12) and folic acid (folate) metabolism are intertwined, and a deficiency in either leads to an alteration in the production of nucleic acids resulting in ineffective erythropoiesis. Niacin is a precursor of NAD and NADP production. Thiamine functions in cellular respiration, providing energy as well as processing carbohydrates, fats, and proteins; nerve signal transmission; and functioning of the heart and muscles.

6. d. The Tensilon test, EMG, NCV, antibody testing, and CT/MRI for thymoma may aid in confirming the diagnosis of myasthenia gravis. Alanine aminotransferase is increased in disease processes that lead to damage/destruction of hepatocytes. CA-125 and carcinoembryonic antigen are tumor markers.

7. c. The lab results reveal a decrease in RBC, Hgb, Hct, MCV, and MCH. The fact that there is a decrease in RBC indicates anemia. The fact that there is a decrease in the size of the RBC (decrease in the MCV value) indicates a microcytic anemia, and the fact that there is a lack of color of the RBC (decrease in the MCH value) indicates a hypochromic anemia. Therefore, the diagnosis of microcytic hypochromic anemia is the correct diagnosis.

8. b. General malaise and high fever should alone indicate bacterial infection. The lab results of an increase in the WBC and seg and accompanying decrease in the lymph and mono values confirm the diagnosis of bacterial infection.

9. a. The only abnormal result of the UA is the 4+ sugar, which can only indicate diabetes.

10. c. Generally, loss of albumin is the first sign of renal disease. Hematuria may occur later and may be caused by conditions other than renal disease. Elevated BUN and creatinine indicates azotemia, often a late finding. Hypoalbuminemia would be seen only after large amounts of albumin are lost in the urine.

11. c. Iron deficiency and thalassemia minor result in a decreased MCV. Acute blood loss results in a normocytic anemia, where the MCV is in the normal range.

12. b. Infarction and many bacterial infections will increase the neutrophil count and decrease the lymphocyte count. Corticosteroids would decrease the lymphocyte count as well.

13. c. In order to answer this question, one must have an understanding of how bilirubin is normally processed. Hemolysis causes increased presentation of unconjugated bilirubin from destroyed red cells to the liver for processing. As the increased amount of bilirubin is conjugated in the liver and released in bile to the intestine, also in increased amounts, intestinal bacteria act on the conjugated bilirubin to produce breakdown products, of which urobilinogen is primary. Urobilinogen is normally found in feces and urine, which means choices "a" and "b" would not be expected in significant hemolysis—both should increase. In this case, the simple destruction of red cells causes increased serum unconjugated bilirubin.

14. b. Recall that the liver both synthesizes substances and processes others for elimination. In cirrhosis, synthetic functions will be depleted, causing reduction in whatever the liver manufactures, and eliminative processes will be affected, allowing an increase in whatever substance the liver was trying to help eliminate. Albumin, globulin, and cholesterol are all substances the liver synthesizes. The liver also makes coagulation cascade proteins. In cirrhosis, these proteins are decreased, making clotting more difficult and thereby prolonging the time it takes to form a clot. Therefore, the prothrombin time is increased or prolonged.

15.   d.   Choice "b" might or might not be changed in pancreatitis and would depend on severity and chronicity of the disease. It is not a direct measure of pancreatic function. Choice "a," of course, is a measure of hepatic inflammation.

Section Seven Recommended Reading

Aminoff MJ, Simon RP, Greenberg DA: *Clinical neurology,* ed 6, New York, 2005, McGraw-Hill.

Anrig C, Plaugher G: *Pediatric chiropractic,* Baltimore, 1998, Lippincott Williams & Wilkins.

Beers M, Berkow R: *The Merck manual of diagnosis and therapy,* ed 17, Whitehouse Station, NJ, 2004, Merck Research Laboratories.

Bickley L: *Bates' guide to physical examination and history taking,* ed 8, Philadelphia, 2004, Lippincott Williams & Wilkins.

Coulehan J, Block M: *The medical interview: mastering skills for clinical practice,* ed 4, Philadelphia, 2001, FA Davis.

Davies N: *Chiropractic pediatrics: a clinical handbook,* Oxford, 2000, WB Saunders.

Giammarco R, Edmeads J, Dodick D: *Critical decisions in headache management,* ed 2, Hamilton, Canada, 2004, BC Decker.

Kasper D, Braunwald E, Fauci A, Hauser S, Longo D, Jameson L, eds: *Harrison's principles of internal medicine, vols. 1-2,* ed 16, New York, 2005, McGraw-Hill.

LeBlond R, DeGowin R, Brown D: *DeGowin's diagnostic examination,* ed 8, New York, 2004, McGraw-Hill.

Liebenson C: *Rehabilitation of the spine: a practitioner's manual,* ed 2, Baltimore, 2005, Lippincott Williams & Wilkins.

Limmer D, O'Keefe M, Grant H, Murray R, Bergeron J: *Emergency care,* ed 10, Upper Saddle River, NY, 2006, Prentice Hall.

Magee DJ: *Orthopaedic physical assessment,* ed 4, Philadelphia, 2005, WB Saunders.

Pagana K, Pagana T: *Mosby's manual of diagnostic and laboratory tests,* ed 2, St Louis, 2002, Mosby.

Patten J: *Neurological differential diagnosis,* ed 2, New York, 1998, Springer.

Ravel R: *Clinical laboratory medicine,* ed 6, St Louis, 1995, Mosby.

Seidel H, Ball J, Dains J, Benedict G: *Mosby's guide to physical examination,* ed 5, St Louis, 2002, Mosby.

Tierney L, McPhee S, Papadakis M, eds: *Current medical diagnosis and treatment,* ed 44, New York, 2005, McGraw-Hill.

Neuromusculoskeletal Diagnosis

*Andre Bussières, Marni Capes, Martin Descarreaux,
Rocco C. Guerriero, Johanne Martel, Michael D. Moore*

CHAPTER 54

Case History

1. A patient presents to your office complaining of posterior neck pain following a car accident. What component of the case history would BEST describe how the tissue was injured?
   a. character of complaint of the symptoms
   b. date of the accident and onset of symptoms
   c. factor that make the symptoms worse
   d. mechanism of injury

2. What component of the case history identifies if the patient's condition is acute, subacute, or chronic?
   a. aggravating factors
   b. character of the complain
   c. date of onset
   d. mode of onset

3. Which of the following is NOT part of the SCORE questionnaire (Simple Calculated Osteoporosis Risk Estimate) for evaluation of osteoporosis risk factors?
   a. patient age over 50
   b. ethnic group or race
   c. history of corticosteroid treatment for immune and inflammatory disorder
   d. BMI <19 kg/m² or weight <57 kg

4. Which of the following choices is NOT an indication for taking radiographs?
   a. persistent localized pain (10 days)
   b. symptoms associated with neurologic signs in the lower extremities
   c. rapidly progressing or atypical scoliosis and other spinal deformities
   d. predisposition for ascending aortic aneurysm

5. Which of the following is NOT an indicator of possible severe underlying pathology?
    a. age over 50
    b. high-risk ligament laxity populations
    c. neck pain in the sagittal plain in the absence of trauma
    d. arm or leg pain with neck movements

6. Which information from the case history is NOT likely a contraindication for manipulation?
    a. peripheral nervous system signs and symptoms
    b. no response to care after 4 to 7 weeks
    c. dysphasia, impaired consciousness
    d. sudden onset of acute and unusual neck pain and/or headache (typically occipital) with or without neurologic symptoms

7. History taking revealed that a patient experienced pain after horseback riding or skating. The pain is located over the anteromedial thigh and is aggravated by resisted abduction. What is the MOST likely preliminary diagnosis?
    a. piriformis syndrome
    b. trochanteric bursitis
    c. adductor longus strain/tendonitis/tendinosis
    d. avascular necrosis

8. A patient has dull posterior hip pain radiating down the leg. He says that he has a limp and that his pain is aggravated by turning his leg outside or with deep pressure near the middle of the right buttock. What is the MOST likely preliminary diagnosis?
    a. piriformis syndrome
    b. trochanteric bursitis
    c. adductor longus strain/tendonitis/tendinosis
    d. avascular necrosis

9. A patient has low back pain of 6 months' duration that is unrelieved by rest. The pain is worse at night. Lying recumbent reduces the pain; standing for long periods of time and walking make the pain worse. When asked to point to the pain, he isolates the location to the L3 vertebral level and is a 8/10 on the pain scale. Using the OPQRST system and the above information, which part of the OPQRST information is MISSING?
    a. quality
    b. radiation
    c. site
    d. palliative

10. A patient has right knee pain. She was working out at the gym when she heard a "pop." The pain is dull and achy. Standing and walking aggravate the knee pain, and on the pain scale the patient circled 8/10. The patient has taken four 200-mg tablets of ibuprofen to reduce the pain. Using the OPQRST system and the above information, which part of the OPQRST information is MISSING?
    a. quality
    b. radiation
    c. site
    d. palliative

11. A male construction worker has low back pain. Symptoms started earlier in the week following lifting a 30-pound box. The pain started as a 7/10 but is now a 10/10 on the pain scale and prevents him from going to work. He states that the pain is isolated around the right L5 vertebral level and down into the right SI joint. Using the OPQRST system and the above information, which part of the OPQRST information is MISSING?
    a. quality
    b. radiation
    c. site
    d. palliative

12. A case history of a whiplash patient should specifically address the following aspects of the accident EXCEPT:
    a. speed of vehicles
    b. road surface condition
    c. fault and legal liability of the patient
    d. head position

13. Which of the following is NOT a red flag for low back pain of pathologic origin?
    a. age under 20 or over 50
    b. radiating pain to the leg
    c. intense nocturnal pain
    d. history of cancer

14. Which of the following is an indicator of functional overlay in low back pain patients?
    a. low back pain on moderate cervical compression
    b. radiating pain to the leg
    c. restricted range of motion
    d. inability to stand for a prolonged period of time

15. Which of the following is NOT considered a red flag?
    a. night pain
    b. previous history of cancer
    c. substantial discrepancy between supine and sitting straight leg raising test
    d. bilateral sciatica, saddle anesthesia, and urinary retention

16. What does the term "yellow flag" mean?
    a. relative contraindication for SMT; proceed with caution
    b. physical barrier to recovery
    c. Waddell's signs
    d. psychosocial barrier to recovery

17. Which information obtained in the case history is NOT a risk factor for osteoarthritis?
    a. Caucasian female
    b. weight of 190 lb in a female measuring 5 ft 5 in
    c. occupation as a farmer
    d. history of a slipped femoral capital epiphysis

18. Which information obtained in the case history will NOT help in differentiating between an inflammatory and a noninflammatory spinal condition?
    a. presence of morning stiffness
    b. pain location
    c. presence of gelling phenomenon
    d. patient's response to exercise

19. Which information obtained in the case history is NOT an indication to obtain osteodensitometry?
    a. personal history of nontraumatic osteoporosis fracture after 40 years of age
    b. familial history of osteoporosis in a second-degree relative
    c. aggressive corticosteroid therapy
    d. early menopause

Answers

1. d. A detailed account of the mechanism that the patient's injured tissue went through in the accident will tell whether the tissue was stretched, compressed, torn, or contused and may help identify the tissue that was injured. This will help provide a differential diagnosis for the patient's condition at the end of the case history.

2. c. If the date of onset is within 72 hours of entering the office for exam, the condition is acute. If the date of onset is greater than 72 hours of entering the office for exam and has never been treated or is an aggravation of a previous condition, it is subacute. If the condition has been present for months or years and the condition was treated and healed, it is chronic.

3. b. The SCORE questionnaire for evaluation of osteoporosis risk factors is a sensitive, reliable, and validated instrument to identify women in need for further testing. It does not include questions pertaining to race. One should also consider if the patient has a history of corticosteroid treatment for immune and inflammatory disorder (>7.5 mg/day × 3 mo), a history of fracture since age 45 (at the hip, rib, or wrist); no history of estrogen use.

4. a. A patient presenting with over 4 weeks of persistent localized pain is unusual and requires plain film radiographs. Specialized imaging is recommended in the presence of a potentially serious pathology as suggested by the patient history, examination, and radiograph or in the absence of clinical improvement after a month of therapy.

5. c. Neck rigidity in the sagittal plane in the absence of trauma may indicate significant underlying pathology, such as discitis, infection, tumor, meningitis, etc. Insidious midline neck pain is usually not a cause for concern.

6. a. Neck pain with nonprogressive peripheral nervous system signs and symptoms is not a contraindication to manual therapy. However, neck pain in the presence of central nervous system signs and symptoms (cranial nerves, pathologic reflexes, long tract signs) requires medical referral and specialized investigation.

7. c. Adductor longus, rectus femoris, and iliopsoas are the muscles typically involved in hip muscle strain/tendonitis/tendinosis. Pain is aggravated by activity or in resistance testing. Adductor strains arise in horseback riders, skiers, and skaters.

8. a. History and type/site of pain are the most important features to direct the examination. Piriformis irritation often presents as dull posterior hip pain radiating down the leg, mimicking radicular symptoms. Limping, pain aggravated by active external rotation, or passive internal rotation on palpation of sciatic notch is a salient feature.

9. a. Quality—which type of pain it is—is not included; for example: dull, achy, sharp, stabbing, gnawing, burning.

10. b. Radiation is missing. Asking open ended questions can reveal this information, such as, "Does the pain go anywhere?" or "Does it travel up or down from the site of pain?"

11. d. Information pertaining to "palliative" is missing. Questions to ask include the following: "What, if anything, makes the pain better?" "Have you used any medications, lotions, physical modalities, exercises, or stretches that make the pain decrease?"

12. c. Secondary gain can influence the chief complaints presentation, but it is not a part of the accident history evaluation. The history of the accident enables the clinician to reconstruct the accident and determine the biomechanics of the injury.

13. b. Radiating pain to the leg is a common low back pain symptom. Leg pain can be observed in different types of low back pain of mechanical origin such as in facet syndrome, sacroiliac syndrome, herniation of nucleus pulposus, muscle syndromes, and lateral and central stenosis.

14. a. Moderate cervical compression will not create important compression or shearing forces in the lumbar region. Low back pain on moderate cervical compression can indicate functional overlay or malingering.

15. c. Night pain and previous history of cancer are red flags and spinal metastasis should be ruled out. Bilateral sciatica, saddle anesthesia, and urinary retention are all symptoms of cauda equina syndrome, which is a red flag and considered a medical emergency. The discrepancy in straight leg raising between sitting and supine is regarded as a nonorganic sign.

16. d. Yellow flags are a psychosocial barrier to recovery. The New Zealand Guidelines report extensively on the many examples of psychosocial barriers to recovery. They are not an absolute contraindication to manipulation.

17. a. Evidence is conflicting regarding racial differences as risk factors for osteoarthritis (OA). At best, the incidence of knee OA might be increased in African-American women compared with Caucasian women. Otherwise, there seems to be no racial difference in the incidence of OA. Other important risk factors for OA include obesity, previous injuries, occupation (as miners, cotton workers, farmers, etc.), developmental anomalies (e.g., Legg-Calvé-Perthes, CHD, SFCE, etc.), other local factors (e.g., joint laxity, quadriceps strength, etc.), sexual hormones (OA is more prevalent in females than in males over 50 years old, less susceptibility in women under estrogen replacement therapy), genetic susceptibility, and systemic factors.

18. b. Major differentiating factors of inflammatory versus noninflammatory joint conditions are morning stiffness, patient's response to exercise, patient's response to anti-inflammatory medication, manifestations other than joints, anomalies in laboratory analyses, and gelling phenomenon.

19. b. Risk factors indicative of a need for osteodensitometry are personal history of nontraumatic osteoporosis fracture after 40 years of age; familial history of osteoporosis in a first-degree relative; corticosteroid therapy (7.5 mg daily or more of prednisone or equivalent during more than 3 months, or Cushing's syndrome); menopause before 45 years of age; small stature (weight less than 57.8 kg or ICM less than 20 kg/m^2); primary hyperparathyroidism; prolonged used of anticonvulsive medication without vitamin D supplements; malabsorption or malnutrition for more than 5 years; chemotherapy; decrease in height; and appearance of kyphosis after menopause.

CHAPTER 55

Posture and Gait Analysis

1. What is the typical posture of a right-handed patient?
   a. low right shoulder, right deviation of the pelvis, high right hip
   b. low left shoulder, left deviation of the pelvis, high left hip
   c. low right shoulder, left deviation of the pelvis, low left hip
   d. low left shoulder, right deviation of the pelvis, high left hip

2. Someone with a steppage gait has a lesion in the:
   a. cerebral cortex
   b. cerebellum
   c. lower motor neuron
   d. spinal cord

3. Which of the following signs is NOT indicative of structural scoliosis?
   a. posterior scapula
   b. trunk muscular asymmetry
   c. positive Adam's position
   d. curvature disappearing in the Adam's position

4. The phases of the gait cycle are the stance phase and the swing phase. During the normal walking cycle, what percentage of time is attributed to the swing phase?
   a. 25%
   b. 30%
   c. 35%
   d. 40%

5. When assessing a patient's posture for an antalgic lean in the lumbar spine from an intervertebral disc protrusion with nerve root entrapment, what do you have to know about the patient's symptoms in order to determine if the disc protrusion is medial or lateral to the nerve root lesion?
   a. where the orthopedic signs are in relationship to the lean
   b. where the neurologic signs are in relationship to the lean
   c. where the symptoms are in relationship to the antalgic lean
   d. where the VSC is in relationship to the antalgic lean

6. Which statement is most likely INCORRECT?
    a. metatarsal pain syndrome, gout, and rheumatoid arthritis may cause a patient to limp
    b. coxarthrosis, septic arthritis, and trochanteric bursitis may cause a patient to limp
    c. sacroiliac syndrome and posttraumatic arthritis may cause a patient to limp
    d. studies show a significant correlation between posture and lower back symptoms

Answers

1. a. The typical posture of a right-handed person is conditioned by lateralization. This posture is typically as follows: low right shoulder compared with the left; mild right deviation of the pelvis; right hip mildly higher than its left counterpart; mild left deviation of the spine; increased left foot pronation compared with the right; right gluteus medius weaker than the left.

2. c. Someone with a steppage gait typically has a lesion with the S1 nerve root. The patient will elevate the whole leg by using their hip flexor, because of a weakness in toeing off.

3. d. Curvature disappearing in the Adam's position is indicative of a mild to moderate functional scoliosis. A positive Adam's position (posterior or anterior) is indicative of a pathologic or structural scoliosis with altered morphology.

4. d. Forty percent of time is dedicated to the swing phase versus 60% in the stance phase.

5. c. In an antalgic lean, the patient will lean in to the side of symptoms when a disc protrusion is medial to the nerve root in order to relax the nerve root around the protrusion to relieve the symptoms. The patient will lean away from the side of symptoms in a lateral disc protrusion in order to pull the nerve root away from the protrusion to relieve symptoms.

6. d. Overall, studies have not shown any significant correlation between posture and lower back symptoms. In addition, even if degenerative changes are diagnosed, the consequences for clinical or therapeutic management are low for uncomplicated low back pain.

Orthopedic Examination

1. Which test is designed to entrap cervical nerve roots by narrowing the IVF and compressing facet joints at the same time?
    a. Bakody's sign
    b. cervical distraction test
    c. Jackson's compression test
    d. Soto Hall test

2. Adson's test, costoclavicular test, and Wright's test assess for vascular occlusion in the thoracic outlet by which sign?
    a. decrease in or loss of the radial pulse amplitude
    b. decrease in radiating symptoms from the shoulder down the arm
    c. increase in radial pulse amplitude
    d. increase in radiating symptoms from the shoulder down the arm

3. A patient is placed prone on an exam bench. The knee is flexed to 90 degrees, loaded axially in a proximal direction, and then the leg is internally rotated (Apley's compression test). This is a test to check the integrity of the:
    a. ACL
    b. lateral meniscus
    c. medial meniscus
    d. PCL

4. For what is Fajersztajn's sign (well leg raise test) indicative of when it reproduces symptoms in the contralateral back and down the contralateral leg and when it relieves symptoms in the contralateral back and down the contralateral leg?
    a. lateral disc protrusion, medial disc protrusion
    b. medial disc protrusion, lateral disc protrusion
    c. medial disc protrusion, subrhizal disc protrusion
    d. subrhizal disc protrusion, lateral disc protrusion

5. Which of the following is NOT part of a screening examination for a rheumatologic condition?
    a. spinal mobility
    b. range of movement of the lower extremity
    c. motion palpation of the spine
    d. gait and postural analysis

6. What is the loose-packed position for the thoracic facet joints?
    a. midway between left and right rotation
    b. midway between flexion and extension
    c. full extension
    d. full flexion

7. Which of the following BEST illustrates a positive straight leg raise?
    a. reproduction of the patient's lower back pain at an angle of 80 degrees of SLR
    b. reproduction of the patient's lower back pain at an angle of 30 degrees of SLR
    c. reproduction of the patient's posterior thigh and leg pain at an angle of 70 degrees of SLR
    d. reproduction of the patient's posterior thigh and leg pain at an angle of 40 degrees of SLR

8. According to the AHCPR Guidelines, which one of the following is NOT an indication for referring a patient with a lumbar disc herniation for decompressive surgery?
    a. acute and debilitating sciatica
    b. acute and debilitating lower back pain
    c. persistent sciatica with no improvement over a 1-month period or rapidly progressive
    d. obvious signs of specific nerve root involvement associated with a disc herniation at the same level and on the same side on imaging

9. You suspect a patient has scoliosis. What evaluation procedure would you do, and what are you looking for?
    a. forward flexion, kyphosis
    b. forward flexion, rib humping
    c. lateral bending, rib pain
    d. lateral bending, rib stiffness

10. Which of the following has the highest specificity rate in diagnosing lumbar disc herniation?
    a. ipsilateral straight leg raising
    b. crossed straight leg raising
    c. quadriceps weakness
    d. sensory loss

11. A 7-month-old infant is brought to your office with a congenital torticollis. Which condition of the hip should also be ruled out in this child?
    a. congenital hip dislocation
    b. transient synovitis
    c. Legg-Calvé-Perthes disease
    d. slipped femoral capital epiphysis

12. What is the normal Q-angle range?
    a. 0 to 5 degrees
    b. 6 to 10 degrees
    c. 12 to 18 degrees
    d. 20 to 30 degrees

13. Which of the following test is LEAST likely to be positive for a shoulder tendonitis?
    a. Dawbarn's sign
    b. Codman's sign
    c. Apley's scratch test
    d. supraspinatus press test

14. In a patient older than 60 years, which two tests are most predictive of a rotator cuff tear?
    a. supraspinatus weakness and external rotation weakness
    b. Codman's sign and Apley's scratch test
    c. Apley scratch test and supraspinatus press test
    d. Dawburn's sign and Codman's sign

15. Noble's compression test would be positive for what condition?
    a. meniscal injuries
    b. anteromedial knee instability
    c. iliotibial band syndrome
    d. patellofemoral syndrome

16. A 22-year-old male tennis player complains of acute right knee pain. He felt a pop in his knee and experienced excruciating pain after his body twisted to the right while his foot was fixed on the ground. He could not continue playing and his knee swelled within 8 hours. What orthopedic tests are likely to be positive?
    a. posterior drawer test
    b. varus stress test
    c. Lachman's test
    d. patellofemoral tests

17. A 7-year-old boy complains of groin and anteromedial knee pain. He had a bad fall some time ago. You noticed he had a slight limp walking into the office. Physical examination is unremarkable but for decreased hip abduction and internal rotation bilaterally and a positive left FABERE (Patrick's test). What is the MOST likely diagnosis?
    a. posttraumatic fracture
    b. congenital hip dysplasia
    c. Legg-Calvé-Perthes
    d. slipped femoral capital epiphysis

18. A 10-year-old boy has had a significant limp for 3 days and does not play with his friends any more. There is no history of a fall, and past medical history is unremarkable except for a mild upper respiratory infection a week ago. Examination reveals limited hip flexion, abduction, and external rotation of the involved side. The remaining orthopedic and neurologic exams are normal. What is the most likely diagnosis?
    a. transient hip synovitis
    b. congenital hip dysplasia
    c. Legg-Calvé-Perthes
    d. slipped femoral capital epiphysis

19. A space-occupying lesion located at the anterior cervical spine could be found when performing which orthopedic test?
    a. foraminal compression test
    b. Halstead's maneuver
    c. Valsalva's maneuver
    d. swallowing test

20. An L4 disc pathology can lead to weakness of which muscle?
    a. peroneus longus
    b. quadriceps
    c. extensor hallicus longus
    d. gluteus maximus

21. A positive result for which test indicates deep vein thrombophlebitis?
    a. Homer's test
    b. Hochman's test
    c. Hoffman's test
    d. Homan's test

22. Which test evaluates the integrity of the menisci of the knee?
    a. Dugas' test
    b. Apley's distraction
    c. McMurray's test
    d. drawer test

23. Which test would not be positive in the presence of symptoms originating from the cervical facets?
    a. pain relief with cervical distraction
    b. positive maximal cervical compression test
    c. positive Jackson's test
    d. pain increasing with cervical distraction

24. Which of these tests would be positive in the presence of L4 radicular symptoms?
    a. spinal percussion test
    b. Yeoman's test
    c. Lasegue's test
    d. Ely's test

25. Which test will most likely be negative in the presence of biceps tendinitis?
    a. transverse humeral ligament test
    b. Codman's sign
    c. Yergason's test
    d. Speed's test

26. Which of the following is NOT a common risk factor for patellofemoral syndrome?
    a. increased Q angle
    b. excessive foot supination
    c. weakness of the vastus medialis obliquus
    d. excessive tightness of the iliotibial tract

27. Which muscle does NOT upwardly rotate the scapula?
    a. upper trapezius
    b. lower trapezius
    c. anterior serratus
    d. rhomboid major

Answers

1. c. Jackson's compression test is a cervical lateral flexion compression test that narrows the IVF and compresses the facet joints on the ipsilateral side of lateral flexion, followed by a strong downward pressure on the top of the head causing further narrowing of the IVF and compression of the facet joints. This will reproduce symptoms of nerve root pathology from compression in the IVF with radiating symptoms or symptoms of facet joint surface pathology from compression, which are local symptoms to the anatomic location of the facet.

2. a. The thoracic outlet consists of the subclavian artery, subclavian vein, and brachial plexus that runs from the anterolateral base of the neck to the anterior shoulder and can be trapped or occluded by the scalene muscles, clavicle, and first rib or the pectoralis minor muscle. The three tests functionally stress the above-mentioned tissue to further compress the thoracic outlet, which can mechanically occlude the artery and decrease the amplitude of the radial pulse or be lost altogether.

3. b. The Apley's compression test runs the lateral meniscus down the lateral condyle of the femur as it is internally rotated and compresses the meniscus onto the condyle at the same time (the heel points to the meniscus being tested). If there is pathology in the lateral meniscus, this procedure will produce internal lateral knee symptoms.

4. b. Fajersztajn's sign (well leg raise test) classically identifies a medial disc lesion to the contralateral nerve root. This reproduces or aggravates symptoms in the back and down the contralateral side of testing while performing a straight leg raise type of test by pulling the nerve root into the disc protrusion. Conversely, the test will pull a nerve root away from a lateral disc protrusion.

5. c. The GALS (gait-arms-legs-spine) examination is suggested for screening when there is suspicion of a rheumatologic condition. This examination is performed in a few minutes and helps determine the extent of joint involvement and which joint to further evaluate.

6. b.   The loose-packed position of a joint is the position of the range of
         motion in which the joint is under the least mechanical stress. It is
         the position used to treat a joint with mobilization. The loose-
         packed position for all segments of the spine is midway between
         flexion and extension. The close-packed position of a joint is the
         position of the range of motion in which the joint has its maximum
         stability. It is used to stabilize a joint when mobilizing an adjacent
         joint. The close-packed position of the facet joints of the spine is
         full extension.

7. d.   A positive SLR is reproducing the patient's radicular pain in the
         lower extremity below 60 degrees of elevation. The biomechanical
         principle underlying this test is that the nerve roots glide freely in
         the intervertebral foramen and, with straight leg raising, the roots
         move outside the intervertebral foramen. This excursion is up to
         12 mm at the level of the L5 nerve root. The tension on the sciatic
         nerve is at its maximum at 60 degrees, at which point it stabilizes.

8. b.   According to the AHCPR Guidelines, the combination of the
         following factors are indications for decompressive surgery in the
         presence of lumbar disc herniation: acute and debilitating sciatica;
         persistent sciatica with no improvement over a 1-month period or
         rapidly progressive; obvious signs of specific nerve root
         involvement associated with a disc herniation at the same level and
         on the same side on imaging. Many patients with severe nerve root
         compromise related to disc herniation will recover within 1 month.
         There is no evidence that the condition of the patient will
         deteriorate if surgery is delayed for this period of time. More than
         80% of patients suffering from lumbar disc herniation for whom
         surgery is indicated will recover, with or without surgery.

9. b.   You would ask the patient to flex forward (Adam's test) and
         observe for any rib humping in the thoracic spine on the side of
         convexity.

10. c.   Deyo reports a specificity level of 99% in one who has quadriceps
         weakness. Crossed SLR also has a high specificity level (i.e., 90%),
         indicating a lumbar disc herniation. Ipsilateral SLR has a good
         sensitivity level of 80% in detecting a lumber disc herniation.

11. a.   Congenital dislocation of the hip should also be suspected in an
         infant with congenital torticollis. Legg-Calvé-Perthes disease is
         more prevalent in boys aged 6 to 8 years. Slipped femoral capital
         epiphysis is more common in the teenage boy.

12. c. The normal Q angle in the knee is 12 to 18 degrees. In the female, it is typically larger as the pelvis is wider in females than in males. Larger Q angle may predispose one to developing patellofemoral dysfunction or even a patellar dislocation.

13. a. The Dawbarn's sign is a well-localized tender area at the subacromial bursa as the examiner palpates the affected shoulder deeply. The pain disappears as the deltoid muscles overlap during abduction.

14. a. Hawkin's test, supraspinatus weakness, and weakness in external rotation can predict a rotator cuff tear. Ultrasound is considered the best specialized investigation for confirmation.

15. c. Pain evoked by repetitive knee flexion, radiation of pain over the lateral joint line, lower extremity misalignment, and palpable tenderness over the lateral femoral condyle indicate probable iliotibial band friction syndrome.

16. c. The mechanism of injury, the popping sound, acute pain, and rapid swelling all point toward an anterior cruciate ligament tear. A positive Lachman's test is almost pathognomonic for an ACL tear (sensitivity of 80% to 99%, specificity of 95%).

17. c. The incidence of Legg-Calvé-Perthes is 1.5 to 5 per 10,000. Boys between the ages of 2 and 13 (most common between 4 and 9 years) are more commonly affected in a ratio of 4:1, and it is bilateral in 10% to 20%. Although the precise etiology is still undetermined, Waldelström has described four stages observed on radiographs. A history of a fall is often present, and hip abduction and internal rotation tend to be restricted. Patrick's FABERE test and Trendelenburg may be positive.

18. a. Transient hip synovitis is the most common hip condition in kids with an incidence of 6.1 and 3.1 per 10,000 boys and girls, respectively. Although the precise etiology is unknown, half describe an upper respiratory infection or recent hip trauma. Physical exam may reveal restricted hip flexion, abduction, and external rotation. Signs of inflammatory disorders are absent.

19. d. A disc problem is usually triggered by some form of trauma. Symptoms can include sudden and severe neck and arm pain as well as paresthesia along the involved nerve root. Neck movements, especially lateral flexion toward the affected side, will typically aggravate the pain.

20. c. L4 disc pathology can affect the L5 nerve root, which may cause weakness to the extensor hallucis longus muscle.

21. d. For this test, the patient is supine with legs extended. The examiner elevates the affected leg to 45 degrees and the calf is squeezed firmly. As the calf pressure is maintained, the examiner dorsiflexes the foot. Deep calf or leg pain during this maneuver indicates thrombophlebitis. When the pain remits quickly, thrombophlebitis is suspected. When the pain persists or lags as an ache, calf strain is suspected.

22. c. For this test, the patient lies supine with the thigh and leg flexed until the heel approaches the buttock. The examiner internally (tests the lateral meniscus) rotates and slowly extends the leg. The same procedure is repeated with the leg externally (tests the medial meniscus) rotated. If at some point in the arc a painful click or snap is heard, then the sign is considered positive.

23. d. Cervical distraction decreases facet compression, and patients presenting with cervical pain originating from the cervical facets should feel relief during this test. Increased local cervical pain during compressions (extension/compression test, Jackson's test, and maximal cervical compression) may indicate pain originating from posterior facet joints.

24. c. Leg elevation with knee extension stretches the sciatic nerve. Increased tension of a trapped or compressed nerve root will reproduce radiating pain in the lower limb. To be considered positive, the Lasegue test must provoke radicular pain before 60 degrees of elevation. Pain elicited from stretching of the hamstrings is not considered a positive Lasegue test.

25. b. Codman's sign is performed to evaluate the integrity of the rotator cuff muscles. In the presence of rotator cuff rupture (most frequently, supraspinatus muscle), the patient will not able to lower the arm smoothly and rhythmically from the abducted position. Transverse humeral ligament test, Yergason's test, and Speed's test are performed to evaluate the integrity of both the long portion of and the biceps transverse humeral ligament.

26. b. Excessive foot supination will potentially create a genu varum deformity, which is not usually considered a risk factor for patellofemoral syndrome. Increased Q angle (associated with genu valgum), weakness of the vastus medialis obliquus, and excessive tightness of the iliotibial tract will affect patellar tracking.

27.   d.   Upper and lower trapezius combined with the serratus anterior upwardly rotate the scapula. The upper trapezius elevates the lateral scapula; the lower trapezius pulls the medial border of the scapula downward. The rhomboid muscles medially stabilize and adduct the scapula toward the spine and act as scapular elevators.

Neurologic Examination

1. Referred pain from nerve roots will demonstrate specific patterns. Which choice below is FALSE?
   a. referred pain from T5 is produced in the areola area
   b. referred pain from T7-8 is produced in the epigastric area
   c. referred pain from T10-11 is produced in the umbilical area
   d. referred pain from T12 is produced in the lower abdominal area

2. Which of the following is FALSE regarding the positive neurologic findings in carpal tunnel syndrome?
   a. sensory deficit present over the palmar and dorsal aspects of the first three digits and the lateral half of the fourth digit
   b. weakness of forearm flexors and pronators
   c. decrease in the brachioradialis deep tendon reflex
   d. atrophy of the thenar muscles

3. According to the AHCPR and other clinical practice guidelines, there is strong evidence that some tests will adequately document the presence of a neurologic deficit in patients with a lumbar disc herniation. Which of the following does NOT do so?
   a. sensory distribution over the dorsal aspect of the foot
   b. Achilles tendon reflex
   c. strength of ankle dorsiflexion
   d. atrophy of the calf

4. What is the difference in testing motor function when evaluating for a nerve root deficit versus a peripheral nerve deficit?
   a. in peripheral nerve deficit, the motor weakness is evident more rapidly when applying resistance compared with nerve root deficit
   b. in nerve root deficit, the motor weakness is evident more rapidly when applying resistance compared with peripheral nerve deficit
   c. in peripheral nerve deficit, the motor weakness is only evident when applying resistance without gravity
   d. in nerve root deficit, the motor weakness is only evident when applying resistance without gravity

5. Which of the following is NOT a typical feature of a L4 nerve root lesion?
    a. diminished knee jerk
    b. diminished resisted foot inversion
    c. diminished resisted knee extension
    d. paresthesia over the medial aspect of the leg and foot

6. Which impairment occurs in carpal tunnel syndrome?
    a. atrophy of the hypothenar eminence
    b. paresthesias over the dorsal aspect of the hand
    c. decreased resisted thumb abduction
    d. decreased resisted forearm pronation

7. Which statement does NOT apply to central lumbar stenosis?
    a. can be caused by anterior longitudinal ligament hypertrophy
    b. presence of neurogenic claudication
    c. night pain and sciatic tension signs are common
    d. is usually relieved by trunk flexion

8. Which anatomic structure is NOT responsible for a thoracic outlet syndrome?
    a. scalenus anterior
    b. pectoralis minor
    c. cervical ribs
    d. scalenus posterior

9. Which of the following is a feature of Bell's palsy?
    a. loss of cutaneous sensation in the frontal region
    b. is caused by a supranuclear contralateral lesion
    c. drooping of the mouth on the affected side
    d. loss of taste sense in the posterior third of the tongue

10. Irritation of the C5 nerve root would likely produce which of the following?
    a. anesthesia of the lateral upper arm, absent biceps deep tendon reflex, and/or increased dermatomal sensation of the lateral upper arm
    b. anesthesia of the lateral upper arm, decreased biceps deep tendon reflex, and/or decreased dermatomal sensation of the lateral upper arm
    c. paresthesia of the lateral upper arm, absent biceps deep tendon reflex, and/or absent dermatomal sensation of the lateral upper arm
    d. paresthesia of the lateral upper arm, increased biceps deep tendon reflex, and/or increased dermatomal sensation of the lateral upper arm

11. Which choice best describes C7 muscle test, deep tendon reflex, and sensory testing?
    a. finger abduction, pectoralis deep tendon reflex, and medial upper arm sensory from the elbow to the axilla
    b. wrist extension, brachial radialis deep tendon reflex, and lateral forearm and digits 1 and 2 sensory from the elbow to the tip of the fingers
    c. wrist flexion, triceps deep tendon reflex, and anterior and posterior middle finger sensory from the wrist to the tip
    d. shoulder abduction, biceps deep tendon reflex, and lateral upper arm sensory from the shoulder to the elbow

12. The L4 deep tendon reflex is elicited at which of the following?
    a. Achilles tendon
    b. femoral tendon
    c. medial hamstring tendon
    d. patella tendon

13. Evaluating foot eversion motor function tests which nerve root?
    a. L3
    b. L4
    c. L5
    d. S1

14. What signs or symptoms help differentiate between cervical spine radiculopathy and cervical spine myelopathy?
    a. radicular pain
    b. weakness in a specific myotome
    c. increased muscle tone
    d. diminished upper extremity deep tendon reflex

15. A 35-year-old man presents with severe, short-lasting acute attacks of unilateral facial pain causing involuntary grimacing of the cheek. These painful attacks may be provoked by chewing, washing his face, or shaving. What is the MOST likely diagnosis?
    a. temporomandibular joint (TMJ) disorder
    b. trigeminal neuralgia
    c. migraine headache
    d. dental neuralgia

16. Which symptoms are classically associated with cervicogenic vertigo?
    a. vertigo and restricted cervical range of motion
    b. constant vertigo and nystagmus
    c. vertigo and recurrent acute episodes
    d. vertigo and hearing loss

17. With regard to central and peripheral vertigo, which of the following is CORRECT?
    a. vertigo intensity tends to be severe in central vertigo and weak in peripheral vertigo
    b. nystagmus appears instantly in central vertigo but within 2 to 10 seconds in peripheral vertigo
    c. nystagmus tends to gradually decrease in central vertigo but is persistent in peripheral vertigo
    d. common causes of central vertigo are labyrhinitis, otitis, and VPPB; common causes of peripheral vertigo include multiple sclerosis and brainstem tumor

18. A 26-year-old woman was involved in a motor vehicle accident on the morning of her visit to your office. She complains of severe neck and right arm pain and noticed her thumb was numb. On examination, she has neck stiffness and decreased range of motion in all directions. Neurologic examination reveals a decreased bicipital deep tendon reflex and diminished pinprick sensations of the first digit on the right. Clonus and plantar reflexes are absent. What is the MOST likely diagnosis?
    a. grade II whiplash (WAD)
    b. brachial plexus neuralgia
    c. thoracic outlet syndrome
    d. cervical spine fracture

19. Which of the following statements is INCORRECT?
    a. rheumatoid arthritis and ankylosing spondylitis patients have a low prevalence of atlantoaxial subluxations
    b. preliminary data do not support the use of the upper cervical flexion test for screening atlantoaxial subluxations in patients with Down syndrome
    c screening (clinically) for high-risk ligament laxity populations has little value for manual therapists
    d. a patient with a 5-year history of rheumatoid arthritis and a recent onset of leg stiffness and arm pain with neck movement should be investigated for possible spinal cord compression

20. A 25-year-old football player fell on his shoulder vertically and violently stretched his neck in the opposite direction. He was later diagnosed with a brachial plexus injury (Erb-Duchenne paralysis). His arm is hanging at his side in medial rotation in the "waiter's tip" position. What results are expected from the neurologic examination?
    a paralysis of the deltoid, triceps, wrist extensors (long and short carpi radialis), and finger extensors
    b. paralysis of all intrinsic muscles of the hand, flexors muscles (claw hand), loss of sensation over C8-T1 dermatomes, and Horner's syndrome
    c. hypesthesia over C5-6 and weakness of the deltoid, supraspinatus and infraspinatus, biceps, and brachioradialis muscles
    d. Klumpke paralysis caused by forced hyperabduction of the arm

21. Concerning upper extremity mononeuropathies, which of the following statements is INCORRECT?
    a. shoulder blade protrusion when pushing against a wall is caused by weakness of the serratus anterior muscle supplied by the long thoracic nerve
    b. wasting of the superior-posterior shoulder blade with difficulty in abducting and externally rotating the arm is associated with scapular nerve neuropathy
    c. difficulty abducting the arm between 15 and 90 degrees and hypesthesia over the deltoid muscle are associated with auxiliary nerve neuropathy (deltoid and teres minor muscles)
    d. wasting of the superior-posterior shoulder blade with difficulty in abducting and externally rotating the arm is associated with rhomboid muscle weakness supplied by the rhomboid nerve

23. Shoulder abduction is a muscle test used to evaluate which nerve root?
    a. C5
    b. C6
    c. C7
    d. C8

23. The L5 dermatome most likely covers which of the following areas?
    a. lateral leg and dorsum of the foot and middle three toes
    b. medial side of the leg and foot and big toe
    c. lateral side of the leg and foot and little toe
    d. posterior aspect of the thigh, popliteal fossa, and posteromedial leg

24. Which deep tendon reflex is associated with weak foot plantarflexion and eversion?
    a. patellar
    b. tibialis anterior
    c. tibialis posterior
    d. Achilles

25. Which reflex is classified as a pathologic reflex?
    a. superficial anal reflex
    b. superficial abdominal reflex
    c. Babinski's reflex
    d. Achilles tendon reflex

26. Which procedure is NOT typically done in the clinical evaluation of cranial nerve III?
    a. observe eyelid position
    b. pupillary response to light
    c. accommodation
    d. testing visual fields

27. Which of the following is NOT typically a symptom for cerebellar disease?
    a. weakness
    b. ataxia
    c. diplopia
    d. atrophy

28. What is stereognosis?
    a. inability to alternate hand movements
    b. inability to hear out of both ears equally
    c. ability to recognize familiar objects placed in one's hand
    d. inability to identify symbols drawn on the skin

29. If you detect ankle clonus in a patient, where is the location of the lesion?
    a. ankle
    b. spinothalamic tract
    c. nerve root
    d. corticospinal tract

30. Which type of sensation is carried in the lateral spinothalamic tract?
    a. light touch
    b. vibration
    c. pain
    d. position

31. If you come across someone who is unconscious, what is the MOST appropriate assessment that should be administered first?
    a. motion palpation
    b. Glasgow Coma Scale
    c. mini-mental status assessment
    d. plain film radiography

32. A patient complains of light sensitivity. He will most likely have a problem with which cranial nerve?
    a. optic
    b. oculomotor
    c. trochlear
    d. facial

Answers

1.   d.   Referred pain from T12 produces pain in the groin area.

2.   c.   The median nerve is compressed in carpal tunnel syndrome (CTS). It innervates the muscles of the thenar eminence and the flexor and pronator muscles of the forearm. There is no deep tendon reflex deficit in CTS because no nerve root is involved, only a peripheral nerve. The sensory deficits of CTS are hypesthesia of the palmar and dorsal aspects of the first three digits and the lateral half of the fourth. The motor deficits of a CTS are weaknesses of the thenar muscles; weakness of thumb opposition, flexion, and horizontal abduction; weakness of grip, especially between the thumb and index; and weakness of forearm pronators and flexors.

3.   d.   According to the AHCPR and other clinical practice guidelines, there is evidence (level B) that the following tests will adequately document the presence of a neurologic deficit when evaluating patients with a possible lumbar disc herniation: Achilles and patellar DTRs; ankle dorsiflexion, hallux extension, foot and toes flexion; and sensory distribution over the medial, dorsal, and lateral aspects of the foot.

4.   a.   A lesion of a peripheral nerve produces a complete paralysis of the muscles innervated by this nerve. Weakness is immediately apparent when testing the motor function. A lesion of a unique nerve root produces paresis of the myotome (group of muscles innervated by a single nerve root) innervated by this nerve root. Some time is necessary for the weakness to become apparent when testing for motor function. The isometric contraction must be held for a minimum of 5 seconds.

5.   c.   While diminished knee jerk, diminished resisted foot inversion and paresthesias over the medial aspect of the leg and foot are typical feature of a L4 nerve root lesion, a decrease in resisted knee extension force is more likely observed in a L3 nerve root lesion.

6.   c.   Atrophy of the hypothenar eminence is a sign of ulnar nerve lesion while paresthesias over the dorsal aspect of the hand are symptoms of radial nerve lesion. Decreased resisted thumb abduction and forearm pronation are signs of median nerve lesion but the motor branches of pronator teres and pronator quadratus arise before the median nerve enters the carpal tunnel.

7. a. Central lumbar stenosis can be caused by ligamentum flavum hypertrophy. The anterior longitudinal ligament is located on the anterior aspect of vertebral bodies and cannot be responsible for a central lumbar stenosis. Neurogenic claudication, night pain, sciatic tension signs and symptoms relief with trunk flexion are typical signs of central lumbar stenosis.

8. d. The neurovascular bundle responsible for thoracic outlet syndrome can be compressed between the scalenus anterior and scalenus medius, between the first rib and clavicle, under the pectoralis minor, and by a cervical rib. Posterior scalenus is not involved in a thoracic outlet syndrome.

9. c. Bell's palsy is an acute lower motorneuron facial paralysis (cranial nerve V). It can also affect the sensation of the posterior third of the tongue. It is characterized by drooping of the mouth, drooling, tearing from the eye, and ptosis on the affected side. Bell's palsy usually follows viral infection and is self-limited in time.

10. d. Nerve irritation causes physiologic facilitation to the nerve, which excites nervous function. Therefore, an excited C5 nerve root from disc, osteophyte, or traumatic irritation will cause the biceps deep tendon to be increased in function. The C5 nerve root carries sensation to the lateral brachium skin surface, which becomes hypersensitive to the pinprick, and the patient may experience paresthesia along the lateral upper arm.

11. c. In Stanley Hoppenfeld's text *Orthopedic Neurology,* he lists the tests for C7 nerve root as 1) wrist flexion for muscle testing, 2) triceps for deep tendon reflex, and 3) dermatome surface as being the third digit of the hand anterior and posterior from the wrist to the tip of the finger for sensory testing.

12. d. According to Hoppenfeld, the patella deep tendon reflex muscles (the quadriceps muscle group) are innervated by the L4 nerve root via the femoral nerve.

13. d. Foot eversion is accomplished by the peroneus longus and brevis muscles. They are innervated by the superficial peroneal nerve, a branch of the sciatic nerve, S1 nerve root. Therefore, this procedure can be used to assess S1 nerve root for motor function.

14. c. Increased muscle tone (spasticity) indicates absent or decreased inhibition of pyramidal tracts (upper motor neuron lesion). Cervical radiculomyelopathy will affect nerve roots exiting at the level of compression as well as the spinal cord, giving both lower and upper motor neuron signs and symptoms.

15. b. Trigeminal neuralgia (tic douloureux) is a very disabling condition aggravated by simple touching or exposure to cold to the trigeminal nerve involved territory (V1, V2, or V3). It affects 4.3 per 100,000 people, with a female predominance (ratio of 3:2).

16. a. A history of neck trauma, muscle spasm, and restricted cervical range of motion are classically associated with cervicogenic vertigo.

17. b. Central vertigo results from central lesions to the vestibular apparatus (vestibular nuclei and their connections). The origins of peripheral vertigo include all conditions of the peripheral vestibular apparatus (labyrinth, vestibular portion of the auditory nerve, or proprioceptive organs of the cervical region).

18. d. Cervical spine fracture with C6 nerve root compression is likely to explain her presentation. This would be a whiplash-associated disorder (WAD) grade IV according to the Quebec task force (Spitzer) classification. A traumatic cervical disc herniation at C5-6 level could also explain the neck and arm pain with associated neurologic changes (WAD grade III).

19. d. Possible causes of atlantoaxial instability include inflammatory arthritis (known RA, psoriatic arthropathy, chronic juvenile RA, AS, enteropathic arthritis, SLE, Reiter's). Indicators from the patient history and physical examination should point to red flags. Panus formation of the atlantoaxial joint may rupture the transverse ligament, causing spinal cord compression.

20. c. The mechanism of injury indicates implication of the superior plexus of C5-6, causing diffuse arm weakness not fitting typical radicular presentation (involvement of one myotome). Nerve regeneration is still possible when only the endonurium and capillary complex are disrupted ("a burner"). However, when the perineurium (funiculus) or epinurium is disrupted (brachial neuropraxia), useful regeneration is not expected. This requires urgent neurosurgical intervention to prevent permanent neurologic deficit.

21. d. Upper extremity mononeuropathies may be caused by carrying heavy objects, strapping of the shoulder, brachial neuropathies, and diabetes. Such events or conditions tend to cause suprascapular neuropathy involving the suprasinatus and infraspinatus muscles and long thoracic neuropathy (serratus anterior muscle). Shoulder dislocations can cause injury to the auxiliary nerve.

22. a. The deltoid muscles are responsible for shoulder abduction and are innervated almost entirely from C5 cord level.

23. a. L4 covers the medial side of the leg, foot, and great toe. L5 covers the lateral leg, dorsum of the foot, and middle three toes. S1 covers the posterior aspect of the leg, lateral side of the foot, and fifth toe.

24. d. Foot plantarflexion and eversion are tested by the peroneus longus and peroneus brevis muscles, which are innervated by S1. Achilles tendon reflex is a deep tendon reflex, supplied predominantly by nerves emanating from the S1 cord level.

25. c. Pathologic reflexes are also superficial reflexes and are mediated through the central nervous system (cerebral cortex). The presence of a pathologic reflex indicates an upper motor neuron lesion and its absence reflects integrity.

26. d. Testing of cranial nerve III involves the assessment of: eyelid position, pupillary response to light, extraocular eye movements, and accommodation. Testing visual fields is done as part of the assessment of cranial nerve II.

27. d. Atrophy is a sign of a lower motor neuron lesion. Cerebellar disease can cause weakness, ataxia, or diplopia because regulation of muscle tone or coordination of movement is affected.

28. c. Stereognosis is one of the discriminative testing protocols. It is used as an alternate to graphesthesia. Place a familiar object in the patient's hand, such as a coin or paperclip, and ask him or her to identify the object.

29. d. Ankle clonus is a sign of an upper motor neuron lesion. Thus, it would be in the corticospinal (pyramidal) tract.

30. c. Pain and temperature sensation are carried in the spinothalamic tract. Light touch, vibration sense, and position sense are carried in the posterior column of the spinal cord.

31. b. Glasgow Coma Scale measures one's level of consciousness out of a score of 15. The mini-mental status assessment measures one's level of cognitive functioning by assessing areas including orientation, registration, attention, and calculation recall and language.

32. b. When a pupil cannot constrict normally in bright light, this causes light sensitivity. The parasympathetic fibers responsible for constriction of the pupil in response to light lie on the surface of cranial nerve III.

Clinical Diagnosis

1. According to the international classification of headache disorders, which of these statements is NOT a typical clinical sign of tension-type headaches?
   a. headache lasting from 30 minutes to 7 days
   b. nonpulsating headache
   c. accompanied by nausea or vomiting
   d. bilateral peripheral cranial pain

2. Which condition may involve atlantoaxial instability?
   a. Reiter's syndrome
   b. cervical spine osteoarthritis
   c. Klippel-Feil syndrome
   d. diffuse idiopathic skeletal hyperostosis (DISH)

3. A 65-year-old woman presents with complaints of localized midthoracic spine pain. The history reveals that the patient is a long-time smoker and alcohol consumer and that she does not exercise at all. Which of the following is the MOST probable diagnosis?
   a. zona (herpes zoster)
   b. intercostal neuritis
   c. pathologic fracture of a thoracic vertebral body
   d. pleurisy

4. Which of the following is NOT a common sign or symptom of chronic arterial occlusive disease of the lower limb?
   a. lower limb pain relieved by rest
   b. lower limb pain relieved by trunk flexion
   c. lower limb paresthesia or numbness
   d. cramping in the calf and foot

5. Which is NOT a common sign or symptom of discogenic pain?
   a. sclerotomal distribution
   b. deep and aching pain
   c. increased pain in sitting posture
   d. not associated with neurologic changes

6. A patient presents with an antalgic positioning toward the right associated with a radiating pain in the left leg. Examination reveals difficulty with toe walking and abolished ankle jerk. Which of the following is MOST likely responsible of the signs and symptoms?
   a. L5/S1 left lateral disc protrusion
   b. L4/L5 right lateral disc protrusion
   c. L5/S1 left medial disc protrusion
   d. L4/L5 left medial disc protrusion

7. An overweight 32-year-old male runner complains of heel pain exacerbated by the first steps in the morning. This pain usually subsides after 5 minutes of walking. During the day, pain decreases with sitting posture. Which of the following is the MOST probable diagnosis?
   a. fifth metatarsal stress fracture
   b. tarsal tunnel syndrome
   c. Achilles tendinitis
   d. plantar fasciitis

8. Which is NOT a typical feature of de Quervain's tenosynovitis?
   a. pain elicited by thumb and wrist motion
   b. most frequently affects men
   c. tender thickening at the radial styloid
   d. positive Finkelstein's test

9. A 34-year-old male patient presents with symmetric muscle weaknesses affecting the lower limbs. The symptoms rapidly evolved in the past 4 days and the patient now has difficulty standing and walking. The patient also noticed a light tingling in both feet. On examination, loss of deep tendon reflex is noticed. Which of the following is the MOST probable diagnosis?
   a. alcoholic polyneuropathy
   b. Guillain-Barré syndrome
   c. Charcot-Marie-Tooth disease
   d. multiple sclerosis

10. An overweight 12-year-old presents with hip pain and weight-bearing difficulties. These symptoms presented rapidly following physical activity. On examination, limping is observed and passive ranges of motion are limited and painful. Which of the following is the MOST probable diagnosis?
    a. Legg-Calvé-Perthes disease
    b. transient hip synovitis
    c. congenital hip dysplasia
    d. slipped femoral capital epiphysis

11. A defining symptom of fibromyalgia is:
    a. fatigue
    b. diffuse pain
    c. regional pain
    d. unexplained weight loss

12. A 30-year-old man presents to your office with recurrent episodes of bilateral sacral pain radiating into the buttock area. Occasional posterior thigh radiation is present. This problem has been recurrent for the past 4 years with increasing frequency. Chiropractic care, including soft tissue and manipulative therapy, has provided equivocal results. What is the primary differential diagnosis?
    a. sacroiliac syndrome
    b. discogenic lower back pain
    c. spinal central stenosis
    d. ankylosing spondylitis

13. Your clinical diagnosis of a 14-year-old female patient is idiopathic scoliosis. Her mother is questioning about the risk of progression of this curvature. Which of the following factors does NOT represent a risk?
    a. menarche at 13 years of age
    b. pattern of the curvature
    c. Risser sign
    d. number of vertebrae involved

14. What are the hallmarks of postmenopausal and aging osteoporosis?
    a. postmenopause osteoporosis predisposes to vertebral fractures and aging osteoporosis predisposes to hip fractures
    b. postmenopause osteoporosis predisposes to hip fractures and aging osteoporosis predisposes to wrist fractures
    c. postmenopause osteoporosis predisposes to vertebral fractures and aging osteoporosis predisposes to wrist fractures
    d. postmenopause osteoporosis predisposes to hip fractures and aging osteoporosis predisposes to vertebral fractures

15. What is the only clinical sign identifying patients suffering from psoriasis who are susceptible to develop an associated arthritis?
    a. extensive dermatologic psoriasis
    b. onset before 20 years of age
    c. ungual involvement
    d. family history of psoriatic arthritis

16. The traditional measures of acute-phase reactant are useful for measuring the inflammatory activity in the joints of patients suffering from which disease?
    a. ankylosing spondylitis
    b. rheumatoid arthritis
    c. fibromyalgia
    d. polymyositis

17. Which one of the following is NOT a criterion for rheumatoid arthritis?
    a. presence of symptoms for at least 10 weeks
    b. morning stiffness
    c. serum rheumatoid factor
    d. arthritis of hands

18. Which does NOT correctly represent a condition and its possible complication?
    a. polymyalgia rheumatica and giant cell arteritis
    b. psoriatic arthritis and arthritis mutilans
    c. systemic lupus erythematosus and nephropathy
    d. reactive arthritis and atlantoaxial instability

19. Which of the following is FALSE regarding septic arthritis?
    a. it mostly affects the small peripheral joints
    b. it is usually monoarticular
    c. preexisting rheumatoid arthritis is a risk factor
    d. it is often caused by gonorrhea

20. A systematic approach to the differential diagnosis of rheumatologic conditions is important in order to reach the proper diagnosis. Which of the following is the PRIMARY category of this approach?
    a. inflammatory versus noninflammatory condition
    b. joint versus nonjoint pain
    c. monoarticular versus polyarticular involvement
    d. localized versus diffuse pain

21. An absent arch in the foot is called:
   a. pes cavus
   b. pes planus
   c. pes valgus
   d. pes varus

22. Morton's neuroma is usually located between which metatarsal heads?
   a. first and second
   b. second and third
   c. third and fourth
   d. fourth and fifth

23. The condition called "housemaid's knee" is an inflammation of which bursa?
   a. superficial prepatellar
   b. infrapatellar
   c. prepatellar
   d. postpatellar

24. Clubbed nails are _____ -shaped and are most commonly the result of a _____ condition?
   a. saucer, respiratory
   b. dome, vascular
   c. dome, respiratory
   d. spoon, vascular

25. Difficulty retracting the scapula may be due to a weak _____ muscle and lead to _____ of the scapula.
   a. serratus anterior, winging
   b. rhomboids, winging
   c. serratus anterior, flaring
   d. rhomboids, flaring

26. Little Leaguer's elbow is also referred to as:
   a. Smith's fracture
   b. medial epicondylar fracture
   c. Colles' fracture
   d. medial supracondylar fracture

27. A 3-year-old boy has exquisite pain over the lateral elbow with no history of trauma or accident to the joint (as reported by his mother). Palpation reveals swelling and a malpositioned radial head. Radiography confirms your palpation findings. What is your INITIAL impression?
    a. nursemaid's elbow
    b. posterior impingement syndrome
    c. lateral epicondylitis
    d. Little Leaguer's elbow

28. A 6-year-old patient complains of hip and groin pain when running and playing. You take an x-ray and see avascular necrosis of the femoral head. Which of the following conditions do you suspect?
    a. avulsion fracture of the ASIS
    b. slipped femoral capital epiphysis
    c. anterior hip dislocation
    d. Legg-Calvé-Perthes disease

29. Which condition presents with pain behind the greater trochanter and extending down the course of the sciatic nerve that is aggravated by internally rotating the hip with the hip and knee in flexion?
    a. obdurator neuropathy
    b. coccydynia
    c. piriformis syndrome
    d. meralgia paresthetica

30. Compression of the lateral femoral cutaneous nerve at or around the inguinal ligament, due to prolonged sitting, is known as:
    a. femoral bursitis
    b. myositis ossificans
    c. avascular necrosis
    d. meralgia paresthetica

31. A 42-year-old woman with a history of recurrent neck pain presents with an acute episode of predominant arm and scapular pain with mild neurologic deficit (hypesthesia over the dorsal aspect of the forearm). She is more comfortable by keeping the involved arm above her head. Spurling's and axial cervical compression aggravate her symptoms. What is the MOST likely diagnosis?
    a. acute cervical spondylotic radiculopathy
    b. cervical radiculomyelopathy
    c. vertebrobasilar artery dissection
    d. acute herniated nucleus pulposus

32. A 35-year-old man complains of significant morning stiffness lasting over an hour. He has had recurrent back pain for the past 10 years with associated stiffness. He has had a low-grade fever for a week and has lost 8 lb dieting. What is the most likely diagnosis?
    a. thoracolumbar vertebral fracture
    b. inflammatory spondyloarthropathy
    c. infection
    d. neoplasia

33. Which are three modifiable risk factors for osteoporosis?
    a. smoking, age, corticosteroid use
    b. excessive consumption of alcohol, smoking, estrogen deficiency
    c. menopause before age 45, age, ethnicity
    d. body mass index <19 kg/m² or weight <57 kg, prolonged bed rest, history of fracture

34. Which is TRUE regarding angular vertebral body fractures?
    a. indicates a pathologic process
    b. in females over age 50, the estimated risk of having osteoporosis-related vertebral fracture some day is 15.5%
    c. plain film radiograph is a reliable instrument for assessment of bone mass changes
    d. typically occur in the lumbar spine

35. With regard to neck pain, which description requires specialized investigation?
    a. a 5-year history of rheumatoid arthritis
    b. sagittal plane neck rigidity in the in the absence of trauma
    c. arm or leg radiation with neck movements
    d. a, b, and c

36. Which of following is NOT considered a risk factor for chronic neck pain in whiplash patients?
    a. prior history of whiplash, neck pain, or headache
    b. initial neck pain and headache intensity
    c. presence of radicular signs and symptoms at onset
    d. high socioeconomic status

37. Factors adversely effecting low back pain recovery in adults include which of the following?
    a. high levels of self-reported functional disability
    b. significant depression
    c. duration of work absence
    d. a, b, and c

38. Physical and psychological risk factors for wrist/hand pain and sickness absence include all EXCEPT which of the following?
    a. prolonged repetitive use (half to most of the time)
    b. activities that frequently flex or extend the elbow
    c. hobbies with repetitive use of thumb (piano playing, sewing, knitting, and weaving)
    d. high perceived job stress

39. According to the Ottawa Ankle/Foot Rule, which of the following is the CORRECT answer?
    a. plain film radiographs are recommended routinely for adult acute ankle and foot injury
    b. radiographs of the ankle are required only if there is pain in the malleolar zone and any of these findings: bone tenderness of distal fibula along 2 cm; bone tenderness of distal tibia along 2 cm; inability to bear weight during eight steps both immediately and in clinic
    c. radiographs of the injured foot are required only if there is pain in the midfoot zone and bone tenderness at the base of the second metatarsal, bone tenderness of the cuboid bone, and unable to bear weight during four steps both immediately and in clinic
    d. radiographs of the ankle are required only if there is pain in the malleolar zone and any of these findings: bone tenderness of distal fibula along 6 cm; bone tenderness of distal tibia along 6 cm; and inability to bear weight during four steps both immediately and in clinic

40. In adult patients with acute knee injuries, the Ottawa Knee Rules recommend to take radiographs only in presence of which of the following signs?
    a. 54 years of age or younger
    b. tenderness of the proximal tibia
    c. isolated tenderness of patella
    d. inability to extend the knee completely

41. A 50-year-old slightly obese man presents with a 1-month history of right hip pain without radiation, a protective limp, and activity-induced symptoms. He improves with rest and has some mild morning stiffness. Examination reveals restricted and painful internal rotation of the hip. What is the MOST likely diagnosis?
    a. inflammatory arthritis
    b. osteoarthritis
    c. osteoporotic hip fractures
    d. iliopsoas tendinosis

42. A patient has tingling pain and burning over the sole of the foot after prolonged standing or walking; it worsens at night. Tinel's sign, nerve compression test, and two-point discrimination are positive. There is hypesthesia of the sole of the foot. What is the MOST likely diagnosis?
    a. tarsal tunnel syndrome
    b. peroneal tendinosis
    c. posterior impingement
    d. L5/S1 lumbar disc herniation

43. A patient presents with right posterolateral neck pain at the level of C5-6 following an extension, right lateral flexion injury. Which test will MOST likely reproduce the symptoms and what are the indications?
    a. foraminal compression test indicating C5 nerve root injury
    b. Jackson's compression test indicating C5-6 facet joint surface injury
    c. passive left lateral flexion range of motion indicating C5-6 joint capsule injury
    d. Soto Hall test indicating C5-6 joint capsule injury

44. A patient has right elbow pain and paresthesia following a fall in which he slipped and landed on the posterior aspect of his flexed elbow. The symptoms are located on the medial aspect of the elbow and radiate down the medial forearm to digits 4 and 5. Radiographs are negative for fracture. Which test would reproduce the symptoms, and what are the indications?
    a. Cozen's sign, indicating lateral epicondylitis
    b. elbow valgus stress test, medial elbow collateral ligament injury
    c. Tinel's sign of the superficial radial nerve, superficial radial nerve injury
    d. Tinel's sign of the ulnar nerve, indicating ulnar nerve injury at the cubital tunnel

45. A patient has neck pain with severe radiation into the arm. If the patient's symptoms were from nerve root pathology, what would motor, reflex, and sensory (MRS) testing likely reveal?
    a. decreased MRS signs
    b. equal bilateral MRS signs
    c. increased MRS signs
    d. the same MRS signs

46. A patient has left anterolateral lower neck pain that radiates into the anterior superior left shoulder and into the lateral arm to the midforearm. Valsalva's maneuver reproduces the patient's symptoms. This indicates that the nerve root is likely compressed by what structure?
    a. cervical sprain
    b. facet joint degeneration
    c. intervertebral disc protrusion
    d. SCM muscle spasm

47. For a patient with a cervical disc herniation, the following tests would likely reproduce the patient's symptoms EXCEPT:
    a. distraction test
    b. foraminal compression test
    c. Jackson's compression test
    d. Spurling's test

48. A patient has thoracic pain, and during the exam you notice that the Adam's sign shows a left posterior rib protrusion from about T10 to T3, and on forward flexion, the protrusion remains. This indicates:
    a. functional scoliosis
    b. negative Adam's sign
    c. normal spine
    d. structural scoliosis

49. A patient slipped and fell on his buttocks and now has achy lumbosacral pain. Range of motion tests reproduce the pain on active extension and a little worse on passive extension with no symptoms on resistive extension. The pain is worsened on standing Kemp's test. Radiographs reveal no fracture or gross pathology. This indicates the patient injured which structures?
    a. facet joint surface
    b. iliolumborum muscles
    c. joint capsule ligament
    d. L5 nerve root

50. A 64-year-old male patient presents with lumbosacral pain that he describes as achy in nature and deep. This patient has had low back pain before but these symptoms are different than before. You examine the patient with range of motion, orthopedic tests, and neurologic testing tests and cannot find the problem. What other differential diagnosis do you most likely need to consider?
    a. appendix problem
    b. colon problem
    c. prostate problem
    d. rectal problem

51. A 28-year-old soccer player injured his right knee 2 weeks ago. While he had his right foot planted to kick the ball with his left leg, he was kicked in the back of the right upper tibia. It resulted in immediate pain, but when the patient comes into your office he is only complaining of the knee clunking while he walks. You perform knee orthopedic tests, and the anterior draw sign demonstrates a 2-cm anterior translation of the tibia, which indicates which of the following?
a. the cruciate ligaments are torn
b. the lateral collateral ligament is torn
c. the medial collateral ligament is torn
d. the menisci are torn

52. A 45-year-old woman presents with left foot pain. She has had this sharp pain for some time. Initially it was an ache, but it recently turned sharp. It is located on the bottom of the ball of the foot in the area of the metatarsal arch. You perform an exam on the foot, and palpation is painful between the first and second metatarsals about midshaft. Morton's test reproduces the sharp pain that radiates distally and indicates:
a. metatarsalgia
b. neuritis
c. neuroma
d. plantar fasciitis

53. What is the point prevalence rate of low back pain?
a. 30%
b. 50%
c. 60%
d. 80%

54. What is the MOST common myofascial pain syndrome of the low back?
a. piriformis
b. quadratus lumborum
c. iliopsoas
d. tensor fascia latae

55. Which of the following types of spondylolisthesis is the MOST common?
a. congenital
b. isthmic
c. degenerative
d. pathologic

56. Which is NOT an indication for normal radiographic investigation in someone presenting with low back pain?
    a. unexplained weight loss
    b. severe back pain
    c. chronic use of corticosteroids
    d. night pain

57. McMurray's test was specifically designed for detecting which of the following?
    a. any meniscal lesion
    b. tears of the anterior horn of the meniscus
    c. tears of the body and posterior horn of the meniscus
    d. coronary ligament tears

58. What is the MOST likely cause of hemarthrosis of the knee is?
    a. PCL injury
    b. ACL injury
    c. meniscal tear
    d. patellar dislocation

59. Which of the following may be considered an urgent medical emergency?
    a. patellar subluxation
    b. tibiofemoral subluxation
    c. patellar fracture
    d. severe anterior thigh contusion

60. The proper term for a "tear in a muscle" is:
    a. rupture
    b. sprain
    c. strain
    d. contusion

61. Which of the following is considered an absolute contraindication to manipulation?
    a. smoking and hypertension
    b. whiplash injury
    c. birth control pills and smoking
    d. acute myelopathy

62. What is the MOST common symptom associated with thoracic outlet syndrome?
    a. weakness and fatigue of the arm
    b. numbness and tingling in the medial forearm and hand
    c. aching pain in the arm
    d. neck pain

63. Which of the following factors will most likely result in the phenomenon called "ramping"?
    a. speeding along a ramp
    b. not wearing a seatbelt
    c. head restraint is too low
    d. head restraint is too far back

Answers

1. c. According to the International Classification of Headache Disorders (*Cephalalgia*, 2004), nausea or vomiting is characteristic of many forms of migraine (without aura), hypnic headache, new daily and persistent headache, postictal headache, and many other kind of headaches caused by a change in intracranial pressure.

2. a. Reiter's syndrome is a seronegative polyarthropathy characterized by the following triad of symptoms: (1) urethritis, (2) conjunctivitis, and (3) polyarthritis. Like rheumatoid arthritis, ankylosing spondylitis, psoriatic arthritis, and enteropathic arthritis, Reiter's syndrome is an arthropathy that can involve atlantoaxial instability.

3. c. The signs of osteoporosis often appear suddenly with the development of a painful kyphosis caused by pathologic fractures of thoracic vertebral bodies. Osteoporosis risk factors include the following: female gender, Causasian or Asian background, early menopause, family history, lean body habitus, lack of exercise, smoking, heavy alcohol consumption, low calcium intake, and vitamin D deficiency.

4. b. The most common cause of arterial occlusion is atherosclerosis. Lower leg and foot cramps, paresthesia, and numbness are common symptoms of vascular diseases. Lower limb pain relieved by trunk flexion is characteristic of neurogenic claudication, whereas lower limb pain relieved by rest and specific activity duration before symptom onset is characteristic of claudication of vascular origin.

5. d. The posterior margin of the annulus is supplied by the sinuvertebral nerve, which is formed by a branch of the ventral rami and a branch of the grey ramus communicans. Discogenic pain is characterized by sclerotomal distribution and a deep and aching pain that increases with intradiscal pressure. Neurologic changes like paresthesia, muscle weakness, and diminished deep tendon reflex are often caused by radicular impairment.

6. a. Difficulty in toe walking (weakness of gastrocnemius, soleus, and posterior tibialis), abolished ankle jerk, and paresthesia in the posterolateral calf and lateral foot are typical signs and symptoms of L5 nerve root impairment. Lateral bending away from the left limb suggests a left lateral disc protrusion.

7.   d.   Plantar fasciitis is one of the most common causes of heel pain in athletes. It is caused by chronic traction of the plantar fascia that often results in microruptures of the aponeurosis. In mild cases, pain may occur only at the onset of training or on the first steps out of bed every morning. In more chronic cases, every step causes pain.

8.   b.   De Quervain's tenosynovitis usually results from overuse of the wrist and thumb and affects women between the ages of 30 and 60. It affects the long abductor and short extensor of the thumb. Differential diagnosis includes entrapment of the superficial branch of the radial nerve and osteoarthritis of the thumb axis.

9.   b.   Guillain-Barré syndrome is a disease known to affect myelin-producing cells. Typically, it affects motor neurons that are well myelinated. The rapid onset and evolution of this syndrome can be explained by the possible infectious and autoimmune origin of the pathology. Patients usually recover within 6 months.

10.   d.   Slipped femoral capital epiphysis is the most common hip condition in adolescent boys (10 to 16 years old). Fifty percent of cases present with a traumatic history. Traumatic slipped femoral capital epiphysis is considered a Salter-Harris type I epiphyseal fracture.

11.   b.   Diffuse pain is a defining criterion of fibromyalgia. According to the American College of Rheumatologists' 1990 criteria for the classification of fibromyalgia, widespread pain must be present for at least 3 months. Pain is considered widespread when all of the following are present: pain in the left side of the body; pain in the right side of the body; pain above the waist; pain below the waist; and axial skeletal pain. Pain in 11 of 18 tender point sites on digital palpation must also be present in order to establish the diagnosis of fibromyalgia.

12. d. In a young male patient with recurrent bilateral sacroiliac pain not responding to chiropractic care, ankylosing spondylitis is the primary differential diagnosis. Typically, the average age of symptoms begins at 26 years of age. The lower back symptoms are usually insidious and have an inflammatory pattern. They are present for longer than 3 months and are aggravated by inactivity and relieved by movement. A morning gelling phenomenon is also usually present. The most common initial presentation is a bilateral symmetrical sacroiliitis with pain often radiating into the gluteal area and the thigh but not below the knee. Typically, the stiffness and discomfort ascends the spine over many years to produce spinal pain and progressive decrease of mobility.

13. d. The factors regarding the risk of progression of an idiopathic scoliosis before osseous maturity are pattern of the curvature (lumbar, double major, etc.), age of the patient, the reaching of menarche, Risser sign, severity of the curvature, and sex of the patient.

14. a. The hallmark of postmenopause osteoporosis is vertebral fractures, and the hallmark of aging osteoporosis is hip fracture, which is the worst consequence of osteoporosis.

15. c. The only clinical sign identifying patients suffering from psoriasis who are susceptible to develop an associated arthritis is ungual involvement. The following factors are indicators of a negative prognosis: family history of psoriatic arthritis, onset of psoriatic arthritis before 20 years of age, presence of HLA-DR3 or HLA-DR4, erosive arthritis or polyarticular arthritis, and extensive dermatologic psoriasis.

16. b. The traditional measures of acute-phase reactant (sedimentation rate and C-reactive protein) are very useful for measuring the inflammatory activity in the joints of patients suffering from rheumatoid arthritis. In the patient suffering from ankylosing spondylitis, these acute-phase reactants are useful to measure the extra-articular activity of the disease and not its joint activity. Patients suffering from polymyositis typically have elevated skeletal muscle enzymes, especially creatine kinase. The sedimentation rate is elevated above 50 mm/hr in only 20% of these patients. As for fibromyalgia, none of these laboratory tests are positive.

17. a. The American Rheumatism Association 1987 revised criteria for classification of rheumatoid arthritis are morning stiffness, arthritis of three or more joint areas, arthritis of the hand joints, symmetrical arthritis, rheumatoid nodules, serum rheumatoid factor, and radiographic changes. The patient must satisfy at least four of the seven criteria, with criteria 1 through 4 being present for at least 6 weeks.

18. d. In polymyalgia rheumatica, up to 40% of patients present with histologic changes of arteritis, although this does not always give rise to symptoms. The symptoms might include headaches, temporal tenderness, intermittent claudication of the jaw, visual manifestations, or visual loss and systemic symptoms such as fatigue, malaise, weight loss, fever, and others. The temporal artery is most often affected. Psoriatic arthritis can cause a rare but very destructive arthritis mutilans of the hands. Systemic lupus erythematosus (SLE) gives rise to renal conditions in up to 50% to 60% of patients, but these conditions are not always symptomatic. In the course of SLE, 30% to 50% of patients will present with hematuria and/or proteinuria. Nephritis is a bad prognostic factor of SLE, and 20% to 30% of lupus patients suffering from nephritis will develop a terminal renal insufficiency. Reactive arthritis does not typically give rise to atlantoaxial instability. The following rheumatologic conditions are associated with atlantoaxial instability: rheumatoid arthritis (20% to 50% of patients with severe disease); psoriatic arthritis (45% of patients with spondylitis); chronic juvenile arthritis (more frequent in patients with RA who were seropositive for the RF in childhood); ankylosing spondylitis (in 2% of patients, usually with longstanding disease).

19. a. Septic arthritis affects the large peripheral joints more frequently than the small ones. It is monoarticular in 80% to 90% of the cases. Its risk factors include age older than 80 years of age, diabetes, preexisting rheumatoid arthritis, presence of a prosthetic device (hip or knee replacement), recent joint surgery, and skin infection. Several diseases should raise the suspicion of a septic arthritis when concomitant with a hot, swollen, red joint with loss of its normal range of motion. Gonorrhea is the most common type of septic arthritis in a young sexually active individual. It is typically associated with migratory arthritis with tenosynovitis and typical prominent cutaneous lesions. Hepatitis B may present as sudden and severe onset of septic arthritis. Hepatitis C shows a triad of arthritis, palpable purpura, and cryoglobulinemia. HIV gives rise to a multitude of musculoskeletal syndromes including reactive arthritis, psoriatic arthritis, or septic arthritis.

20. b. A systematic approach to the differential diagnosis of rheumatologic conditions is important in order to reach the proper diagnosis. The first question to ask oneself in the presence of such a condition is, Is the problem joint or nonjoint pain?

21. b. Flat foot = pes planus. The talar head displaces medially and plantarward from under the navicular and stretches the spring ligament and tibialis posterior, resulting in the loss of the medial longitudinal arch.

22. c. A painful neuroma in the space between the third and the fourth metatarsal heads is a Morton's neuroma.

23. c. The prepatellar bursa overlies the anterior portion of the patella. Inflammation of the bursa can be caused by excessive kneeling and leaning forward, which is referred to as "housemaid's knee."

24. c. Clubbed nails are domed and much broader and larger than normal. Most often they are due to hypertrophy of the underlying soft tissues, but it may also indicate respiratory or congenital heart problems.

25. d. Retraction of the scapula is performed by the rhomboid muscles. When strong, they prevent flaring of the scapulae, such that the inferior angle of the scapula(e) present abnormally with lateral deviation.

26. b. This is an injury occurring in children and adolescents in which the medial epicondyle is inflamed and there is partial separation of the apophysis.

27. a. Nursemaid's elbow is radial head dislocation in a distal direction, which may follow a forceful traction to the forearm.

28. d. Legg-Calvé-Perthes disease is usually seen in the age range of 4 to 8 years and then in teenage years. It is an avascular necrosis of the femoral head with resultant collapse and resorption of sequestered bone. This condition is characterized by chronic hip and groin pain with pain occasionally traveling to the thigh or knee.

29. c. With piriformis syndrome, the patient complains of buttock and posterior leg pain with a nontraumatic onset. Direct palpation of the piriformis may cause a referred pain pattern down the back of the leg.

30. d. Symptoms of meralgia paresthetica may be worse with direct pressure on the lateral femoral cutaneous nerve where it is most superficial. Increased symptoms include passive hip extension or forced hip flexion causing traction and compression.

31. d. Cervical disc herniation tends to present between the age of 35 to 55 with predominant arm and scapular pain presenting with or without neurologic deficit (specific weakness and/or hypesthesia and/or hyporeflexia). Provocation tests (Spurling's, axial compression) and nerve root tension signs (Bakody, shoulder depression, brachial-plexus compression, median nerve, and medial cord stretch test) may be present. Intrathecal pressure (Dejerine's triad/Valsalva) may be increased.

32. b. The following signs or symptoms should alert the clinician to probable inflammatory spondyloarthropathy: significant morning stiffness (>1 hour) and persisting motion restriction, peripheral joint involvement, gradual onset before age 40, and history of UTI, urethral discharge, iritis, and/or skin rash.

33. b. Age, sex, ethnicity, and some endocrine disorders are known risk factors for osteoporosis that cannot be modified. However, excessive consumption of alcohol, soft drinks and caffeine, smoking, estrogen deficiency, insufficient physical activity, and low calcium consumption are risk factors that can be modified.

34. b. In females over 50 years of age, the estimated risk of having osteoporosis-related fractures someday is 40% (vertebrae, 15.5%; wrist, 16%; hip, 17.5%). Although compression fractures can be visualized on plain films, radiography is unreliable for assessment of bone mass changes until there is at least a 30% loss.

35. d. Atlantoaxial subluxation develops relatively early (within 4 years) in the course of RA; these patients have a higher mortality rate compared with RA patients with no atlantoaxial subluxation. Neck rigidity in the sagittal plane in the absence of trauma is suggestive of meningitis and possibly atlantoaxial subluxation secondary to C1-2 congenital anomalies. Arm or leg radiation with neck movements is suggestive of cervical myelopathy and radiculomyelopathy.

36. d. Lower socioeconomic status may be associated with chronicity in whiplash patients. Of interest, an important association exists between a history of a whiplash-associated disorder, pain intensity, and disability and co-morbidity, including headache, low back pain, and digestive and cardiovascular disorders.

37. d. Other psychological factors include self-report of extreme pain and constant pain in multiple body areas; history of prolonged sick-listing after previous injuries; prior history of absenteeism or delays/obstacles in work reentry process; patients who believe they will never return to work; adversarial attitude toward employer; and longstanding history of psychiatric distress or maladjustment.

38. b. Prolonged repetitive use (half to most of the time) is a risk factor for nonspecific forearm pain. Activities that frequently flex or extend the wrist, jobs with repetitive forceful gripping, high force and high frequency of repetition, and vibration tools are all risk factors for carpal tunnel syndrome. Hobbies with repetitive use of the thumb (piano playing, sewing, knitting, and weaving) are risk factors for de Quervain's tenosynovitis.

39. d. The Ottawa Ankle (and foot) Rule is a highly sensitive (89% to 100%) and validated clinical decision tool for fractures.

40. c. The Ottawa Knee Rule is a highly sensitive (98% to 100%) and validated clinical decision tool for fractures. Radiographs are therefore not routinely recommended, but AP supine and lateral views of the injured knee are necessary if one or more signs are present: 55 years of age or older; tenderness at head of fibula; isolated tenderness of patella; inability to flex knee >90 degrees; inability to bear weight both immediately and at presentation (four steps). Radiographs are warranted if obvious deformity or mass is present.

41. b. Patients older than 40 years of age with a new episode of hip pain presents evidence of osteoarthritis in 44% of cases. Restricted and painful internal rotation is highly suggestive of osteoarthritis, and three-plane range of motion limitation is less sensitive but more specific.

42. a. Signs and symptoms are localized to the foot only. L5/S1 lumbar disc herniation generally has a history of low back pain with nerve root tension signs, possible loss of sensation (lateral foot), loss of motor power (plantar flexion and ankle eversion), and diminished Achilles tendon reflex. Peroneal tendinosis and posterior impingement are not associated with sensory alteration.

43. b. Your patient's mechanism of injury involved compressing the right C5-6 facets together and injuring the joint surface. Jackson's compression test would reproduce the symptoms of that injury.

44. d. The patient's fall onto the elbow apparently compressed the ulnar nerve at the cubital tunnel and injured the nerve, causing pain and paresthesia. For Tinel's sign, the physician would use a reflex hammer to tap over the ulnar nerve at the cubital tunnel to reproduce or aggravate the symptoms.

45. a. In nerve root pathology, the nerve function is depressed and would likely show muscle test to be in the corresponding myotome, the corresponding deep tendon reflex to be decreased or absent, and the corresponding dermatome to exhibit hypo- or anesthesia.

46. c. The Valsalva's maneuver and Dejerine's triad increase the volume of cerebrospinal fluid in the subarachnoid space, which will cause the dura mater to expand in the spinal canal. These procedures will also compress the spine and increase the intradiscal pressure causing a disc protrusion to enlarge, entrapping the nerve root and reproducing the symptoms.

47. a. Spurling's, foraminal, and Jackson's are compression tests and will increase the intradiscal pressure and cause a disc protrusion to entrap a nerve root; they will narrow the intervertebral foramen and the spinal canal. A distraction test will decrease intradiscal pressure and may relieve a disc protrusion, enlarge the intervertebral foramen and spinal canal, and may decrease the patient's symptoms or at least not aggravate the symptoms.

48. d. In scoliosis, the spine usually rotates the vertebral bodies toward the convexity of the curve and pushes the back posteriorly on that side, indicating a scoliosis. If the posteriority remains in flexion, it indicates a structural scoliosis (positive Adam's sign).

49. a. A fall on the buttocks like this would result in the facet joint surface being jammed together and injuring the joint surface. Any extension-type maneuver would cause the facet surfaces to be compressed together and produce the patient's symptoms.

50. c. Due to the patient's age and the location and type of pain, the referred pain of a prostate problem is the most likely differential to consider for this patient. The anatomic location of the prostate gland is anterior and inferior to the sacrum and refers to the lumbosacral and sacral area.

51. a. The cruciate ligaments stabilize anterior and posterior translation; this type of injury will stress the anterior cruciate and, if torn, may injure the posterior cruciate. With the drawer sign, there should be no play or translation. Excessive translation (>5 mm) indicates torn cruciates. This much play with no symptoms indicates that both cruciates are avulsed.

52. c. The nerves of the plantar aspect of the foot that run between the metatarsal bones can develop benign tumors known as Morton's neuromas. They can develop from wearing too small of shoes compressing the metatarsal bones together and irritating the nerves, which then can develop the tumors.

53. a. Point prevalence is the rate of low back pain at any given point in time. Lifetime prevalence is equivalent to incidence rate, which is typically a higher value.

54. b. Travell and Simons report that myofascial pain syndrome of the quadratus lumborum muscle is the most common myofascial pain syndrome of the lower back.

55. b. Type II (isthmic) spondylolisthesis is the most common and typically affects the L5 vertebra.

56. b. Unexplained weight loss, chronic use of corticosteroids, and night pain are all red flags. Radiographic investigation is needed in these cases to rule out spinal metastasis or a compression fracture.

57. c. McMurray's test typically stresses the posterior horn of the menisci when internal or external rotation is applied. This is the most common location of a meniscal tear.

58. b. In 75% of cases of hemarthrosis of the knee, the ACL is torn. Rapid effusion occurs within 24 hours. A PCL injury, a peripheral meniscal tear, or a patellar dislocation can also cause hemarthrosis of the knee, but these are not as common as the ACL tear.

59. b. The only medical emergency involving the knee is a tibiofemoral subluxation. This can damage the popliteal artery and/or the common peroneal nerve. A patient with patellar fracture or subluxations and severe anterior thigh contusions may also have to be seen in the hospital emergency department, but these are not considered potentially serious injuries.

60. c. A strain is an injury to the muscle belly or tendon. A sprain is an injury to a ligament. A contusion typically involves a blow to a muscle belly, causing bruising.

61. d. Acute myelopathy is considered an absolute contraindication to manipulation. This may be seen in cervical spondylotic myelopathy. Smoking, hypertension, and use of birth control pills are considered risks for vertebrobasilar insufficiency.

62. b. Numbness and tingling affecting the ring and little finger is the most common symptom in thoracic outlet syndrome (100%). Aching pain in the forearm and hand is also reported in 75% of cases.

63. c. Ramping is a phenomenon that occurs in a rear-end collision when the head restraint is not positioned correctly (too low). The head restraint acts as a fulcrum, and hyperextension of the neck is accentuated.

Section Eight Recommended Reading

Aminoff MJ, Simon RP, Greenberg DA: *Clinical neurology,* ed 6, New York, 2005, McGraw-Hill.

Beers M, Berkow R: *The Merck manual of diagnosis and therapy,* ed 17, Whitehouse Station, NJ, 2004, Merck Research Laboratories.

Cipriano J: *Photographic manual of regional orthopaedic and neurological tests,* ed 4, Philadelphia, 2003, Lippincott Williams & Wilkins.

Cramer G, Darby S: *Basic clinical anatomy of the spine, spinal cord and ANS,* ed 2, St Louis, 2005, Mosby.

Evans R: *Illustrated orthopedic physical assessment,* ed 2, St Louis, 2001, Mosby.

Foreman S, Croft A: *Whiplash injuries: the cervical acceleration/deceleration syndrome,* ed 3, Baltimore, 2002, Lippincott Williams & Wilkins.

Haldeman S: *Principles and practice of chiropractic,* ed 3, New York, 2005, McGraw-Hill.

Herkowitz H, Rothman R, eds: *Rothman-Simeone: the spine,* ed 4, Philadelphia, 1999, WB Saunders.

Hoppenfeld S: *Orthopaedic neurology: a diagnostic guide to neurologic levels,* Philadelphia, 1977, Lippincott-Raven.

Hoppenfeld S: *Physical examination of the spine and extremities,* New York, 1976, Appleton-Century-Crofts.

Klippel J: *Primer on the rheumatic diseases,* ed 12, Atlanta, 2001, Arthritis Foundation.

Magee D: *Orthopedic physical assessment,* ed 4, Philadelphia, 2002, WB Saunders.

Panjabi M, White A: *Biomechanics in the musculoskeletal system,* New York, 2001, Churchill Livingstone.

Patten J: *Neurological differential diagnosis,* ed 2, London, 1998, Springer.

Reid D: *Sports injury assessment and rehabilitation,* Philadelphia, 1992, Churchill Livingstone.

Simons D, Travell J: *Travell & Simons' myofascial pain and dysfunction: the trigger point manual,* ed 2, Baltimore, 1999, Lippincott Williams & Wilkins.

Skinner H, ed: *Current diagnosis & treatment in orthopedics,* ed 3, Norwalk, Conn, 2003, Appleton & Lange.

Waddell G: *The back pain revolution,* ed 2, Oxford, 2004, Churchill Livingstone.

Weinstein S, Buckwalter J: *Turek's orthopaedics: principles and their application,* ed 6, Philadelphia, 2005, JB Lippincott.

Wilson-Pauwels L, Akesson E, Stewart P, Spacey S: *Cranial nerves in health and disease,* ed 2, Toronto, Canada, 2002, BC Decker.

Diagnostic Imaging

John M. Bassano, Julie-Marthe Grenier,
Norman W. Kettner, Lawrence H. Wyatt, Kenneth J. Young

X-ray Technology

1. Which of the following BEST defines "radiographic contrast"?
   a. difference in gray scale between adjacent regions on a radiograph
   b. difference between the darkest and lightest areas on a radiograph
   c. difference between number of photons that strike the anode
   d. difference between the number of photons that strike the cathode

2. Filtration is used in diagnostic radiography to:
   a. absorb low-energy x-rays
   b. remove high-energy x-rays
   c. restrict the useful beam to the body part imaged
   d. manufacture gonad shields

3. Variations in power distribution to the x-ray machine are corrected by the:
   a. full-wave rectifier
   b. high voltage transformer
   c. line voltage compensator
   d. automatic exposure control

4. The cathode side of the tube should be toward which part of the patient?
   a. upper
   b. lower
   c. right
   d. left

5. X-ray quantity increases in direct proportion to increases in:
   a. filtration
   b. kVp
   c. distance
   d. mAs

6. If one changes the technique from 70 kVp at 200 mAs to 70 kVp at 400 mAs, then the optical density on the radiograph will:
   a. remain the same
   b. double
   c. triple
   d. quadruple

7. The smallest particle of any type of electromagnetic radiation is called a(n):
   a. electron
   b. neutron
   c. neutrino
   d. photon

8. What type of interaction in the target generates the most x-rays?
   a. Compton
   b. characteristic
   c. Bremsstrahlung
   d. photoelectric

9. Decreasing kVp will lead to:
   a. increased scatter in the patient
   b. increased optical density on the film
   c. increased contrast on the film
   d. shorter wavelengths in the beam

10. Increasing what will make more electrons hit the target, thereby creating more x-rays in the beam without changing its penetrating power?
    a. mAs
    b. kVp
    c. thermionic emission
    d. collimation

11. During a plain film diagnostic study, where is most of the Compton-type scatter that affects the film generated?
    a. in the collimator
    b. in the patient
    c. in the grid
    d. in the screens

12. Intensifying screens reduce patient dose because:
    a. they partially block scatter radiation
    b. they remove harmful "soft" x-rays
    c. they eliminate the need for shielding
    d. film is more sensitive to light than to x-rays

13. Which of the following factors does NOT detract from image
    sharpness and resolution?
    a. patient movement
    b. scatter radiation
    c. high-detail film/screen combinations
    d. quantum mottle

14. Grid cut-off is usually the result of:
    a. patient motion during the exposure
    b. focal film distance out of range of the grid
    c. improper air-gap technique
    d. too high a kVp value for the area of the body being radiographed

15. When taking radiographs of the lumbar spine of an obese patient, the
    PA lumbar film comes out underexposed and foggy. Which of the
    following will NOT improve film quality?
    a. increasing the mAs
    b. increasing the kVp
    c. using a compression device
    d. using collimation

16. Grid ratio is determined by:
    a. the height of the lead strips divided by the thickness between the
        lead strips
    b. the height of the lead strips divided by the thickness of the lead
        strips
    c. number of lead strips per inch
    d. the net weight of the lead to the total weight of the grid

17. What type of x-ray machine provides the LEAST amount of absorbed
    dose to the patient?
    a. single phase
    b. triple phase
    c. full wave rectification
    d. high frequency

18. What is the electric charge of an x-ray photon?
    a. positive (+1)
    b. positive (+2)
    c. negative (−1)
    d. no charge (0)

19. Which component can be found only in an intensifying screen?
    a. phosphor layer
    b. polyester base
    c. adhesive section
    d. emulsion coating

20. The number of electrons accelerated across an x-ray tube is determined by the:
    a. anode speed
    b. focal spot size
    c. filament current
    d. x-ray–to–filtration ratio

21. Radiographic film used for diagnostic purposes in chiropractic offices is defined as:
    a. double emulsion film
    b. duplicating film
    c. direct exposure film
    d. subtraction film

22. Which choice represents the two major parts of the cathode?
    a. stator and rotor
    b. target and focal spot
    c. filament and focusing cup
    d. glass envelop and oil

23. The target of an x-ray tube used for orthopedic purposes is usually composed of:
    a. copper
    b. molybdenum
    c. tungsten
    d. lead

24. The law of Bergonie and Tribondeau explains which concept?
    a. cells with rapid turnover are more sensitive to ionizing radiation
    b. the distance between a source and an object is proportional to the radiation intensity
    c. the higher the temperature of the filament, the more electrons are emitted
    d. radiographic film speed is proportional to emulsion thickness

25. The major site of radiation damage leading to cell death is:
    a. endoplasmic reticulum
    b. mitochondria
    c. Golgi apparatus
    d. nucleus

26. The damaging effects of ionizing radiation are enhanced in the presence of:
    a. nitrogen
    b. carbon dioxide
    c. carbon monoxide
    d. oxygen

27. The initial interaction between radiation and tissues occurs at what level?
    a. atomic
    b. molecular
    c. subcellular
    d. cellular

28. The most sensitive time during pregnancy for radiation induction of neonatal death is estimated to be:
    a. first 7 days
    b. 1 to 2 weeks
    c. 3 to 5 weeks
    d. 6 to 9 weeks

29. Which one of the following cell types is the most radiosensitive:
    a. osteocytes
    b. nerve cells
    c. chondrocytes
    d. lymphocytes

30. Which of the following is most radiosensitive:
    a. DNA
    b. mRNA
    c. tRNA
    d. cell membrane

Answers

1. a. Radiographic contrast is the difference between subtle shades of gray as seen on the radiograph. The less contrast (more shades of gray) on a radiograph, the better is the delineation, of tissues, primarily between soft tissue shadows.

2. a. Filtrations, usually in the form of aluminum, is used to reduce the number of low-energy x-rays that reach the radiographic film. These x-rays degrade the image and result in lower-quality radiographs. Restricting the useful beam to the body part being imaged is termed "collimation."

3. c. Electricity coming into a building has natural variations in power, both above and below what is most desirable. These fluctuations result in heterogeneous x-ray beams that might degrade the radiographic image. The line voltage compensator brings the voltage to the correct level, resulting in more consistency in the x-ray suite.

4. b. The x-rays produced at the anode are not uniform across the tube, as the anode is angled, which produces the anode heel effect. Installing the x-ray tube with the cathode down (anode up) in the x-ray suite produces the most desirable situation for radiography, as the higher energy x-rays are thereby directed to the thicker parts of the patient.

5. d. The number of x-rays produced is directly proportional to the milliamperage and time allotted for a particular radiograph, as these control the number of electrons produced. Kilovoltage, while having an effect on film density, is more useful for controlling radiographic contrast.

6. b. From a practical standpoint, there is a proportional relationship between increasing mAs and film density. In other words, if one doubles the number of x-rays produced, by doubling the mAs, the film becomes twice as dense (black). By the same token, if one cuts the mAs in half, only half as many x-rays are produced and the resulting film is only half as dense (black) as the original. Kilovoltage, on the other hand, creates logarithmic changes in film density secondary to the "16-20 rule."

7. d. A photon is the smallest particle of any type of electromagnetic radiation, which includes radio waves, visible light, x-rays and gamma rays. The other choices are all subatomic particles.

8. c. Bremsstrahlung, or "braking," radiation is created when electrons from the cathode enter the target (the anode) and slow down, losing energy as they pass near atomic nuclei. Due to the law of conservation of energy, that kinetic energy is transformed and released in the form of an x-ray photon. Characteristic radiation is produced only in small amounts in the diagnostic range, and the other choices are interactions of photons with matter.

9. c. Decreasing kVp increases the average wavelength of photons in the beam, which leads to a less penetrating beam, with fewer photons reaching the film and increased contrast, because the more dense structures are never penetrated by the resultant softer beam.

10. a. mAs (milliamp seconds) is the measure of the number of electrons that are emitted from the cathode, therefore controlling the number of x-ray photons that are generated. kVp also affects the number of photons to a degree, but its major effect is to change the penetrating power of the beam. Collimation alters the shape of the x-ray beam. Thermionic emission is the effect of like charges repelling each other and is not under the control of the operator.

11. b. The shape of the beam is altered by the collimator, which block the exit of radiation from the tube. Once the beam hits the patient, a variety of interactions, most importantly Compton scatter, cause radiation to scatter in all directions. The grid stops much of the scatter from hitting the cassette, and the remnant radiation beyond the grid hits crystals in the screens to expose the film.

12. d. The vast majority of film exposure is due to light generated by the rare earth element crystals within intensifying screens when exposed to x-radiation. Screens are fixed into cassettes into which the film is then placed. The cassettes are placed behind the patient and therefore do not eliminate the need for shielding. They do not block scatter or remove soft x-rays.

13. c. High-detail film/screen combinations will improve image quality.

14. b. Due to the angled grids used, there is an optimal range with regard to tube film distance. Typically, the range is within 40 to 72 inches. If the distance is exceeded, then grid cut-off will result.

15. b. Increasing the kVp would create more scatter radiation, causing the underexposed and foggy appearance.

16. a. Grid ratio is defined as the height of the grid strips divided by the thickness of the interspace.

17. d. High-frequency generators provide the lowest amount of absorbed dose to the patient.

18. d. One of the fundamental properties of an x-ray photon is that it has no charge.

19. a. The purpose of a screen is to transform the incoming x-ray photon into visible light. For each x-ray photon transform, a larger amount of light photon is emitted, thus, the name of intensifying screen. This phenomenon occurs in the phosphor layer. The other components can be found in radiographic film.

20. c. The number of electrons traveling from the cathode to the anode is directly proportional to the filament current. This current heats the filament to high temperatures leading to thermionic emission of electrons. The higher the temperature, the more electrons are produced.

21. a. Film used in most diagnostic imaging procedure is called double emulsion film. Emulsion is coated on both sides of the plastic base. This type of film is designed to be used with a cassette system using two intensifying screens.

22. c. The cathode is formed by the nickel focusing cup and two tungsten filaments. The other components of an x-ray tube are the anode and the glass envelope.

23. c. Tungsten is the material of choice for the target of the anode. In other types of imaging, mammography, for example, the target is made from molybdenum or rhodium.

24. a. In 1906, the two scientists observed that radiosensitivity was a function of the metabolic rate of the cells. Stems cells are the most affected by radiations. In the adult, cells of the gastrointestinal tract and blood cells are some of the most sensitive.

25. d. Ionizing radiation produces biological damage by depositing energy and triggering free radical formation. Genetic information is stored in the nucleus and regulates all cell function; sufficient damage to the nucleus can cause cell death.

26. d. The damaging effects of ionizing radiation are enhanced by O_2 which generates reactive oxygen species. These reactive species damage cellular macromolecules, including DNA, lipids, and proteins. Dietary antioxidants are radioprotective.

27. a. The x-ray photons of ionizing radiation transfer energy to the orbiting electrons of an atom. The energized electrons interact with electrons of other atoms producing additional ionization.

28. c. The effects of radiation on the embryo and fetus include prenatal death, growth retardation, congenital malformation, and mental retardation. Exposure during organogenesis can cause death.

29. d. The most radiosensitive cells and tissues are the most rapidly proliferating. These include lymphoid, spermatids, and bone marrow stem cells. Nerve cells are not radiosensitive.

30. a. The DNA carries the code for all metabolic activity in the cell. Double-strand breaks are the most dangerous injury to this critical macromolecule. Repair mechanisms of radiation induced DNA injury are limited.

Radiographic Positioning and Normal Anatomy

1. A right anterior oblique view of the cervical spine BEST demonstrates:
   a. right pars interarticularis
   b. left pars interarticularis
   c. right intervertebral foramina
   d. left intervertebral foramina

2. A well-defined, 5-mm ovoid ossification is visualized just lateral to the cuboid bone. What is the name of this normal variant?
   a. os peroneum
   b. os trigonum
   c. os tibiale externum
   d. os subfibulare

3. Why is a posterior-to-anterior chest view taken at a focal film distance of 72 inches?
   a. to make the spine less visible
   b. to partially erase the ribs for better visualization of the lungs
   c. to minimize magnification of the heart
   d. to decrease radiation dose

4. What is the BEST view for demonstrating the pisiform?
   a. posterior to anterior
   b. ulnar flexion
   c. medial oblique
   d. ball catcher's

5. A patient with an injured shoulder reports to your office. You decide that the trauma was sufficient to warrant obtaining plain films. The acromioclavicular space measures 7 mm. What should you do next?
   a. refer to an orthopedic surgeon
   b. take a radiograph of the opposite shoulder
   c. nothing, this is a normal measurement
   d. refer for magnetic resonance imaging (MRI)

6. What is the normal ADI (atlantodens interval) in adults?
   a. less than 1 mm
   b. 1 to 3 mm
   c. 3 to 5 mm
   d. 1 to 5 mm

7. The right cervical intervertebral foramen are best visualized on which of the following projections?
   a. lateral
   b. left anterior oblique (LAO)
   c. right anterior oblique (RAO)
   d. APLC

8. You should use lead shielding on a patient:
   a. whenever a radiation-sensitive body region is in the primary beam
   b. only on x-rays of the spine
   c. whenever it does not obscure the region of clinical interest
   d. all of the time

9. A knee measures 20 cm for the AP view. What is the appropriate technique?
   a. 40 FFD with a nonbucky technique
   b. 72 FFD with a bucky technique
   c. 40 FFD with a bucky technique
   d. 72 FFD with a nonbucky technique

10. A lateral lumbar spine radiograph is taken at which of the following techniques?
    a. 72 FFD at 80 kVp
    b. 72 FFD at 90 kVp
    c. 40 FFD at 80 kVp
    d. 40 FFD at 90 kVp

11. What shoulder view BEST demonstrates the greater tubercle?
    a. external rotation
    b. internal rotation
    c. baby arm
    d. transthoracic

12. What structure is the tangential view of the elbow (Jones) taken to better visualize?
    a. coronoid
    b. capitellum
    c. olecranon process
    d. lateral epicondyle

13. On an AP external rotation shoulder radiograph, one can see the lesser tuberosity:
    a. overlapping with the glenoid fossa
    b. overlapping with the greater tuberosity
    c. overlapping the acromion process
    d. overlapping the greater trochanter

14. Fascial plane lines, or fat pads, are what compared with bone?
    a. radiolucent
    b. radiopaque
    c. equivalent in density
    d. radiodense

15. What is the BEST radiographic view to see a fat-blood interface (FBI sign) after severe knee trauma?
    a. AP knee
    b. intercondylar view
    c. sunrise view
    d. cross-table lateral

16. The popliteus tendon groove is an anatomic landmark found on which aspect of the femur?
    a. medial
    b. lateral
    c. anterior
    d. posterior

17. What is the utility of the "Risser sign"?
    a. categorize the severity of avulsion fractures in the pelvis
    b. determine the location of fractures about the elbow joint
    c. assess the level of skeletal maturity
    d. quantify the amount of rotation in congenital torticollis

18. What is the advantage of a PA wrist view with ulnar deviation?
    a. better visualization of the pisiform
    b. accurate measurement of the radioulnar joint
    c. visualize the metacarpal heads looking for early erosions due to rheumatoid arthritis
    d. elongation and better visualization of the entire length of the scaphoid

19. Which of the following cells are normally found in a Howship's lacunae?
    a. giant cell
    b. osteoblast
    c. osteocyte
    d. osteoclast

20. Ligament and tendon attachment sites on a bone are known by which term?
    a. entheses
    b. synarthroses
    c. metaphysis
    d. amphiarthrosis

21. Which radiographic projection of the cervical spine will exclude overhang of the lateral masses of C1?
    a. flexion
    b. AP open mouth
    c. oblique
    d. extension

22. Which of the following specialized radiographic projections is used to provoke intersegmental instability in the lumbar spine?
    a. traction-compression
    b. Kasabach's view
    c. Water's projection
    d. 25- to 30-degree obliques

23. The presence of instability in the symphysis pubis is optimally detected by which of the following examination?
    a. flamingo (stork) view
    b. 5-degree upward tube tilt
    c. oblique views
    d. frog-eg views

24. Select the appropriate positioning for a lateral thoracic spine in a scoliotic patient:
    a. cranial 5-degree tube tilt
    b. caudal 5-degree tube tilt
    c. concavity toward bucky
    d. convexity toward bucky

25. The typical tube tilt for an AP lower cervical spine radiograph is:
    a. 0 degrees
    b. 15 degrees
    c. 45 degrees
    d. 70 degrees

26. The normal angle of obliquity for a mortise view of the ankle is _____ degrees medially.
    a. 0
    b. 20
    c. 45
    d. 75

27. The pars interarticularis in the lumbar spine is best seen on which view?
    a. AP
    b. lateral
    c. oblique
    d. lateral flexion

28. The greater tuberosity of the humerus is best seen on which view?
    a. neutral AP
    b. internal rotation
    c. external rotation
    d. oblique swimmer's

29. Which of the following describes the proper normal anatomy of the proximal carpal row, from lateral to medial?
    a. capitate, lunate, triquetrum, pisiform
    b. lunate, trapezium, capitate, hamate
    c. scaphoid, lunate, triquetrum, pisiform
    d. scaphoid, hamate, lunate, capitate

Answers

1. b. With a right anterior oblique view of the cervical spine, the patient is positioned facing 45 degrees with the right shoulder toward the cassette, which positions the intervertebral foramen in the orientation of the primary beam, and a 15-degree caudal tube tile is used for optimum visualization. Lumbar spine oblique views demonstrate the pars.

2. a. A few of the accessory ossicles that occur in the ankle are common and should form part of the anatomic knowledge base of chiropractors. The os peroneum is a sesamoid bone in the peroneus longus tendon and appears just lateral to the cuboid on dorsoplantar foot radiographs. Os trigonum is posterior to the talus, os tibiale externum is just medial to the tarsal navicular, and os subfibulare is just inferior to the distal fibula.

3. c. Because the heart is an anterior structure, positioning the patient posterior-to-anterior will place it closer to the cassette will minimize its magnification and distortion. This allows for a standardized measurement method of heart size through the cardiothoracic ratio, which, in normal patients is 1:2 or less. The high kVp used for chest films is what makes the spine and ribs less visible, due to the decreased contrast, and the radiation dose is dictated by the beam factors necessary to produce a properly exposed film, not the focal film distance.

4. d. The ball catcher's view is taken with the posteromedial side of the hand against the cassette; this allows the anteromedially placed pisiform to be visualized without any overlapping osseous structures.

5. b. While the usual measurement of the acromioclavicular joint is 2 to 4 mm, a distance of up to 8 mm may be normal, as long as the contralateral side is within 2 mm. The best way to determine this is to take one view of the opposite shoulder.

6. b. The ADI, which is a measure of upper cervical stability, is normally 1 to 3 mm in adults. A measurement less than 1 mm may occur in degenerative disease, and a measurement greater than 3 mm is seen with damage to the transverse ligament (ruptured, stretched, eroded, or congenitally absent), leading to forward movement of the atlas on the axis and potential compression of the spinal cord. Children may have an ADI of up to 5 mm, due to normal ligamentous laxity.

7. c. The right-sided intervertebral foramen are positioned so they are closest to the film in the oblique projection.

8. c. Lead shielding is used to protect the areas of the body that are very sensitive to radiation. If the shielding obscures the area of clinical interest, then the study would need to be repeated without the shielding, thus increasing unnecessary exposure to the patient.

9. c. For the knee (or any extremity), the film focal distance is 40 inches. However, if an extremity measures greater than 16 cm (thicker than average), then a bucky technique is used to reduce scatter from fogging the film.

10. d. The appropriate technique for a lateral lumbar radiograph is 40 FFD at 90 kVp.

11. a. Due to the anatomic location of the greater tubercle, external rotation positions it in profile for best visualization.

12. c. The tangential or Jones view of the elbow is taken to visualize the olecranon process in the coronal plane.

13. b. The lesser and greater tuberosity will overlap on an AP view of the shoulder with external rotation. The lesser tuberosity will project over the glenoid fossa on a view of the shoulder with internal rotation.

14. a. Radiolucent structures allow x-rays to be transmitted and reach the film. Radiopaque structures prevent or significantly attenuate the x-ray beam. The amount of attenuation is characteristic to each tissue, particularly its density and atomic number.

15. d. Cross-table lateral views or horizontal beam radiographs allow for settling of fat and blood within the joint capsule. The line becomes visible when the x-ray beam is parallel to the interface between the two fluids. If seen, this sign indicates an intra-articular fracture with bleeding and marrow fat seeping into the joint.

16. b. The popliteus tendon groove is used to identify the lateral aspect of the femur on knee radiographs. It is especially useful when the fibular head is collimated out or on coronal magnetic resonance images when the fibula is not in the field of view.

17. c. Skeletal maturity is an important factor to consider when managing patients with scoliosis. The Risser sign refers to the level of ossification of the secondary center of the iliac crest. The Risser sign is graded into five stages.

18. d. With ulnar deviation (flexion), the scaphoid will appear elongated because of the rotation in a plane parallel to the film. It will also allow for better visualization of the waist of the scaphoid and distraction of fracture fragments.

19. d. These multinucleated cells responsible for bone resorption are located in resorptive cavities termed Howship's lacunae.

20. a. The osseous insertion sites of ligaments and tendons are metabolically active and may undergo pathologic changes known as enthesopathy. This radiographic finding is seen in seronegative arthropathy and hyperparathyroidism.

21. b. The upper cervical complex is best seen with the AP open mouth projection. Fractures of the C1 ring (Jefferson's) will displace the lateral masses to produce an abnormal "step off" defect with the superior articular process of C2. Up to 2.0 mm of "step off" is normal.

22. a. Traction-compression radiography of the lumbar spine will trigger anterior or posterior translation of an unstable segment. Segmental instability may complicate spondylolytic spondylolisthesis or degenerative spondylolisthesis.

23. a. The flamingo view is a PA collimated view of the symphysis pubis performed with the right leg hanging and the contralateral leg is supported. Then a second view flexes the right leg at the knee with the hip neutral and the left leg is supportive.

24. d. Scoliotic thoracic spines should be positioned with the convexity of the curve toward the bucky. This will allow normal beam divergence to optimize disc and vertebral body visualization.

25. b. The 15-degree cephalic tube tilt used in an AP lower cervical film helps to align the x-ray beam with the disc spaces and creates a better picture of the anatomy of the lower cervical spine in the coronal plane.

26. b. The 20-degree medial angulation of the ankle produces a beautiful image of the ankle mortise (tibiotalar joint), while the 45-degree angle does not.

27. c. The pars interarticularis is best seen on the oblique view, where the classic "Scotty dog" appearance of the neural arch structures is seen. It can also be seen on the AP and lateral views but not with the definition seen on oblique views.

28. c. The greater tuberosity of the humerus is seen best on the external rotation view, as it is now seen *en profile,* rather than *en face.* The lesser tuberosity is best seen on the internal rotation view.

29. c. This is the normal anatomy, lateral to medial of the proximal row of the carpus. The distal row, lateral to medial, is the trapezium, trapezoid, capitate, and hamate.

X-ray Diagnosis

1. Which of the following is the MOST common primary skeletal malignancy?
   a. osteosarcoma
   b. multiple myeloma
   c. metastasis
   d. chondrosarcoma

2. Which if the following is the MOST common form of skeletal metastasis?
   a. lytic
   b. blastic
   c. mixed
   d. telengectatic

3. Which of the following is the MOST commonly fractured bone in the human body?
   a. C2
   b. clavicle
   c. femur
   d. scaphoid

4. Intracapsular fractures tend to heal slowly secondary to the lack of what within the joint capsule of MOST joints?
   a. osteoblasts
   b. osteoclasts
   c. periosteum
   d. synovium

5. Osteopenia is MOST commonly secondary to:
   a. ischemia
   b. hyperemia
   c. osteonecrosis
   d. osteosclerosis

6. The MOST commonly fractured bones in the cervical spine are _____ and _____.
   a. C1, C2
   b. C1, C5
   c. C2, C7
   d. C2, C6

7. Paget's disease of a vertebra results in which of the following?
   a. enlargement with spinal canal stenosis
   b. enlargement of the spinal cord
   c. malignant degeneration in most cases
   d. retrolisthesis of the affected vertebra

8. Which is the MOST common type of spondylolisthesis?
   a. congenital
   b. isthmic (spondylolytic)
   c. traumatic
   d. pathologic

9. Hyrdoxyapatite deposition disease is MOST common in which body region?
   a. ankle
   b. hip
   c. shoulder
   d. knee

10. Which is the MOST common form of joint disease of the spine?
    a. rheumatoid arthritis
    b. ankylosing spondylitis
    c. infectious spondylitis
    d. degenerative joint disease

11. What is the anomaly in patients with Chiari malformation?
    a. elevated, hypoplastic, and rotated scapula with an omovertebral bone
    b. multiple block segmentation
    c. calcification of the stylohyoid ligament
    d. herniation of the cerebellar tonsils through the foramen magnum

12. A patient's radiographs demonstrate marked, widespread, osseous sclerosis with undertubulation of the bones of the extremities. Which of the following is a well-known complication of this disease?
    a. mental retardation
    b. absence of the clavicles and diastasis of the pubic symphysis
    c. frequent pathologic fractures
    d. abnormally large height

13. Which of the following radiographic features helps differentiate osteomalacia from osteoporosis?
   a. insufficiency fractures and increased atlantodental interval
   b. osteopenia
   c. pseudofractures and bowing deformities
   d. resorption of the secondary trabeculae and insufficiency fractures

14. A patient presents with fever and radiographs reveal unilateral sacroilitis. The best differential diagnosis is:
   a. degenerative joint disease
   b. an inflammatory arthropathy such as ankylosing spondylitis
   c. septic arthritis
   d. a metabolic joint disease such as gout

15. Which is a radiographic sign of bone marrow hyperplasia?
   a. acro-osteolysis
   b. increased bone density
   c. undertubulation of bone
   d. sclerosis of the calvarium

16. Which disease may be caused by chronic renal disease?
   a. osteomalacia
   b. hypothyroidism
   c. thalassemia
   d. hypercortisolism

17. Radiographs of a 30-year-old man demonstrate generalized osteopenia, compression fractures, atherosclerotic plaque, and early signs of avascular necrosis in the right femoral head. The patient MOST likely suffers from:
   a. osteomalacia
   b. hyperparathyroidism
   c. hypercortisolism
   d. reflex sympathetic dystrophy

18. A radiograph demonstrates decreased bone density, coarse trabeculation, bowing deformities, and pseudofractures in an adult patient with chronic malabsorption syndrome. The best differential diagnosis is:
   a. osteogenesis imperfecta
   b. osteoporosis
   c. osteomalacia
   d. osteopetrosis

19. A radiograph of the thoracolumbar spine demonstrates multiple levels of vertebral body destruction, a focally increased kyphosis, a paraspinal mass, and a psoas abscess. The MOST likely diagnosis is:
    a. cellulitis
    b. tuberculosis
    c. thalassemia
    d. sickle cell anemia

20. A patient presents with extremely severe burning pain in the foot for the past 6 months. Her foot is red and very swollen. The patient cannot remember any trauma and does not have any other symptoms. The radiographs demonstrate patchy osteopenia localized to the area. The MOST likely diagnosis is:
    a. hyperparathyroidism
    b. reflex sympathetic dystrophy
    c. acute osteomyelitis
    d. Kohler's disease

21. The earliest radiographically visible site of skeletal destruction from rheumatoid arthritis is the:
    a. articular cartilage
    b. synovial linings
    c. bare area
    d. articular capsule

22. Early degenerative disease in the knee is MOST likely to affect which of the following?
    a. patellofemoral joint
    b. lateral tibiofemoral joint
    c. medial tibiofemoral joint
    d. a and c

23. Interspinous fusion is MOST commonly encountered as a result of which condition?
    a. ankylosing spondylitis
    b. DISH
    c. rheumatoid arthritis
    d. Reiter's disease

24. The cause of the "sausage digit" appearance in psoriatic arthritis is:
    a. intra-articular swelling
    b. cellulitis
    c. tenosynovitis
    d. periostitis

25. What compartment of the hip joint is affected by early degenerative disease?
   a. axial
   b. superior
   c. medial
   d. posterior

26. The MOST likely diagnosis for an individual who demonstrates periarticular erosions with sclerotic margins, maintenance of the joint spaces, and bone density, as well as soft tissue swelling that is asymmetrical around the affected joints, is:
   a. rheumatoid arthritis
   b. psoriatic arthritis
   c. CPPD
   d. gout

27. The joint erosions of systemic lupus erythematosus are:
   a. inflammatory
   b. mechanical
   c. crystal
   d. degenerative

28. The Andersson lesion is seen in which of the following diseases?
   a. scleroderma
   b. neuropathic joint
   c. rheumatoid arthritis
   d. ankylosing spondylitis

29. Which of the following BEST describes the spinal, bony proliferation typically seen in psoriatic arthritis?
   a. bamboo spine
   b. syndesmophytes
   c. parasyndesmophytes
   d. flowing ossification

30. "Carrot stick" fractures in ankylosing spondylitis are MOST frequently encountered in which of the following locations?
   a. lumbar spine
   b. femur
   c. lower cervical spine
   d. thoracic spine

31. What is the full name given to pathologic deposition of calcium in the insertions of tendons and ligaments?
    a. calcium pyrophosphate deposition disease (CPPD)
    b. synovial osteochondrometaplasia
    c. sodium urate deposition disease
    d. hydroxyapatite deposition disease (HADD)

32. An adolescent male complains of thoracolumbar pain. Radiographs reveal multiple focal indentations in the vertebral end-plates of that area, mild anterior wedging of the vertebral bodies of T11 and T12, and mild hyperkyphosis. What is the diagnosis?
    a. compression fractures
    b. Scheuermann's disease
    c. Legg-Calve-Perthés disease
    d. Schmorl's nodes

33. Which of the following choices is typical of the radiographic findings in degenerative joint disease?
    a. marginal erosions, uniform loss of joint space, osteophytes
    b. marginal erosions, nonuniform loss of joint space, steophytes
    c. subchondral cysts, nonuniform loss of joint space, osteophytes
    d. subchondral cysts, uniform loss of joint space, osteophytes

34. A 60-year-old man with neck pain and dysphagia reports to your office. Physical exam reveals mild loss of range of motion globally in the cervical spine and joint play restrictions. Routine urinalysis reveals the presence of glucose. Plain films demonstrate large anterior nonmarginal spondylophytes throughout the cervical spine and maintenance of the intervertebral disc spaces and facet articulations. What is the MOST likely diagnosis?
    a. ankylosing spondylitis
    b. enteropathic arthritis
    c. Reiter's disease
    d. diffuse idiopathic skeletal hyperostosis

35. In what order do the following spinal changes due to ankylosing spondylitis occur?
    a. Romanus lesion, shiny corner sign, marginal syndesmophytes, bamboo spine
    b. shiny corner sign, Romanus lesion, marginal syndesmophytes, bamboo spine
    c. marginal syndesmophytes, shiny corner sign, Romanus lesion, bamboo spine
    d. marginal syndesmophytes, bamboo spine, Romanus lesion, shiny corner sign

36. Which two types of degenerative disease MOST commonly lead to compromise of the intervertebral foramina in the cervical spine?
    a. degenerative disc disease, spondylosis deformans
    b. uncinate arthrosis, degenerative disc disease
    c. spondylosis deformans, uncinate arthrosis
    d. uncinate arthrosis, facet arthrosis

37. Abnormal proliferation of histiocytes, creating a well-defined, lucent lesion in the femur, is characteristic of:
    a. hyperparathyroidism
    b. eosinophilic granuloma
    c. hemophilia
    d. ochronosis

38. A 23-year-old female patient reports sudden onset of chest pain and shortness of breath. A PA chest film reveals a thin, thread-like, curvilinear opacity paralleling the left upper and lateral chest wall, 2 cm medial to it, and absence of lung markings between the opacity and chest wall. What is the MOST likely diagnosis?
    a. pneumonia
    b. pneumoperitoneum
    c. pneumothorax
    d. pneumatocele

39. A patient with a severe ankle inversion injury should also be investigated for a possible fracture in the:
    a. proximal tibia
    b. proximal fibula
    c. distal femur
    d. patella

40. Radiographs of a 15-year-old boy with unrelenting knee pain demonstrate a spiculated periosteal response with a permeative pattern of bone destruction in the metaphysis of the femur. What is the MOST likely diagnosis?
    a. osteoblastoma
    b. chondrosarcoma
    c. fibrosarcoma
    d. osteosarcoma

41. The findings of a low posterior hairline, short neck, and limitation of cervical ranges of motion describe the classic triad of:
    a. Tay-Sachs disease
    b. Turner's syndrome
    c. Klippel-Feil syndrome
    d. Kleinfelter's syndrome

42. The presence of an os odontodium indicates:
    a. basilar invagination
    b. block vertebrae
    c. possibility of upper cervical instability
    d. no clinical significance

43. Arnold-Chiari malformation type I is frequently associated with:
    a. syringomyelia
    b. Klippel-Feil syndrome
    c. toliomyelitis
    d. Paget's disease

44. Which classification of spondylolysis and spondylolisthesis is congenital in nature?
    a. dysplastic
    b. isthmic
    c. degenerative
    d. traumatic

45. Which of the following is an intramedullary tumor?
    a. astrocytoma
    b. neurofibroma
    c. meningioma
    d. osteoma

46. The MOST common spinal complication of achondroplasia is:
    a. unilateral facet dislocation
    b. central canal stenosis
    c. bilateral facet dislocation
    d. spina bifida occulta

47. Which of the following is a cause of an ivory vertebra?
    a. hyperparathyroidism
    b. Paget's disease
    c. steroid therapy
    d. alcoholism

48. Select a generalized disorder of connective tissue associated with a deficiency of osteoblasts in which (1) a white ring surrounds the cornea, (2) the long bones are slender and overconstricted, and (3) there is defective enamel formation and obliteration of root canals.
    a. progeria
    b. osteogenesis imperfecta
    c. Pyle's disease
    d. Weismann-Netter syndrome

49. The H-shaped vertebra is suggestive of:
    a. thalassemia
    b. spherocytosis
    c. osteoporosis
    d. sickle cell

50. Radiographs of a 48-year-old man revealed an osteolytic lesion in the sacrococcygeal region. There is a soft tissue mass with multiple calcific foci. The patient's chief complaint is vague low back pain and incontinence. Your choice for diagnosis is:
    a. aneurysmal bone cyst
    b. chondroblastoma
    c. metastatic prostate carcinoma
    d. chordoma

Answers

1. b. Multiple myeloma is the most common *primary* skeletal malignancy, while metastases is the most common malignancy overall. Osteosarcoma is the second most common primary skeletal malignancy.

2. a. Lytic metastasis from lung cancer is most common overall. Blastic metastases (e.g., prostate, breast) is second most common, and mixed metastases is third. Telengectatic is a description of a form of primary malignancy.

3. b. The clavicle is the most commonly fractured bone in the body. The scaphoid bone, femur, and C2 are also commonly fractured but lag behind the clavicle.

4. c. Inside the capsule of synovial joints, the periosteum is essentially replaced by synovium. Without periosteal bone formation, fractures heal more slowly.

5. b. Hyperemia of bone results in increased resorption of bone, which, in turn, leads to osteopenia. Avascular necrosis (e.g., ischemia) results in bone sclerosis.

6. d. The odontoid process and the neural arch/vertebral body of C6 are the most commonly fractured bones in the cervical spine.

7. a. Paget's disease of bone results in an increase in the size of the affected bone. When a vertebra is affected, this often results in spinal canal narrowing. While malignant degeneration of Pagetic bone is possible, it is unusual.

8. b. Of the five types of spondylolisthesis (congenital, traumatic, isthmic, degenerative, pathologic), isthmic is the most common, while degenerative is second most common.

9. c. HADD can affect any tendon, bursa, or ligament in the body, but the shoulder joint (e.g., subacromial bursa, rotator cuff tendons) is the most common location. Other common locations include the knee and the hip.

10. d. Degenerative joint disease is the most common form of arthropathy. It is seen commonly throughout the spine and weight-bearing joints. Rheumatoid arthritis is seen more commonly in the hands, with the upper cervical spine being the second most common location for this disease.

11. d. Chiari malformations can be diagnosed on brain and cervical magnetic resonance imaging. The inferior aspect of the cerebellum will extend below the level of the foramen magnum. Associated abnormalities may include syringomyelia and block vertebrae.

12. c. Osteosclerosis and undertubulation of bones are characteristic findings of osteopetrosis. In this condition, the osteoclasts are dysfunctional resulting in faulty bone remodeling. The lack of remodeling and accumulation of crystals in the bone make it brittle and predisposes the patient to fracture.

13. c. Pseudofractures are a collection of nonmineralized osteoid (bony matrix) along the trabeculations. They are seen in many bone-softening diseases such as osteomalacia and Paget's disease. Bowing along the weight-bearing bone is another classic finding of osteomalacia. In osteomalacia, the ratio between crystal and matrix is altered, the quality is decreased, and bone becomes soft. Osteoporosis affects bone quantity only while preserving the ratio between matrix and crystal. Osteoporotic bone does not bend; it breaks.

14. c. Fever is a classic sign of infection. It is not present in gout, ankylosing spondylosis, or joint disease unless it is associated with an underlying condition. Gout and DJD are not frequently seen in the sacroiliac joints. AS typically presents bilaterally.

15. c. There are multiple causes of bone marrow hyperplasia such as hemolytic anemias, lipid storage disorders, and chronic hypoxic states. It presents on radiographs as widening of the diaphysis due to the marrow expansion.

16. a. Proper kidney function is essential to proper calcium-phosphate balance. With chronic renal disease, calcium is excreted in large amounts, leading to an overall deficit. This may result in secondary hyperparathyroidism or osteomalacia.

17. c. Hypercortisolism, whether from an endogenous or exogenous cause, will present with osteoporosis and increased fracture risk. The altered lipid metabolism will also lead to atherosclerosis and avascular necrosis.

18.   c.   Patients with malabsorption syndromes will be deficient in most nutrients. They will present with a multitude of signs of nutritional deficiencies, such as osteomalacia. Osteogenesis imperfecta and osteopetrosis present with fractures but no increased risk for AVN. Both diseases are genetic and are due to collagen abnormality and defective osteoclasts, respectively.

19.   b.   Tuberculosis usually reaches the spine via the circulation; however, it extends to multiple levels through subligamentous spread. Suppurative osteomyelitis involves only one motion segment. Paraspinal and psoas abscess develop as a result of slow development of granulomatous material. *Cellulitis* is a term used for infection of the soft tissues.

20.   b.   RSD, complex regional pain syndrome, Sudeck's atrophy, or causalgia refers to a group of neurologic syndromes characterized by severe burning pain, skin alterations, and rapid bone density changes. The exact mechanisms and etiologies are not known. Acute osteomyelitis usually presents with fever. Kohler's disease is avascular necrosis of the navicular and is more common in children.

21.   c.   The bare area is the region within the joint that is not protected by hyaline cartilage.

22.   c.   The medial tibiofemoral joint is the weight-bearing portion of the knee and is first to be affected by the degenerative process.

23.   a.   Characteristic of AS is enthesopathy and ligamentous fusion including the supraspinous and interspinous ligaments.

24.   c.   Psoriatic arthritis causes an inflammatory reaction at the synovium, including the synovium located at the tendon sheaths that lubricate the tendons at the feet and hands. Once inflamed, they give the characteristic "sausage digit" appearance.

25.   b.   The medial compartment is involved in late degenerative disease, and the axial compartment is involved with inflammatory arthritides such as rheumatoid.

26.   d.   Gout is the only periarticular disease presented. The others affect the articular components.

27.   b.   The repetitive dislocations and relocations result in mechanical destruction or erosion of the articular components in lupus.

28. d. Hypermobility through a fractured, previously ankylosed segment is the Andersson lesion that is seen in ankylosing spondylitis.

29. c. Parasyndesmophytes or nonmarginal syndesmophytes are typically seen with psoriatic arthritis.

30. c. "Carrot stick" fractures occur at the cervicothoracic junction in ankylosing spondylitis.

31. d. The mineral deposited in the insertions of tendons and ligaments is calcium hydroxyapatite. Calcium pyrophosphate is deposited in hyaline and fibrocartilage, under different pathologic circumstances. Synovial osteochondrometaplasia is the transformation of fragments of synovium into cartilage within a joint space, and sodium urate is deposited inside and outside joints in gout.

32. b. Multiple Schmorl's nodes, vertebral end-plate irregularity, anterior wedging of the bodies in the thoracolumbar region, and increased kyphosis of the thoracic spine are the classic finding of Scheuermann's disease. No history of trauma or bone mineral density reduction were given to indicate compression fracture as the diagnosis, Legg-Calve-Perthés disease is osteochondrosis of the femoral epiphysis, and Schmorl's nodes alone is an insufficient diagnosis for all of the findings described.

33. c. Although not all are found in every case, the typical findings of degenerative joint disease include nonuniform loss of joint space, subchondral sclerosis, subchondral cyst formation, osteophyte formation, and asymmetrical distribution in the body. Marginal erosions and uniform loss of joint space are generally indicative of inflammatory arthropathy.

34. d. The typical radiographic findings of ankylosing spondylitis and enteropathic arthritis include marginal syndesmophytes, which are thin, vertically oriented osseous excrescences. Spondylophytes, or osteophytes on vertebral bodies, are oriented transversely at the attachment to the body and then often curve toward the disc space. Unlike DISH, Reiter's syndrome is not associated with diabetes, although it may demonstrate large nonmarginal syndesmophytes, which could be confused for osteophytes.

35. a. Inflammatory changes lead first to erosions at the corners of the vertebral bodies that appear as lucencies known as Romanus lesions. Transient, reactive bone repair then occurs, giving the appearance of a radiopaque or "shiny" corner as seen on plain films. Marginal syndesmophytes then begin to form, and when extensive, they make the spine resemble a stalk of bamboo.

36. d. The uncinate processes form part of the anterior border of the IVF, and when they hypertrophy with degenerative disease, they grow into the IVF. The facets form part of the posterior border of the IVF, and when they hypertrophy with degenerative disease, they also grow into the IVF. The combination of these two types of degeneration leads to the characteristic "figure eight" appearance of an impinged cervical IVF.

37. b. Although usually considered with tumors, the Langerhans cell histiocytoses do not involve true metaplasia but rather an area of overgrowth of normal histiocytes. And, although usually benign appearing, eosinophilic granuloma, now often referred to as unifocal Langerhans cell histiocytosis, may appear with ill-defined borders and laminated periosteal response, mimicking an aggressive lesion.

38. c. Pneumothorax, or the presence of air in the chest cavity but outside the lung, allows demonstration of the visceral pleural membrane separate from the chest wall, and the invading air is indirectly visualized as an absence of the lung vasculature, which should normally be seen within 1 cm of the chest wall. Pneumonia is seen as an area of opacity within the lung, pneumoperitoneum is air in the abdominal cavity, and a pneumatocele is a thin-walled, gas-filled cyst within the lung parenchyma, most commonly occurring secondarily to pneumonia.

39. b. The forces involved in ankle inversion injuries pull on the fibula and may create a fracture of the proximal metadiaphyseal area. This is known as a Maisonneuve fracture. It is not infrequent for this injury to be missed at initial examination, due to the overriding severity of the ankle pain, which masks the pain below the knee unless directly palpated. A long bone tibia/fibula radiograph should be considered in these circumstances.

40. d. The described appearance is clearly aggressive in nature; therefore, osteoblastoma is an unlikely choice. Although fibrosarcoma can occur at any age, the typical appearance is of a lytic lesion with a large soft tissue mass; spiculated periosteal reaction is not common. Chondrosarcoma is typically seen in adults over 40 years of age and often demonstrates calcification within the tumor matrix.

41. c. Klippel-Feil patients are characterized by a congenital constellation of osseous abnormalities. There are typically segmentation defects in two or more cervical vertebrae. Anomalies in other organ systems are also reported. Minor cervical spine injury may result in neurologic sequelae.

42. c. Os odontodium may be asymptomatic even if unstable. Neurologic compromise, however, if present, may be devastating. Operative fixation is recommended for symptomatic cases.

43. a. Nontraumatic syringomyelia often occurs in association with Arnold-Chiari malformation. The malformation is the descent of the cerebellar tonsils below the foramen magnum. Osseous anomalies of the posterior fossa, craniovertebral junction, and spinal cord cavitation (syringomyelia) are demonstrated.

44. a. Up to 20% of all spondylolisthesis is of the dysplastic type. It is usually asymptomatic in children, becoming symptomatic in adolescence.

45. a. Astrocytoma and ependymoma are the most common intramedullary tumors. MRI and CT are capable of detecting these uncommon but morbid disorders. Extradural and intradural-extramedullary are the other categories of spinal tumors.

46. b. Spinal stenosis with neurogenic claudication is an important neurologic manifestation of this skeletal dysplasia. The most common cause of spinal stenosis is degenerative spondylosis.

47. b. Paget's disease, Hodgkin's lymphoma, and metastatic prostate carcinoma all display homogeneous osteoblastic activity that opacifies a vertebral body (ivory vertebrae). The other distractors provoke osteopenia.

48. b. Osteogenesis imperfecta is a genetic disorder characterized by reduced bone mass, bone fragility, and associated connective tissue abnormalities. Many clinical types have been described. Treatment uses bone-sclerosing agents (bisphosphonates).

49. d. Sickle cell anemia produces vaso-occlusive complications in the vertebral body, resulting in infarction. The infarction collapses the central vertebral body and end-plate, resulting in the "H" appearance.

50. d. Chordoma is a rare tumor arising from the primitive notochord. It is a locally aggressive malignant tumor with a predilection for the sacrum and clivus.

Methods of Interpretation

1. Shenton's line is used to evaluate for which of the following:
   a. hip dislocation
   b. fracture of the talar dome
   c. basilar invagination
   d. central canal stenosis

2. The acromiohumeral joint space has a range between 7 and 11 mm. A measurement less than 7 mm can indicate which of the following:
   a. dislocation
   b. joint effusion
   c. supraspinatus rupture
   d. glenohumeral degenerative joint disease

3. In measurement of the thoracic kyphosis, a line is drawn across the T1 superior endplate projecting anteriorly. A second line is drawn across the T12 inferior end-plate, again projecting anteriorly. Intersecting lines perpendicular to these lines are drawn. What angle is the limit of normal?
   a. 20
   b. 55
   c. 30
   d. 10

4. What is the mean for the basilar angle?
   a. 100 degrees
   b. 110 degrees
   c. 200 degrees
   d. 137 degrees

5. The normal measurements for the retropharyngeal and retrotracheal interspaces are _____ mm and _____ mm, respectively, in a normal adult patient.
   a. 3, 5
   b. 3, 7
   c. 7, 14
   d. 7, 21

6. Which of the following should be included in the differential diagnosis for a decreased Boehler's angle?
   a. basilar invagination
   b. calcaneal fracture
   c. platybasia
   d. scaphoid fracture

7. A 13-year-old girl who stepped into a hole reports to your office with dull left hip pain and reduced range of motion. You suspect slipped femoral capital epiphysis and take AP pelvis and left frog-leg views, which at first appear unrewarding. What measurement would be MOST helpful at this point?
   a. Klein's line
   b. Shenton's line
   c. femoral angle
   d. acetabular angle

8. Which anatomic structure(s) are BEST when assessing the presence of vertebral rotation?
   a. spinous process
   b. pedicles
   c. transverse processes
   d. vertebral body

9. A patient presenting with coxa vara demonstrates which of the following?
   a. increased femoral angle
   b. decreased femoral angle
   c. increased iliac angle
   d. decreased iliac angle

10. Boehler's angle is used to assess the integrity of which structure?
    a. acetabulum
    b. navicular
    c. calcaneus
    d. tibia

Answers

1. a. Shenton's line is a curvilinear line constructed along the undersurface of the femoral neck and continued across the joint to the inferior margin of the superior pubic ramus. This line is used to evaluate for hip dislocation, femoral neck fracture, and slipped femoral capital epiphysis.

2. c. A measurement of less than 7 mm indicates a rotator cuff tear or degenerative tendonitis caused by the unopposed action of the deltoid muscle, allowing for axial migration of the humerus.

3. b. Osteoporotic vertebral fractures are often the etiology for a thoracic kyphosis. Disturbances in pulmonary function are increased as the kyphosis exceed 55 degrees.

4. d. This angle measures the relationship between the anterior skull and the base. Beyond 152 degrees, platybasia is present with elevation of the skull base. Platybasia may be congenital or acquired.

5. d. The space between the anterior inferior corner of C2 and the posterior aspect for the pharyngeal air shadow normally measures 7 mm or less, and the space between the anterior inferior corner of C6 and the posterior aspect of the tracheal air shadow normally measures 21 mm. Enlargements of these measurements suggest a space-occupying lesion in the region (e.g., posttraumatic hematoma).

6. b. Boehler's angle (calculated by measuring the angle between lines drawn tangent to the anterior and middle tubercles of the calcaneus and the middle and posterior tubercles of the calcaneus) should measure between 28 and 40 degrees. Measurements less than 28 degrees suggest compression fracture of the calcaneus.

7. a. The best line to draw to help determine the presence or absence of SFCE is Klein's line, which may be used on AP or frog-leg views. This is a straight line tangential to the outer margin of the femoral neck. It should intersect the lateral margin of the femoral epiphysis. Although some authors do not advise placing a patient with suspected SFCE in a position of external rotation and abduction of the hip, frog-leg views are often more revealing than AP, because the usual direction of slippage of the epiphysis is posteromedial. Shenton's line may also be used but is not as specific.

8. b. Although commonly advocated by some chiropractic systems, the use of spinous processes to determine vertebral rotation is unreliable, due to common, normal asymmetry. Transverse processes are also commonly asymmetrical in size and shape. The roundness of the vertebral body would make it a poor reference to determine rotation. Nash and Moe created a system for relative measurement of vertebral rotation using the pedicles as reference points.

9. b. The normal femoral angle values range from 110 to 130 degrees. Coxa vara refers to the deformity of the femur when the angle is decreased. In the reverse situation, the term coxa valga is used. Fractures and bone-softening diseases can lead to both deformities.

10. c. Boehler's angle is used to assess the integrity of the articular surfaces of the calcaneus. The normal values range from 30 to 35 degrees. When the angle is decreased, it is a sign of burst fracture of the calcaneus. An axial (tangential) view or computed tomography can be useful to assess the location of the fracture.

Specialized Imaging Procedures

1. Which of the following is the BEST imaging modality to determine whether a spondylolysis is active or inactive?
   a. computed tomography
   b. fluoroscopy
   c. bone scan
   d. SPECT (single-photon emission computed tomography)

2. What is the BEST imaging modality for detecting the changes in the articular cartilage seen with chondromalacia patella?
   a. plain film radiography
   b. bone scan
   c. MRI (magnetic resonance imaging)
   d. CT (computed tomography)

3. Which of the following is BEST for the earliest detection of avascular necrosis?
   a. diagnostic ultrasound
   b. magnetic resonance imaging
   c. computed tomography
   d. bone scan

4. Which of the following imaging modalities does NOT give a radiation dose to the patient?
   a. magnetic resonance imaging
   b. computed tomography
   c. mammography
   d. bone scan

5. Barium is used as a contrast agent for which of the following imaging techniques?
   a. gastrointestinal imaging
   b. arthroscopy
   c. discography
   d. magnetic resonance imaging

6. Which of the following imaging modalities utilizes hydrogen protons as a signal source?
    a. magnetic resonance imaging
    b. computed tomography
    c. ultrasonography
    d. plain film radiography

7. High signal intensity in a lesion seen on T1-weighted MRI is indicative that the lesion is composed of what kind of tissue?
    a. bony
    b. cartilaginous
    c. fatty
    d. watery

8. Radionuclide bone scanning is used to help differentiate which of the following types of lesions?
    a. benign and malignant
    b. infectious and malignant
    c. ischemic and osteonecrotic
    d. trauma and malignant

9. An axial CT bone window section through L4 at the level of the pedicle reveals bilateral lucent defects with sclerotic margins. What is the MOST likely diagnosis?
    a. spondylolysis
    b. spondylosis
    c. spondylitis
    d. spondylophyte

10. A 24-year-old woman reports 3 weeks of bilateral numbness and tingling in her hand. MRI of her brain yielded numerous foci of periventricular white matter hyperintensities. What is the MOST likely diagnosis?
    a. multiple sclerosis
    b. thoracic outlet
    c. basilar arterial aneurysm
    d. Graves' disease

Answers

1. d. To describe a spondylolysis as "active" means that microfractures are still occurring, and therefore the patient has a chance to stop the pathologic process before complete fracture occurs. Neither CT nor fluoroscopy will determine the metabolic activity of a lesion. While a standard bone scan will identify metabolic activity, SPECT, which gives multiplanar bone scan–type images, is best for demonstrating the exact location of the affected area as well as its metabolic activity. MRI will demonstrate edema and other changes associated with active spondylolysis with sensitivity equal to SPECT but was not a choice offered in this example.

2. c. While direct visualization of articular cartilage is possible with both MRI and CT, MRI gives better resolution and detail. Neither bone scan nor plain film radiography will show the cartilage.

3. b. MRI can detect bone death from an avascular event in approximately 24 to 48 hours.

4. a. MRI does not provide any form of radiation to the patient.

5. a. Barium sulfate is a heavy metal solution use to outline the gastrointestinal tract. It can be administered orally for the evaluation of the esophagus and stomach and rectally for visualization of the colon. Arthroscopy is direct visualization of the joint through an incision and insertion of a small camera. Discography is a contrast study of the intervertebral disc performed using an iodinated contrast agent. Although MRI is often performed without contrast, gadolinium administered intravenously or inside the joint capsule can be used in certain situations.

6. a. CT and plain film radiography both use an x-ray source to produce an image. A high-frequency sound wave is used for ultrasonography. MRI is based on the signal or frequency emitted by hydrogen protons when submitted to a large magnetic field and radiofrequency pulses.

7. c. Fatty tissues, secondary to short relaxation times, are seen as very bright on T1-weighted MRI. One may think of T1-weighted images as "fat images" and T2-weighted images as "water images," where the brightest signal intensity represents fat for T1-weighted MRI or water for T2-weighted MRI.

8. a. Radionuclide bone scanning is a very sensitive, but poorly specific, form of imaging. It finds very subtle lesions but does not easily determine the nature of a lesion (e.g., malignancy and osteomyelitis can look identical on a bone scan) that determines the amount of vascular activity in bone. Because malignant bone lesions tend to be very vascular, they appear as "hot spots" (e.g., black) on bone scans.

9. a. The presence of bilateral defects in the pedicle on an axial CT indicates spondylolysis. Defects in the pars can simulate apophyseal joints, but joints are not at the level of the pedicle.

10. a. Multiple sclerosis (MS) is the most common demyelinating disease. MRI of the brain can confirm the diagnosis of clinically definite MS. Periventricular white matter T2 hyperintensities is the typical presentation of an MRI exam.

Section Nine Recommended Reading

Boone R: *Pocket guide to chiropractic skeletal radiography,* Norwalk, Conn, 2001, Appleton & Lange.

Bushong S: *Radiologic science for technologists: physics, biology and protection,* ed 8, St Louis, 2004, Mosby.

Guebert G, Pirtle O, Yochum T: *Essentials of diagnostic imaging,* St Louis, 1995, Mosby.

Marchiori D: *Clinical imaging: with skeletal, chest and abdomen pattern differentials,* ed 2, St Louis, 2005, Mosby.

Taylor J, Resnick D: *Skeletal imaging: atlas of the spine and extremities,* Philadelphia, 2000, WB Saunders.

Wyatt L: *Differential diagnosis of neuromusculoskeletal disorders,* Sudbury, Mass, 1994, Jones and Bartlett.

Wyatt L: *Handbook of clinical chiropractic care,* ed 2, Sudbury, Mass, 2005, Jones and Bartlett.

Yochum T, Rowe L: *Essentials of skeletal radiology: (vols 1-2),* ed 3, Baltimore, 2004, Lippincott Williams & Wilkins.

Principles of Chiropractic

Carol Claus, Carl S. Cleveland III, Jason Flanagan,
Thomas M. Redenbaugh, David Seaman

CHAPTER 64

Evolution of Chiropractic Principles

1. In 1996, the _____ was published, representing a series of statements describing the nature of chiropractic and its professional attributes. It has been widely adopted by the ACA, the ICA, the World Federation of Chiropractic, and most state chiropractic organizations, making it one of the foundational documents by which the professional organizations can agree to pursue common goals and objectives.
   a. Manga Report
   b. Agency for Health Policy and Research Report
   c. Consortium for Chiropractic Research Consensus Statement
   d. Association of Chiropractic Colleges' Chiropractic Paradigm

2. A _____ suggests that a "life force" concept explains the existence of living organisms, while _____ implies that life can be explained in strictly physical terms.
   a. vitalist/materialist
   b. spiritualist/atheist
   c. mechanist/vitalist
   d. atomist/theosophist

3. The Latin term *vis medicatrix naturae* may be defined as:
   a. healing power of nature
   b. natural vitalism
   c. innate intelligence
   d. natural state of wellness

4. The chiropractic equivalent of *vis medicatrix naturae* is defined as:
   a. healing power of nature
   b. natural vitalism
   c. innate intelligence
   d. natural state of wellness

5. The chiropractic analytic system in which clinical manifestations or symptoms are considered in terms of "zones" or "meres" representing body sections segmentally innervated by a pair of spinal nerves is termed:
    a. metamerism
    b. meta-analysis
    c. meric analysis
    d. meric recoil

6. Salon Massey Langworthy rejected Palmer's "bone out of place" concept and presented his theory known as:
    a. axonal aberration-trophic model
    b. decreased axoplasmic transport model
    c. visceral disease simulation model
    d. motion restriction–joint fixation model

7. Choose the traditional chiropractic philosophical doctrine that focuses on the modulating function of the nervous system in the self-healing of the human organism.
    a. rationalism
    b. vitalism
    c. holism
    d. naturalism

8. An early manual diagnostic procedure, which followed a tender nerve from its spinal origin to some inflammatory/pathologic zone or from a tender inflammatory zone back to its spinal exit, was known as which of the following?
    a. kinetic palpation
    b. motion tracing
    c. nerve tracing
    d. malpositional palpation

9. Who pioneered the use of thermography in chiropractic?
    a. Langworthy
    b. B. J. Palmer
    c. Roentgen
    d. Korr

10. The practice of chiropractic includes:
    a. establishing a diagnosis
    b. facilitating neurologic and biomechanical integrity through appropriate case management
    c. promoting health
    d. a, b, and c

11. Spinography or weight-bearing x-rays were first introduced to the profession around 1910 by:
    a. D. D. Palmer
    b. Virgil Strang
    c. B. J. Palmer
    d. Leon Coelho

12. B. J. Palmer posited that the adjustment functioned to relieve pressure on spinal nerves, which allowed for the appropriate flow of mental impulses, an expression of innate intelligence. Which of the following is consistent with Palmer's view of the nature of innate intelligence?
    a. electrical impulse or action potential
    b. spiritual force
    c. quantum mechanical expression of intelligence
    d. energy that is similar to the "Qi" that is posited to flow along the acupuncture meridians

13. Which of the following early chiropractic authors perpetuated the theory that subluxations would reduce the flow of mental impulses from brain cell to tissue cell?
    a. Dr. Solon Langworthy
    b. Dr. Ralph W. Stephenson
    c. Dr. Oakley Smith
    d. none of the above

14. Which popular theory of the nervous system was in use at the time Palmer developed the theory that subluxations acted to compress spinal nerves and cause nerve interference?
    a. neuron theory
    b. synaptic theory
    c. reticular theory
    d. axoplasmic theory

15. From a review of B. J. Palmer's writings, it has been suggested that his primary reason to hold firm to innate philosophy was to:
    a. contrast chiropractic and medicine
    b. provide a legal defense
    c. reject contemporary mechanistic theory
    d. prove the validity of subluxation

16. What discipline did D. D. Palmer attempt to merge with science that became the early foundation of vitalism?
    a. osteopathy
    b. occultism
    c. metaphysics
    d. naprapathy

17. D. D. Palmer defined "intelligence that controls all bodily functions" as:
    a. individualized
    b. personalized
    c. rationalized
    d. generalized

Answers

1.   d.   The paradigm's significance is its utility as a platform for communicating the identity of chiropractic. As a position statement, it holds wide endorsement from within the profession. Representing a consensus of the chiropractic academic leaderships and built on a foundation that chiropractic is a science, a philosophy, and an art, the paradigm establishes the profession's purpose: *to optimize health*, its principle: *the body's innate recuperative power is affected by and integrated through the nervous system*, and its practice: *establish a diagnosis, facilitate neurologic and biomechanical integrity through appropriate chiropractic case management, and promote health*. For additional reading related to the ACC Paradigm, see Chapter 2, Redwood and Cleveland III, *Fundamentals of Chiropractic,* Mosby, 2003.

2.   a.   *Vitalism* is an explanatory model that suggests the body requires a "vital energy," something greater than physical and chemical processes to function. In chiropractic, proponents of the vitalist approach attribute the effects of adjustment or manipulation to restoring the flow of life force (i.e., innate intelligence) as it may be affected by correction of vertebral subluxation, whereas those advocating a materialist (or *mechanist)* position attribute the effect of manipulation to physical phenomena, such as reducing nerve compression, increasing joint range of motion or affecting aberrant spinal reflexes. It is noted that fundamental chiropractic principle acknowledges that the body's innate recuperative power (vitalism) is affected by and integrated through the nervous system and that the biomechanical manifestations (mechanism) of vertebral subluxation adversely affect the expression of nerve function and good health.

3.   a.   V*is medicatrix naturae* means the "healing power of nature." *Vis* = energy, strength or force; *medicatrix* = medicine or healing; *naturae* = nature.
      This is expressed in the context of the body's inherent ability to heal and restore health. This phrase is equivalent to the concept of "innate intelligence" or "wisdom of the body."

4. c. Innate intelligence refers to the inborn or intrinsic biologic ability of an organism to react physiologically to the changing condition of the external and internal environments; this term is also referred to as the *wisdom of the body* or equivalently as the *vis medicatrix naturae (healing power of nature)*. It is a fundamental chiropractic principle that the body is a self-regulating and self-healing organism and that the body's innate recuperative power is affected by and integrated through the nervous system.

5. c. The reference to "mere" or "meric" pertains to the term *segment*. In this context, *meric analysis* (also termed *neuromeric analysis*), refers to the clinical assessment process that acknowledges the body's characteristic *segmental innervation* as observed and reflected in the *dermatome, myotome,* and *autonomic nervous system charts.* Correlation of specific vertebral segment dysfunction, associated spinal cord segments (spinal cord and spinal nerves), and symptoms observed within the distribution of segmentally innervated pathways is termed *meric* or *neuromeric analysis.*

6. d. Langworthy suggested that subluxation did not necessitate a fixed or abnormal position of a vertebra. He thought that the difference between a "simple" subluxation and a "normal" vertebra would be its field of motion and the center of the field of motion.

7. b. Vitalism was referred to by Dr. Palmer as the body's *innate intelligence.* It is a philosophy relating to the body having an innate capacity to heal and resist disease.

8. c. This was an early method of analysis or diagnosis of autonomic dysfunction. Other early methods included static palpation and manual palpation of heat differentials known as "hot boxes" as further indicators of disturbance of autonomic tone.

9. b. Thermography was introduced into the chiropractic profession as a method of detecting vertebral subluxation by B. J. Palmer in 1924.

10. d. Chiropractic has evolved from the time of D. D. Palmer into a complete health system that recognizes the chiropractor as a primary health care physician who is able to diagnose, treat, and recommend strategies that promote health and the prevention of disease.

11. c. Spinography is the term for radiographs taken while the patient is standing upright. B. J. Palmer pioneered its use as one of the first purchasers of x-ray equipment sometime between 1908 and 1911, installing a Sheidel-Western at Palmer School of Chiropractic.

12. b. B. J. Palmer's view of innate intelligence, which is expressed in the human body via mental impulses, is distinctly spiritual. We are told this throughout the writings of Palmer in his so-called Green Books.

13. d. Despite what many might think, Stephenson did not advocate the notion that subluxations reduce the flow of mental impulses/innate intelligence. On page 275 of the *Chiropractic Text Book*, he states: "The writer (Stephenson) is emphasizing these points, for it is the curse of Chiropractic, one of the things that have done much to corrupt the science, that students of Chiropractic will persistently forget that the nerve cell is a living thing, very sensitive and delicate, and mental impulses are immaterial messages and not a material something which ca be damned back in the nerve by an interference, as by the flood."

14. c. There is no such thing as the synaptic or axoplasmic theory. The neuron theory was put forth by Santiago Ramon y Cajal, which posited that nerve cells were individual units and they communicated with one another via their close contact, eventually referred to as a synapse. The term "reticulum" refers to a netlike structure. The reticular theory posited that the anatomy of the nervous system was much like that of our circulatory system, a continuous network. When describing the nervous system from the perspective of the reticulary theory, neuroanatomists liken the nervous system to a syncytium or a multinucleated mass of cytoplasm that is not separated into individual cells. With this view of the nervous system in mind, it is not surprising how our original chiropractic theories were developed.

15. b. B. J. Palmer wrote a pamphlet just before his death warning readers that "straying" from innate philosophy would "spell the very death" of chiropractic.

16. c. As a student of metaphysics, D. D. Palmer attempted to merge science and metaphysics while practicing magnetic healing around 1890.

17. a. In his 1910 text, D. D. Palmer defined innate as "the individualized intelligence which runs all the functions of the body."

Concepts of Subluxation and Spinal Lesions

1. Which component of the hierarchic organization of the vertebral subluxation complex is the "central goal" in chiropractic clinical practice?
    a. neuropathology
    b. myopathology
    c. kinesiopathology
    d. histopathology

2. Which one of the following statements concerning joint mobilization is NOT true?
    a. joint mobilization restores normal joint function
    b. joint mobilization restores normal joint physiology
    c. joint mobilization restores joint histologic architecture
    d. joint mobilization restores cross-bridging of collagen fibers

3. What is the central theme of neurodystrophic hypothesis, which can modify the immune system and alter nerve function?
    a. chemical irritation
    b. lowered tissue resistance
    c. converging pain fibers
    d. referred pain

4. According to the intervertebral encroachment theory, which one of the following clinical signs is NOT the result of decreased neural activity?
    a. numbness
    b. muscle weakness
    c. dry skin
    d. vasoconstriction

5. Which one of the following is a long lever arm procedure description?
    a. force is applied distal to the axis of rotation
    b. force is intended to increase capsular elasticity
    c. force produces a greater translatory glide
    d. force is minimally absorbed by the soft tissues

6. Which one of the following is NOT a component of the nerve complex?
   a. nerve root
   b. posterior root ganglion
   c. intervertebral foramen
   d. dura mater

7. An infectious process resulting in ligamentous laxity and atlantoaxial subluxation, where patients complain of unrelenting throat and neck pain is known as:
   a. Grisel's syndrome
   b. juvenile onset diabetes mellitus
   c. mucopolysaccharidosis type VII
   d. Reiter's syndrome

8. Mild neurologic complications occur secondary to cervical manipulation in 1 of _____ cases.
   a. 400
   b. 4,000
   c. 40,000
   d. 400,000

9. Which one of the following statements is NOT true of the helper T cell response?
   a. B cells proliferate and become plasma cells
   b. T cells synthesize antibodies
   c. antibodies are Y-shaped proteins
   d. the shaft of the antibody attaches to macrophages

10. Which one of the following statements about axoplasmic transport is TRUE?
    a. anterograde transport moves products toward cell bodies
    b. retrograde transport moves products toward the cell terminals
    c. intracellular movement in neurons is similar to that in prokaryotic cells
    d. whether fast or slow, axoplasmic transport constituents move in both directions inside nerve fibers

11. Which researcher is credited with laying the groundwork for the subluxation theory that chiropractors call the "proprioceptive insult hypothesis"?
    a. Irvin Korr
    b. Major DeJarnette
    c. C. O. Watkins
    d. Willard Carver

12. Which of the following is the appropriate term to use when spinal dysfunction leads to changes in cardiovascular function?
    a. proprioceptive insult
    b. somatosomatic reflex
    c. somatovisceral reflex
    d. viscerosomatic reflex

13. Which of the following terms BEST describes the nature of the vertebral subluxation?
    a. lesion or condition that chiropractors adjust
    b. theory of spinal dysfunction
    c. spinal misalignment
    d. fixated spinal joint

14. Pain and inflammation are typically associated with spinal subluxation. What is the term used to describe the state in which C-fibers and local tissue cells perpetuate inflammation?
    a. acute inflammation
    b. chronic inflammation
    c. neurogenic inflammation
    d. reflex sympathetic dystrophy

15. Which neurologic concept related to vertebral subluxation is INACCURATE and MISLEADING?
    a. neurocompression
    b. altered afferent input
    c. somatovisceral
    d. proprioceptive insult hypothesis

16. Which of the following are considered to be subluxation syndromes?
    a. intervertebral disc syndrome
    b. sacroiliac syndrome
    c. facet syndrome
    d. all of the above

17. Which term is used to describe a putative mechanism by which a neurocompressive spinal subluxation will influence the nervous system?
    a. altered axoplasmic transport
    b. proprioceptive irritation
    c. somatovisceral reflex
    d. disc herniation

18. Which is the appropriate term to describe the physiologic nature of pain caused by sacroiliac dysfunction/subluxation?
    a. neuropathic pain
    b. nociceptive pain
    c. mechanical pain
    d. nonspecific back pain

19. Which of the following terms is used to describe a physiologic mechanism by which spinal subluxation can influence the central nervous system in a general fashion and lead to nonpain symptoms such as clumsiness, depression, and fatigue?
    a. brain hibernation
    b. psychosomatic responses
    c. neurodystrophy
    d. dystopia

20. Which of the following is the MOST accurate statement to describe a reduction of pain after a spinal adjustment?
    a. a subluxation has been corrected
    b. mechanoreceptors were stimulated, leading to segmental nociceptive inhibition
    c. nerve interference has been corrected
    d. the chiropractic encounter can often result in an analgesic response

21. Aberrant activity of the sympathetic nervous system associated with trauma at various spinal levels has been implicated as centrally excitatory in somatovisceral reflex disorders resulting in end-organ dysfunction. Choose the name associated MOST with this clinical entity.
    a. viscerosomatic reflex
    b. nerve compression hypothesis
    c. somatosomatic reflex
    d. facilitative lesion

22. Palmer's earliest concept of subluxation etiology centered upon this idea.
    a. joint fixation
    b. nerve compression
    c. aberrant motion
    d. hypermobility

23. Name the mechanism associated with articular structural dysfunction capable of mimicking the signs and symptoms of internal organ disease.
    a. viscerosomatic reflex
    b. facilitative lesion
    c. simulated visceral disease model
    d. primary visceral dysfunction

24. Which is NOT considered to be a result of joint fixation?
   a. change in nociceptive reflexes
   b. pain
   c. regenerative change
   d. muscle spasticity

25. The *neuropathophysiologic* component of the Faye model of vertebral subluxation complex is MOST associated with:
   a. irritation/compression
   b. muscle spasticity
   c. joint hypomobility
   d. histamine/prostaglandin changes

26. Which of the terms below would NOT be used in a *static* definition of vertebral subluxation?
   a. retrolisthesis
   b. extension malposition
   c. segmental hypomobility
   d. altered intersegmental spacing

27. Which one of these x-ray lines of mensuration is most often used to assess the spinal lesion known as spondylolisthesis?
   a. Chamberlain's method
   b. gravitational line of L3
   c. McNab's line
   d. Meyerding's classification

28. Cervical subluxation at what level is most often associated with cerebrovascular accident or stroke?
   a. C0-C1
   b. C3-C4
   c. C5-C6
   d. C7-T1

29. Name the third stage of spinal degeneration.
   a. stabilization
   b. hypomobility
   c. instability
   d. dysfunction

30. Which concept below would be considered a *trophic model* of subluxation?
   a. fixation from adhesion
   b. aberrant axoplasmic transport
   c. motion segment buckling
   d. spinal cord traction

31. The component of vertebral subluxation complex (VSC) that is most directly associated with *hypomobility* is termed:
    a. neuropathology
    b. kinesiopathology
    c. myopathology
    d. histopathology

32. The vertebral subluxation complex (VSC) component most directly associated with the concept of *facilitation* or sustained receptor hyperactivity is:
    a. neuropathophysiology
    b. kinesiopathology
    c. myopathology
    d. histopathology

33. Which one of the vertebral subluxation complex (VSC) components would MOST DIRECTLY be identified with inflammation and swelling associated with joint dysfunction?
    a. neuropathophysiology
    b. kinesiopathology
    c. myopathology
    d. histopathology

34. The hypothesis in which subluxation is proposed to irritate somatic afferent nerves resulting in the mimicry of visceral disease is referred to as:
    a. decreased axoplasmic transport
    b. neurodystrophic
    c. disease simulation model
    d. joint dysafferentation

35. According to what hypothesis, spinal biomechanical insult to nerves may affect intraneuronal axoplasmic transport mechanisms and, in turn, affect the quality of trophic influences and molecular (chemical) changes in the cells?
    a. nerve compression
    b. aberrant spinal reflex
    c. somatosomatic reflex
    d. neurodystrophic

36. Which subluxation hypothesis is BEST described by the phrase "lowered tissue resistance is the cause of disease?"
    a. decreased axoplasmic transport
    b. neurodystrophic
    c. disease simulation model
    d. joint dysafferentation

37. The earliest of chiropractic explanations or hypotheses regarding the proposed effects of vertebral subluxation on nerve function and chiropractic case management is the:
    a. nerve compression
    b. aberrant spinal reflex
    c, somatosomatic reflex
    d. decreased axoplasmic transport

38. It has been demonstrated that prolonged nerve excitability, sustained hyperactivity of afferent receptors, and aberrant reflex response were associated with movement restriction in the spine. It is proposed that joint subluxation can alter spinal reflexes adversely. The heightened reflexive reactivity at spinal cord levels associated with palpable spinal characteristics is BEST termed:
    a. visceral disease simulation
    b. aberrant spinal reflex
    c. facilitated lesion
    d. decreased axoplasmic transport

39. Identify the component of the PARTS acronym that is most closely associated with the *histopathologic* component of vertebral subluxation complex.
    a. pain and tenderness
    b. asymmetry
    c. range of motion abnormality
    d. tissue tone, texture, and temperature abnormality

40. Identify the component of the PARTS acronym that is most closely associated with the *neuropathophysiologic* component of vertebral subluxation complex (VSC).
    a. pain and tenderness
    b. asymmetry
    c. range of motion abnormality
    d. tissue tone, texture, and temperature abnormality

41. All of the following are associated with segmental dysfunction EXCEPT:
    a. loss of normal motion
    b. signs of neuromuscular dysfunction
    c. misalignment of the motion segment
    d. point tenderness or altered pain threshold

42. According to Gatterman, this was the first person to describe the characteristics of the subluxation as "...a lessened motion of the joints, by slight change in position of the articulating bones and pain... ."
    a. D. D. Palmer
    b. Andrew Still
    c. Hieronymus
    d. Galen

43. An aggregate of signs and symptoms that relate to pathophysiology or dysfunction of spinal and pelvic motion segments or to peripheral joints is:
    a. subluxation complex
    b. subluxation syndrome
    c. manipulable subluxation
    d. vertebral subluxation

44. The unified model of vertebral subluxation complex does NOT include which phase?
    a. phase of segmental dysfunction
    b. phase of rehabilitation
    c. phase of instability
    d. phase of stabilization

45. The neurodystrophic hypothesis states that neural dysfunction is stressful to the visceral and other body structures and this lowered tissue resistance:
    a. can modify the nonspecific immune responses
    b. can modify the specific immune responses
    c. can modify the nonspecific and specific immune responses
    d. cannot modify the immune response and disease ensues

46. Which two components of the vertebral subluxation complex are common to concepts of subluxation? (select 2)
    a. kinesiopathology
    b. myopathology
    c. histopathology
    d. neuropathology

47. What happens to the diameter of the IVF during flexion and extension?
    a. the IVF increases with extension and decreases with flexion
    b. the IVF increases with flexion and decreases with extension
    c. the IVF decreases with either flexion or extension
    d. there is no change in the diameter of the IVF during flexion or extension

48. Tropism refers to an anomalous condition in which:
    a. the superior and inferior endplates of a vertebra form a 60-degree angle
    b. there is fusion of the vertebrae from T10 to T12
    c. there is asymmetrical articular facings of the facets
    d. there is fusion of the sacrum and L5

49. Clinical features of facet syndrome usually present with all of the following EXCEPT:
    a. hip pain
    b. buttock pain
    c. calf pain
    d. back pain

50. The mobility of a given motion unit (segment) that is excessive but not so extreme as to be life-threatening or require surgery BEST describes:
    a. hypermobility
    b. hypomobility
    c. instability
    d. double-jointed

Answers

1. c. Restoration of motion is the central goal of chiropractic clinical practice.

2. d. Joint mobilization disrupts collagen fiber cross-bridging, where adhesions develop following the inflammatory process as the result of trauma to the joint.

3. b. Lowered tissue resistance is the result of neural dysfunction; stress to viscera and body structures modifies the immune response and alters the function of nerves.

4. d. Pressure on the contents of the intervertebral foramen produces either an increase or decrease in neural activity. Vasoconstriction is a sign of increased neural activity.

5. a. All of the descriptions are for short lever arm adjusting except choice "a." Applying a force distal to the axis of rotation is a long lever arm procedure, much like many osteopathic osseous manipulation procedures.

6. c. A nerve complex is composed of a nerve root, dorsal root ganglion, spinal nerve, and connective tissue covering.

7. a. Grisel's syndrome is a form of compressive myelopathy. Differential diagnoses include Down syndrome and os odontoideum.

8. c. A survey among the Swiss Society for Manual Medicine revealed mild neurologic complications occurring secondary to cervical manipulation in one of 40,000 cases. Serious complications occurred in 1 of 400,000 cervical spine manipulations.

9. b. T cell lymphocytes destroy viral or malignant cells. Helper T cells secrete substances to mobilize other components of the immune system.

10. d. Anterograde transport moves products from the cell body to the cell terminals, as opposed to retrograde axoplasmic transport that moves products from the cell terminals to the cell body. Intracellular movement is similar to that seen in eukaryotic cells.

11. a. Irvin Korr, PhD, was one of the pioneering researchers for the osteopathic profession and part of his research focus was proprioceptive mechanisms.

12. c. Students often find that the terminology used to describe spinal reflexes is confusing. Spinal tissues are somatic tissues, and so when nociceptive irritation within spinal tissues leads to a visceral response, the term *somatovisceral reflex* is often used.

13. b. The term *vertebral subluxation* represents a chiropractic theory of spinal dysfunction. In this context, subluxation is posited as a lesion or condition that is corrected by adjusting/manipulation. However, an appropriate operational definition of subluxation has yet to be developed. Vertebral subluxation is also used in a general sense by chiropractors when referring to a broad range of spinal pathology.

14. c. When C-fibers (group IV afferents and gray rami) and local tissue cells participate in driving the inflammatory process, it is referred to as "neurogenic inflammation." Activated group IV afferents release substance P locally, which excites local inflammatory cells to release their inflammatory mediators. Group IV afferents also ultimately lead to the excitation of gray rami, which subsequently perpetuates group IV excitation. Gray rami release catecholamines and prostaglandins in the region of the group IV afferent, which leads to additional excitation and substance P release.

15. d. The term "insult" connotes a noxious stimulus of sorts. Proprioceptors, or mechanoreceptors, as they are most commonly referred to today, are not activated by noxious stimuli. Only nociceptors encode noxious stimuli, so the term "nociceptive insult hypothesis" would be more appropriate.

16. d. The intervertebral disc syndrome, sacroiliac syndrome, facet syndrome, and costovertebral joint syndrome are all considered subluxation syndromes. This illustrates how chiropractors use the term "subluxation" as a general descriptor for dysfunction of joint complex structures. The use of "subluxation" in this fashion is identical to the use of the term "mechanical pain" that has become popularized in recent years.

17. a. Axoplasmic transport is a complex process that brings substances from the neuron cell body to the peripheral and central terminals of sensory neurons and to the peripheral terminals of motor neurons. However, to date, no research has demonstrated changes in axoplasmic flow with spinal or soft tissue manipulation.

18. b. Nociceptive pain refers to any pain that is caused by the damage or irritation of somatic or visceral tissues. Neuropathic pain is that which results from nervous system injury, either peripheral neuronal injury or spinal cord injury. Mechanical pain is a general term that is used to describe pain that is not caused by a "red flag" condition. Nonspecific back pain is used synonymously with mechanical pain.

19. a. Brain hibernation, cerebral dysfunction syndrome, and diachisis are terms used to describe a theory in which a reduction of cerebral blood flow can occur in regions of the brain that are healthy and intact. Two medical doctors are credited with the development of this theory. Each noticed that spinal manipulation was able to improve nonpain symptoms such as dizziness, fatigue, slurred speech, glare distress, and many others. Chiropractors can suggest that spinal dysfunction/subluxation may lead to an alteration of cerebral blood flow and promote brain hibernation.

20. d. To date, we do not specifically know why pain reduction occurs after an adjustment. Numerous factors can lead to an analgesic response, such as patient expectations, stress reduction, and the somatosensory stimulation that occurs with an adjustment; however, we do not know which is most active in a given patient encounter.

21. d. A "facilitated" segment may be the source of sympathetic nervous system signals. The irritable spinal cord segment causes a greater response to a stimulus than that degree of stimulation would ordinarily warrant. *Facil* is a French word that means "easy." In this case, think of it as being "easy" to stimulate the nerve.

22. b. Palmer's original theory grew out of a *static* model of subluxation, a positional, bone on bone theory of compression. The dynamic, or *motion,* theories came later.

23. c. Sensory fibers that carry nociceptive impulses from somatic structures converge with sensory fibers that transmit stimuli from visceral structures in the same neuronal pool. It may be impossible to distinguish signs and symptoms that mimic visceral disease from their somatic neural origin.

24. c. Joint fixation results in degenerative change on many levels, but it is not an agent of regeneration.

25. a. Irritation, compression, and decreased axoplasmic transport are ways in which subluxation causes neuropathophysiologic change in the Faye model. Muscle spasticity, joint hypomobility, and histamine/prostaglandin changes are associated with myopathological, kinesiopathological, and biochemical changes, respectively.

26. c. Hypomobility is a concept associated with the *dynamic* definition of subluxation, as it pertains to joint motion. Static definitions refer to position and do not include motion attributes.

27. d. Meyerding's determines the degree of anterior displacement in a spondylolisthesis. Chamberlain's, gravitational line, and McNab's relate to sacroiliac motion, flexion-extension of the lumbar spine, and imbrication of the zygapophyseal joints, respectively.

28. a. The mechanism of stroke from cervical adjustment relates to injury of the vertebral artery as it passes through foramen transversarii in the upper cervical area. Hard rotation may traumatize the artery at C0-C1 or C1-C2.

29. a. In the first phase, there is dysfunctional movement, which becomes increasingly mobile and unstable in phase two. In the third phase, restabilization takes place by means of ankylosis or fusion of the hypermobile or unstable segments.

30. b. Fixation, buckling, and traction are structural concepts, while axoplasmic transport is the movement of trophic substance through the axon for growth, development, and maintenance functions in the end organs.

31. b. In chiropractic, *kinesiopathology* is a component of VSC associated with hypomobility, diminished or absent joint play, or compensatory segmental kinematic hypermobility. Lack of appropriate joint motion is proposed to be associated with nociceptive and mechanoreceptive reflex activity. In addition, an early manifestation of chronically fixated vertebral articulations is the shortening of ligaments as an adaptation to limited range of motion.

32. a. Biomechanical dysfunction is proposed to affect neural function in three forms, individually or in combination, to include:
    (1) *Irritation (sustained hyperactivity)* of nerve receptors or nerve tissue resulting in *facilitation* (lowering threshold of excitability of afferent nerve cells, i.e., dysafferentation)
    (2) *Compression* or mechanical insult (pressure, stretching, angulation, or distortion) to neural elements in or about the intervertebral foramina

(3) *Decreased axoplasmic transport* affecting intra-axonal transport mechanisms for neurotrophic substance to end organs. Such decrease affects development, growth, and maintenance of cells or structures dependent on this *trophic* (growth) influence expressed via the nerve. More specifically, in the context of this question, joint fixation (hypomobility) is proposed to produce *facilitation* or the characteristics of the *facilitated lesion* resulting in sustained hyperexcitability of afferent neurons, thus contributing to altered efferent responses, to include excitation of alpha-motoneurons (resulting in muscle spasm) and excitation of preganglionic sympathetic neurons (resulting in vasoconstriction). For additional reading related to the ACC Paradigm, see Chapter 8, Redwood and Cleveland III, *Fundamentals of Chiropractic*, Mosby, 2003.

33. d. The histopathologic component is associated with inflammation, including pain, heat, and swelling, and may result from trauma or joint dysfunction or occur as part of the repair process.

34. c. Somatic dysfunction or vertebral subluxation may often simulate, or mimic, the symptoms of visceral disease. The concept of visceral disease simulation proposes that afferent nociceptive signals generated from dysfunctional spinal joints (or from deep somatic structures) can often result in referred pain patterns and equally misleading autonomic reflex responses. These reflex responses have been shown to simulate (rather than cause) true visceral disease due to these somatic afferent neuronal convergence on the same segmental spinal cord neuronal pools that also receive afferent input from segmentally innervated internal organs. The *visceral disease simulation hypothesis* is offered as a potential explanation for certain patient response to perceived visceral conditions under chiropractic case management.

35. d. The neurodystrophic hypothesis is the proposition that neural dysfunction is stressful to viscera and other body structures, which may modify immune responses and alter trophic function of involved nerves. In the most basic form, the concept may be reduced to D. D. Palmer's assertion that "lowered tissue resistance is the cause of disease."

36. b. The neurodystrophic hypothesis proposes that interference with the quality or quantity of axonal transport mechanisms adversely affects conveyance of trophic substances that are responsible for growth, development, and maintenance of the end organs (target cells). *Trophic* refers to growth. Depriving an end organ structure of trophic materials results in lack of growth or atrophy of these structures.

37. a. Among D. D. Palmer's early theories, he proposed, "The relationship existing between bones and nerves…especially those of the vertebral column, cannot be displaced without impinging upon adjacent nerves." Although contemporary research has demonstrated that other mechanisms of spinal dysfunction may be responsible for inducing neuronal disturbances, the clinical significance of *nerve compression* should not be discounted.

38. c. The clinical research of Irwin Korr provides evidence of heightened reflexive reactivity at spinal cord levels association with palpable spinal lesions (movement restriction) and observed reliable increases in galvanic skin response readings at specific cord levels. This is termed *facilitation*, the *facilitated segment*, or the *facilitated lesion*. Normalization of segmental spinal restrictions is proposed to address the prolonged and sustained hyperreflexive activity.

39. d. As with other aspects of patient examination, the doctor of chiropractic uses observation, palpation, percussion, and auscultation when identifying the adjustive lesion (subluxation). The the acronym PARTS provides the clinician with a pattern of five diagnostic criteria (Pain and tenderness; Asymmetry; Range-of-motion abnormality; Tissue tone, texture, and temperature abnormality; and Special tests) for identifying joint subluxation or dysfunction. The *histopathologic* component of VSC is associated with tissue response to injury, including the characteristics of inflammation, including pain, heat, and swelling, and can result from trauma or joint dysfunction or occur as part of the repair process.

40. a. As with other aspects of patient examination, the doctor of chiropractic uses observation, palpation, percussion, and auscultation when identifying the adjustive lesion (subluxation). The the acronym PARTS provides the clinician with a pattern of five diagnostic criteria (Pain and tenderness; Asymmetry; Range-of-motion abnormality; Tissue tone, texture, and temperature abnormality; and Special tests) for identifying joint subluxation or dysfunction. The *neuropathophysiologic* component of VSC is associated with the first component of the PARTS acronym, pain and tenderness.

41. c. Leach defines *segmental dysfunction* as a common spinal lesion recognized by lessened or otherwise altered mobility, altered pressure threshold to pain, and signs of neuromuscular dysfunction.

42. c. Hieronymus identified these characteristics in 1746. D. D. Palmer founded chiropractic in 1895. Andrew Still founded the principles of osteopathy based on treating the body to improve its natural functions without drugs around 1889. Galen of Pergamum (ca. 130 to 200), a Greek physician considered second only to Hippocrates, did not comment on subluxation.

43. b. Leach defines *subluxation syndrome* as an aggregate of signs and symptoms that relate to pathophysiology or dysfunction of spinal and pelvic motion segments or to peripheral joints.

44. b. The unified model for phases of vertebral subluxation complex includes only three phases: the phase of segmental dysfunction, the phase of instability, and the phase of stabilization.

45. c. The neurodystrophic hypothesis is aimed at the interaction between the central nervous system function and immunity. Research has substantiated that neural dysfunction is stressful to the visceral and other body structures, and this "lowered tissue resistance" can modify the nonspecific and specific immune responses and alter the trophic function of the involved nerves.

46. a and d. In the integrated physiologic model of the vertebral subluxation complex, common to all concepts of subluxation is some form of kinesiologic dysfunction and some form of neurologic involvement.

47. b. During flexion of the spine, the diameter of the intervertebral foramen increases slightly as the inferior facets of the superior vertebra move away from the superior facets of the inferior vertebra. During extension, the facets move toward each other and the diameter decreases.

48. c. Tropism refers to an anomalous condition in which the articular facings of the lumbar facets are asymmetrical. The upper lumbar facets are normally situated more in a sagittal orientation, while the lower facets assume a more coronal presentation.

49. c. Classic lumbar facet pain includes hip, buttock, and back pain. Calf pain is part of a differential diagnosis that helps eliminate facet involvement and favors disc problems.

50. a. The terms *instability* and *hypermobility* are not synonymous. The clinical and therapeutic approaches to treatment will not be the same. Instability is loss of the ability of the spine under physiologic loads to maintain relationships between vertebrae in such a way that there is neither damage nor subsequent irritation to the spinal cord; this means there is damage and may require surgery.

Basic Science Concepts in Chiropractic

1. The posterior aspect of the intervertebral discs is innervated by:
    a. recurrent meningeal
    b. medial branch of the posterior primary division (dorsal ramus)
    c. the lateral branch of the anterior primary division
    d. vagus nerve

2. Three pathways for pain are considered discriminative. The primary of these pathways for the transmission of nociception is:
    a. paleospinothalamic tract
    b. neospinothalamic tract
    c. nociceptothalamic tract
    d. thalamoreticular tract

3. Reliability is a measurement of all of the following EXCEPT:
    a. reproducibility
    b. accuracy
    c. consistency
    d. sameness

4. Algometry refers to the measurement of:
    a. angles
    b. temperature
    c. pain
    d. force

5. Which type of complex nerve endings is MOST common within the joint capsules and nearby ligaments?
    a. Golgi tendon organs
    b. muscle spindles
    c. Ruffini-type endings
    d. coiled end organs

6. According to Giles, which of the following structures is NOT innervated?
   a. zygapophyseal joint
   b. synovial fold
   c. ligamentum flavum
   d. intervertebral disc

7. The process whereby macromolecules are conveyed through the axon from the nerve cell body to the terminal ending is termed:
   a. axoplasmic transport
   b. neurodystrophic process
   c. disease simulation
   d. joint dysafferentation

8. What materials are manufactured in the nerve cell body and are transported via intra-axonal transport mechanisms to the neuron's terminal ending for liberation into the synaptic gap? Such materials then influence the growth, development, and maintenance of the innervated tissues or end organs supplied by the nerve.
   a. endorphin
   b. nociceptive irritant
   c. bradykinin
   d. trophic

9. Reflexes whose afferent and efferent pathways are somatic nerve fibers would be termed:
   a. somatosomatic
   b. viscerovisceral
   c. somatovisceral
   d. viscerosomatic

10. Reflexes whose afferent and efferent pathways are visceral sensory fibers and autonomic nerve fibers would be termed:
    a. somatosomatic
    b. viscerovisceral
    c. somatovisceral
    d. viscerosomatic

11. Reflexes whose afferents are somatic sensory fibers and whose efferents are autonomic efferent fibers are termed:
    a. somatosomatic
    b. viscerovisceral
    c. somatovisceral
    d. viscerosomatic

12. Reflexes whose afferents are visceral sensory fibers and whose efferents are somatic motor nerve fibers are termed:
    a. somatosomatic
    b. viscerovisceral
    c. somatovisceral
    d. viscerosomatic

13. An explanation for the adaptive behavior used to distract the nervous system from the perception of pain through such acts as rubbing an elbow that has just been bumped, scratching an itch, or "shaking off" a traumatized joint is:
    a. stimulus-induced parasthesia
    b. somatosympathetic reflex
    c. efferent inhibition
    d. gate-control theory

14. What is the relationship in size of the cervical intervertebral foramina to the nerves and nerve roots in that region?
    a. nerves and nerve roots completely fill the anteroposterior diameter of the cervical IVF
    b. the IVF is 5 to 6 times the diameter of the spinal nerves
    c. nerves and nerve roots completely fill the vertical diameter of the cervical IVF
    d. the IVF is approximately 12 times the diameter of the spinal nerves

15. Sharpless, in an effort to test the vulnerability of spinal nerve roots to compression, demonstrated that what amount of pressure could decrease conduction up to 60% in 30 minutes?
    a. 5 mm Hg
    b. 10 mm Hg
    c. 20 mm Hg
    d. 30 mm Hg

16. According to this law, bone is shaped by the forces applied to it, or by the lack of force applied during immobilization of a joint.
    a. Newton's law
    b. Hilton's law
    c. gravitational law
    d. Wolff's law

17. A nerve that includes preganglionic and postganglionic fibers would be:
    a. visceral afferent
    b. visceral efferent
    c. somatic afferent
    d. somatic efferent

18. These two vertebral ligaments are likely the MOST stabilizing in preventing or decreasing hyperflexion in the cervical spine.
    a. ligamentum nuchae/ligamentum flavum
    b. anterior longitudinal/posterior longitudinal ligaments
    c. supraspinous ligament/ligamentum nuchae
    d. intertransverse ligament/anterior longitudinal ligament

19. Which one of the following vertebral ligaments contains a predominance of elastic fibrous connective tissue?
    a. supraspinous
    b. intervertebral disc
    c. posterior longitudinal
    d. ligamentum flavum

20. What structure forms the floor of the intervertebral foramen (IVF)?
    a. pedicle of the vertebrae above
    b. pedicle of the vertebrae below
    c. vertebral body of the vertebra below
    d. vertebral body of the vertebra below

21. Which one of the following structures does NOT traverse the IVF?
    a. mixed spinal nerve
    b. lymphatic channels
    c. communicating veins between the internal and external vertebral venous plexuses
    d. gray communicating ramus

22. An increased sensitivity to pain is known as:
    a. hypertropism
    b. hypotropism
    c. hyperalgesia
    d. hypoalgesia

23. Which one of the following statements identifies type III receptor nerve endings?
    a. unmyelinated nerve endings weaving throughout the capsule; nociceptors
    b. larger joint ligament corpuscles; thinly encapsulated mechanoreceptors
    c. fibrous capsule containing conical corpuscles in the deep layers; thickly encapsulated mechanoreceptors
    d. globular corpuscles in the fibrous capsule; thinly encapsulated mechanoreceptors

24. Which one of the following statements about "spinal learning" is TRUE, according to Patterson and Steinmetz?
    a. complete spinal fixation occurred in anesthetized rats if cord section occurred after 35 minutes
    b. cerebral cortex and brainstem are necessary for observed alterations in spinal reflex excitability
    c. direct stimulation of the hind limb producing reflex flexion of the limb showed fixation within 90 to 120 minutes
    d. alterations from spinal fixations are due to changes in spinal reflex circuits and peripheral inputs

25. According to the Gatterman/Goe model of segmental dysfunction, the release of platelets and serotonin does what to nerve endings?
    a. sensitizes
    b. desensitizes
    c. liberates
    d. depletes

26. Of the afferent fibers innervating musculoskeletal tissues, which is the MOST abundant?
    a. group I (A-alpha fibers)
    b. group II (A-beta fibers)
    c. group III (A-delta fibers)
    d. group IV (C-fibers)

27. Which of the following nerve fibers function to regulate local tissue homeostasis?
    a. group Ia afferents
    b. C-fibers
    c. A-beta fibers
    d. group IV afferents

28. After a patient is adjusted, he or she explains that awareness of where he or she is in space is better. Which of the following afferent pathways was likely to be activated by the adjustment?
    a. dorsal columns
    b. dorsal spinocerebellar tract
    c. ventral spinocerebellar tract
    d. anterolateral system

29. The posterior aspect of the intervertebral disc is innervated by which of the following?
    a. dorsal ramus
    b. sinuvertebral nerve
    c. group II, III, and IV afferents and gray rami
    d. A fibers and C fibers

30. When inflammatory substances are applied to the spinal nerve sheath, pain can develop. What term is used to describe the "nerves that innervate nerves"?
    a. vasa recti
    b. vasa nervorum
    c. nervi vasorum nervorum
    d. nervi nervorum

31. What is the process by which sacroiliac dysfunction/subluxation generates the experience of pain?
    a. first-order group III, IV neurons from the sacroiliac joint synapse with second-order neurons in the lumbosacral cord dorsal horn; second-order neurons ascend to the thalamus in the contralateral anterolateral pathway and synapse in the ventral posterolateral nucleus of the thalamus; third-order thalamocortical neurons travel to the sensory strip and limbic system
    b. first-order group III, IV neurons from the sacroiliac joint enter the ipsilateral fasciculus gracilis and synapse with second-order medial lemniscal neurons in the nucleus gracilis; second-order neurons ascend to the thalamus in the medial lemniscus and synapse in the ventral posterolateral nucleus of the thalamus; third-order thalamocortical neurons travel to the sensory strip and limbic system
    c. first-order group III, IV neurons from the sacroiliac joint synapse with second-order neurons in the lumbosacral cord dorsal horn; second-order neurons ascend to the thalamus in the ipsilateral anterolateral pathway and synapse in the ventral posterolateral nucleus of the thalamus; third-order thalamocortical neurons travel to the sensory strip and limbic system
    d. first-order group III, IV neurons from the sacroiliac joint enter the contralateral fasciculus gracilis and synapse with second-order medial lemniscal neurons in the nucleus gracilis; second-order neurons ascend to the thalamus in the medial lemniscus and synapse in the ventral posterolateral nucleus of the thalamus; third-order thalamocortical neurons travel to the sensory strip and limbic system

Answers

1. a. The outer third of the annulus fibrosus receives both sensory and vasomotor innervation. Posterior aspect of the disc receives its innervation from the recurrent meningeal nerve. The posterolateral aspect of the disc receives both direct branches from the anterior primary division and also branches from the gray communicating rami of the sympathetic chain.

2. b. The primary pathway in the spine for nociceptive sensation is the lateral spinothalamic system (neospinothalamic tract). Although other tracts are functional in nociception, the three discriminative pathways are the neospinothalamic tract, the dorsal column system, and the spinocervicothalamic tract.

3. b. Reliability in basic science is the reproducibility or consistency of measurement or diagnosis. It is the extent to which a test can produce the same result on repeated attempts.

4. c. Algometry refers to measurement of pain. Algometry quantifies two specific assessments. One is pressure tolerance (the amount of pain a patient can withstand), and the other is pressure-pain threshold (the minimum force that causes discomfort or pain).

5. c. Spray or Ruffini-type endings are the most common complex nerve endings within the joint capsules and nearby ligaments. Golgi tendon-type receptors are sometimes found in ligaments near the joint. Simple coiled end organs are found in the adventitia of blood vessels.

6. c. Chiropractic anatomist L. G. F. Giles in his text *Anatomical Basis of Low Back Pain* (Williams & Wilkins, 1989) demonstrated paravascular myelinated fibers in synovial folds and encapsulated nerve fibers in zygapophyseal joints but found no neural structures in the ligamentum flavum.

7. a. An intracellular transport system carries large molecules formed in the nerve cell body the full length of the axon to the nerve fiber terminals. The transported materials exert a *trophic influence* affecting the development, growth, and maintenance of the end organs supplied by the nerve.

8. d. *Trophic* = growth. Trophic nerve influence affects those interactions between nerves and other cells that initiate or control molecular modification in the other cells. Restated, trophic nerve supply affects chemical process related to development, growth, and maintenance of end organs (target cells) supplied by the nerve. In addition to the impulse-based function of the nerve (the conveyance of nerve membrane action potentials), a non–impulse-based function includes nerve cell body synthesis of macromolecular trophic substances, the axoplasmic transport of these products to the terminal nerve ending, and the liberation of these chemicals at the synapse. Such chemicals exert a neurotropic effect on the postsynaptic cell (end organ supplied via the nerve). Deprivation of an end organ of its trophic influence may result in *atrophy* of such target cells.

9. a. Except for skilled movements, body functions are largely reflexive. These include somatosomatic, viscerovisceral, somatovisceral, and viscerosomatic reflexes. In the context of the specific spinal reflexes, various hypotheses have been constructed to explain the observed clinical response to chiropractic procedure. Such hypotheses propose that vertebral subluxation induces aberration of the various spinal reflex activities that are associated with a variety of clinical manifestations.

10. b. Except for skilled movements, body functions are largely reflexive. Examples include heartbeat, respiratory movements, digestive activity, and postural adjustments. Reflexive responses to stimuli include muscular contraction and glandular secretion. Spinal reflexes, which are involuntary responses to stimuli, are purposeful and exist to regulate physiologic function. Reflexes can be divided into four types based on the contributions of somatic and autonomic nerves to efferent and afferent pathways of the reflexes.

11. c. Except for skilled movements, body functions are largely reflexive. Examples include heartbeat, respiratory movements, digestive activity, and postural adjustments. Reflexive responses to stimuli include muscular contraction and glandular secretion. Spinal reflexes, which are involuntary responses to stimuli, are purposeful and exist to regulate physiologic function. Reflexes can be divided into four types based on the contributions of somatic and autonomic nerves to efferent and afferent pathways of the reflexes. These include somatosomatic, viscerovisceral, somatovisceral, and viscerosomatic reflexes. In the context of the specific spinal reflexes, various hypotheses have been constructed to explain the observed clinical response to chiropractic procedure. Such hypotheses propose that vertebral subluxation induces *aberrant* spinal reflex activities that are associated with a variety of clinical manifestations.

12. d. Except for skilled movements, body functions are largely reflexive. Examples include heartbeat, respiratory movements, digestive activity, and postural adjustments. Reflexive responses to stimuli include muscular contraction and glandular secretion. Spinal reflexes, which are involuntary responses to stimuli, are purposeful and exist to regulate physiologic function. Reflexes can be divided into four types based on the contributions of somatic and autonomic nerves to efferent and afferent pathways of the reflexes. These include somatosomatic, viscerovisceral, somatovisceral, and viscerosomatic reflexes. In the context of the specific spinal reflexes, various hypotheses have been constructed to explain the observed clinical response to chiropractic procedure. Such hypotheses propose that vertebral subluxation induces *aberrant* spinal reflex activities that are associated with a variety of clinical manifestations.

13. d. The gate-control theory by Melzck and Wall proposed that mechanical intervention (e.g., rubbing a painful area) activates large, fast-conducting A-fibers (mechanoreceptors), which in turn inhibit the synaptic transmission of the smaller pain conveying C-fibers, therefore suppressing the signals of pain. This concept is also referred to as the *gate theory, afferent inhibition,* or *stimulus-induced analgesia* and has been proposed in part as an explanation for the pain relief experienced from the mechanical effects of an adjustive procedure.

14. a. In the cervical spine, the nerves and nerve roots completely fill the AP diameter of the IVF, making it highly susceptible to compression. It is the lumbar IVF that is approximately 5 to 6 times the diameter of the spinal nerve.

15. b. Spinal nerve roots are at much greater risk of compression than peripheral nerves. Sharpless' study decreased nerve conduction by 60% in 30 minutes, but function was restored in most nerves in about 20 minutes after decompression. Rydevik determined that venous flow to nerve roots was blocked with 5 to 10 mm Hg.

16. d. Wolff's law suggests that structure follows function. This is why weight-bearing exercise is recommended to postmenopausal women and anyone prone to osteopenia, because trabecular patterns in bone change when the bones are subjected to weight-bearing stresses.

17. b. Preganglionic and postganglionic fibers are autonomic or visceral efferent nerves, which synapse in the sympathetic ganglion, hence the terms "preganglionic" and "postganglionic." Neither visceral afferent nor somatic afferent or efferent nerves have presympathetic and postsympathetic ganglionic fibers.

18. c. The supraspinous and nuchal ligaments are situated most posteriorly on the spinal column. The nuchal ligament in the cervical region and the supraspinous ligament continue in the thoracic and lumbar regions. Flexion is an anterior motion closing the anterior angle; therefore, these two ligaments work to prevent hyperflexion in the spine.

19. d. The word *flavum* means "yellow," as in yellow *elastic* fibrous connective tissue. Both ligamentum flavum and nuchae have more yellow elastic fibrous connective tissue than the other common vertebral ligaments. The others are composed primarily of white, inelastic, fibrous connective tissue.

20. b. The pedicle of the vertebrae forms the roof. The pedicle of the vertebrae below forms the floor. Both vertebral bodies form the anterior wall of the IVF.

21. d. The gray communicating ramus is a communicating branch between the sympathetic chain and the ventral spinal nerve before traversing the IVF.

22. c. Hyperalgesia is an increased sensitivity to pain. The CNS implores several mechanisms to create hyperalgesia; damaged tissue remains hypersensitive until healing has occurred.

23. b. Type III receptor nerve endings are characterized by their large corpuscles and thinly encapsulated mechanoreceptors.

24. d. Choice "a" would be true if complete spinal fixation were changed to partial spinal fixation. Cerebral cortex and brainstem are *not* necessary for observed alterations in spinal reflex activity, and direct stimulation of the hind limb produced reflex flexion within 35 to 40 minutes.

25. a. Release of platelets, serotonin, and breakage of mast cells containing histamine sensitize nerve endings.

26. d. Group IV afferents are, by far, the most abundant afferent fibers that innervate joints and muscles.

27.   b.   C-fibers are the smallest of our nerve fibers. Group IV afferents are of the C-fiber size, and postganglionic sympathetic gray rami are motor fibers of the C-fiber size. Group IV afferents and gray rami work in concert with the neuroendocrine system to regulate local tissue homeostasis. For example, they help to drive tissue healing or chronic inflammation, depending on the needs of the local tissue environment and the biochemical health of the individual.

28.   a.   Part of dorsal column function is to provide us with the realization of where we are in space, which is referred to as proprioception or kinesthetic awareness.

29.   c.   This is somewhat of a trick question. We typically refer to nerves as innervating various target tissues; however, a "nerve" is the vascularized connective tissue tube that carries nerve fibers to and from the spinal cord to innervate a given tissue. Nerve fibers actually do the innervating, not nerves. In the case of connective tissues such as the disc or ligaments, we find only group II, III, and IV afferents and gray rami. Group I afferents innervate muscle spindles and Golgi tendon organs. The only motor fibers to connective tissue are the gray rami, which innervates the local blood vessels. There is no skeletal muscle in connective tissue, so there is no innervation by alpha-, beta-, or gamma-motoneurons, which are all A-fibers.

30.   d.   Vasa recti are the blood vessels that parallel the loops of Henle. Vasa nervorum are blood vessels within nerves. Nervi vasorum nervorum are the nerve fibers that innervate the blood vessels within nerves. And nervi nervorum are the nerve fibers that innervate the connective tissue of the nerve sheath. Research suggests that local inflammatory processes can stimulate the group III and IV afferents and lead to nonradicular pain that is similar in nature to muscle and joint pain.

31.   a.   No matter where pain occurs in the musculoskeletal system, the neurologic pathway is generally the same. First order nociceptive neurons synapse in the ipsilateral dorsal horn. Second order spinothalamic neurons enter the contralateral anterolateral system and terminate in the ventral posterolateral thalamic nucleus, and synapse with third order thalamocortical neurons. The only difference among "pains" is the location of the initial nociceptive stimulus and the location they arrive in the sensory homunculus in the parietal lobe.

CHAPTER 67

Applied Chiropractic Principles

1. Postural analysis dictates that a lateral plumb line in the normal erect spine should go through the mastoid process, greater trochanter of the femur, and pass:
    a. slightly posterior to the lateral malleolus
    b. slightly anterior to the lateral malleolus
    c. through the lateral malleolus
    d. through the calcaneous

2. The typical diversified adjustment is best described as a _____ thrust.
    a. high-velocity, low-amplitude
    b. low-velocity, low-amplitude
    c. high-velocity, high-amplitude
    d. low-velocity, high-amplitude

3. Cavitation takes place in the:
    a. physiologic zone of movement
    b. paraphysiologic zone of movement
    c. psychological zone of movement
    d. pathologic zone of movement

4. The common palpatory/observable characteristics of a PI ilium include:
    a. higher iliac crest (standing)
    b. functionally shorter leg (sitting)
    c. superior PSIS
    d. functionally long leg (sitting)

5. Which of the following disc herniations would you expect to respond MOST favorably to traction therapy?
    a. medial to the nerve root
    b. lateral to the nerve root
    c. anterior to the nerve root
    d. posterior to the nerve root

6. If a patient presents with vertebobasilar artery insufficiency after an adjustment, you should NOT:
    a. cease manipulation
    b. refer if symptoms do not subside
    c. adjust on the side opposite that caused the symptoms
    d. observe the patient to see if the symptoms subside

7. You obqserve that a standing patient is leaning to the patient's right. The left iliac crest palpates higher than the right. Which leg would you expect to find shorter than the other one when the patient is prone on the adjusting table?
    a. left
    b. right
    c. neither, the legs are even and the pelvis is uneven
    d. neither, the legs are even and the sacrum is uneven

8. When adjusting the pediatric spine, what consideration must be given for the size and age of the patient?
    a. decrease the depth of the thrust
    b. increase the degree of specificity of the segmental contact
    c. avoid taking the joint to tension due to relative "laxity" of pediatric ligaments
    d. a, b, and c

9. When delivering a high-velocity, low-amplitude thrust to the upper cervical spine, which combined ranges of motion should be avoided as much as possible?
    a. flexion/extension
    b. extension/rotation
    c. lateral flexion/extension
    d. flexion/rotation

10. Increasing the tension significantly on the table pads before performing a drop table–assisted adjustment will change the delivery of the adjustment in what way?
    a. requires less force utilization by the adjuster
    b. patient experiences decreased application of force by the adjuster
    c. requires greater force utilization by the adjuster
    d. patient experiences no difference in the force applied by the adjuster

11. Why is it important to rule out cervical spine subluxation on a patient displaying leg length inequality before adjusting for a PI ilium?
    a. leg length growth is not always bilaterally symmetrical
    b. the PI ilium may cause cervical subluxation
    c. leg length inequality may be physiologic and not anatomic
    d. cervical subluxation may cause leg length inequality

12. Why is leg length inequality often an unreliable indicator of subluxation in a pediatric patient?
    a. leg length growth is not always bilaterally symmetrical
    b. the PI ilium may cause cervical subluxation
    c. leg length inequality may be physiologic and not anatomic
    d. cervical subluxation may cause leg length inequality

13. This segmental contact should not be used in the lumbar spine:
    a. mammillary process
    b. spinous process
    c. transverse process
    d. lamina

14. A right rotational malposition at the level of T7 would contraindicate a posterior-to-anterior thrust on which segmental contact?
    a. right transverse process
    b. left transverse process
    c. spinous process
    d. right lamina region

15. Which of the following statements describes the connective tissue component of the vertebral subluxation complex?
    a. plays the central role as mediator of all subluxation effects
    b. synovial fluid undergoes fibrofatty consolidation
    c. disuse atrophy is a consequence of immobilization
    d. retrograde venous flow can bring toxins to the site of immobilization

16. Which nucleus serves to explain the neuroanatomic basis of headache referred from the neck?
    a. trigeminocervical nucleus
    b. nucleus ambiguous
    c. red nucleus
    d. nucleus gracilis

17. Which one of the following symptoms is NOT associated with reflex sympathetic dystrophy?
    a. spontaneous burning pain
    b. hyperpathia
    c. peripheral tissue dystrophic changes
    d. hypoalgesia

18. Panjabi and White have shown that a 10.8 mph rear-end collision with impact duration of 0.1 second will accelerate the lead vehicle _____ times the force of gravity.
    a. 2
    b. 3
    c. 4
    d. 5

19. Which one of the following is a description for a lateral flexion injury on the flexion side?
    a. tearing of the capsules of the intervertebral joints
    b. traction of the nerve roots
    c. facet jamming
    d. superior subluxation of the first rib

20. Which one of the following symptoms of thoracic outlet syndrome is NOT an initial management indication for surgical consultation?
    a. chronic pain
    b. vascular ischemia
    c. embolic complication
    d. muscle wasting

21. Which one of the following terms is INCONSISTENT with an intervertebral disc?
    a. herniation
    b. degeneration
    c. inflammation
    d. exostosis

22. Which nucleus receives nociceptive input from cervical structures innervated by the upper/mid cervical nerves and can lead to cervicogenic headache?
    a. nucleus cuneatus
    b. central cervical nucleus
    c. trigeminocervical nucleus
    d. substantia gelatinosa

23. The term "facilitated segment" is used in relation to spinal dysfunction. Which of the following is synonymous with "facilitated segment"?
    a. central sensitization
    b. neurogenic inflammation
    c. central excitatory state
    d. hyperexcitable segment

24. When pain extends down the leg and into the foot, which of the following has been demonstrated to be a possible cause?
   a. spinal misalignment
   b. disc herniation
   c. facet syndrome
   d. b and c

25. The atlas was adjusted and pain in the right hand, left foot, and low back improved. Which of the following antinociceptive mechanisms can explain this outcome?
   a. facilitated segment
   b. central sensitization
   c. diffuse noxious inhibition
   d. allodynia

26. Which of the following is an example of a neuroendocrine response to nociception that may influence subluxation processes?
   a. hypercortisolemia
   b. substance P release
   c. opiate release from white cells
   d. cytokine release from histiocytes and fibroblasts

27. Which of the following "theoretic models" of subluxation can represent a medical emergency that should be referred for a surgical consult?
   a. dysafferentation
   b. spinal cord compression
   c. somatovisceral reflex
   d. IVF encroachment

28. If substance P is found in the disc, joint capsule, or spinal ligament, this indicates that the tissue is innervated by which of the following nerve fibers?
   a. group II afferents
   b. group III and IV afferents
   c. group I and IV afferents
   d. indicates white blood cell infiltration and not afferent fiber innervation

29. A procedure in which the hands directly contact the body to treat the articulations or soft tissues is termed:
   a. manual therapy
   b. mobilization
   c. manipulation
   d. adjustment

30. Movement applied singularly or repetitively within or at the physiologic range of joint motion, without imparting a thrust or impulse, with the goal of restoring joint mobility is termed:
    a. manual therapy
    b. mobilization
    c. manipulation
    d. adjustment

31. A manual procedure that involves a directed thrust to move a joint past the physiologic range of motion without exceeding the anatomic limit is termed:
    a. manual therapy
    b. mobilization
    c. manipulation
    d. adjustment

32. A chiropractic clinical procedure that uses controlled force, leverage, direction, amplitude, and velocity directed at specific joints or anatomic regions is termed:
    a. manual therapy
    b. mobilization
    c. manipulation
    d. adjustment

33. The temporary immobilization of a joint in a position that it may normally occupy during any phase of normal movement is best termed:
    a. joint dysfunction
    b. joint play
    c. joint accessory motion
    d. joint fixation

34. The term _____ is applied to an imbalance in afferent input such that an increase in nociceptor input and a reduction in mechanoreceptor input occur.
    a. dysafferentation
    b. afferentation
    c. deafferentation
    d. dysponesis

35. Margaret Wislowska of the Institute of Clinical Medicine in Warsaw, in a study on the contribution of pain to segmental muscular contraction and subsequent rotation of vertebrae in the origin and pathogenesis of lateral spinal curvature, determined that irritation of the nervous system resulting in pain in the abdominal cavity from kidney stones may reflexively cause symptomatic rotation of the lumbar vertebrae. Such an example may be associated with which aberrant spinal reflex hypothesis?
    a. aberrant somotosomatic reflex hypothesis
    b. visceral disease simulation
    c. aberrant somatovisceral reflex hypothesis
    d. aberrant viscerosomatic reflex hypothesis

36. Karel Lewit, in a review of vertebrovisceral relations, cites examples where changes in spinal function (joint blockage or hypomobility) are linked to tachycardia (abnormally rapid heart rate). Therefore, it was observed that when mobility of the spinal column is normalized, heart rhythm also becomes normal and remains so as long as no relapse occurs in the spinal column dysfunction. Such clinical observation may BEST be associated with the following contemporary hypothesis:
    a. aberrant somatosomatic spinal reflex hypothesis
    b. aberrant somatovisceral spinal reflex hypothesis
    c. aberrant viscerosomatic spinal reflex hypothesis
    d. visceral disease simulation

1. b. The plumb line should pass slightly anterior to the lateral maleolus in the normal erect spine. Posterior to the lateral maleolus or through the lateral maleolus or calcaneous would cause the center of gravity to be positioned too far posterior, as may result from excessive lordosis.

2. a. The chiropractic adjustive thrust is a high-velocity, low-amplitude force designed to induce joint distraction and cavitation without exceeding the limits of anatomic joint motion.

3. b. Three zones of physiologic movement are recognized when adjusting a joint, according to Sandoz: the zone of physiologic movement where active and passive range of motion occurs, the paraphysiologic zone of movement—the zone of joint play where the high-velocity thrust suddenly separates the articular surfaces (manipulation) and results in the sound (cavitation), and the pathologic zone of movement where strain/sprain occurs.

4. d. The common palpatory/observable characteristics of a PI ilium include a lower iliac crest (standing), a prominent and inferior PSIS, and a functionally shorter leg supine, prone, and standing; however, it presents as a functionally longer leg sitting.

5. b. When the disc is in the axilla of the nerve root (medial), axial traction may irritate the problem.

6. c. Vertebral basilar artery insufficiency subsequent to an adjustment is a very serious event. You should immediately cease manipulation and observe the patient and seek medical assistance if the symptoms do not subside. Do not adjust on the other side in an attempt to balance things out.

7. b. The right leg would be functionally shorter in the prone position. They have a right PI ilium with the common finding of a lower iliac crest (standing), and the functionally longer leg on the left would cause the lean to the right.

8. d. Due to the size of the pediatric patient, the depth of thrust and the amount of force must be significantly decreased to avoid injury. The size of the adjuster's hand is great compared with the size of the vertebrae, therefore, single digit or very specific contacts are necessary. Pediatric ligaments are soft and pliable, and it is easy to overrotate if taking a joint to tension.

9. b. Cerebrovascular accidents, or strokes, while rare, are documented as having been associated with rotation and/or rotation and extension of the upper cervical spine. Vigorous rotation may traumatize the vertebral artery. Cervical extension activities such as stargazing, overhead work, and beauty parlor syndrome are also associated vertebrobasilar and cerebrovascular accidents.

10. c. Increasing the tension of the drop pads requires increased force to drop the pads. Ideally, the adjuster would set the drop tension to a degree that accounts for both the weight of the patient and the individual amount of preadjustive force used by the adjuster. In this way, any forward motion, or thrust, would activate the drop mechanism.

11. d. Romer Derefield developed the leg length inequality association to cervical syndrome when a short leg evened out as the patient turned his head to speak on the telephone. Cervical subluxation may cause leg length inequality, often associated with a PI ilium. It is important, therefore, to rule out the cervical syndrome before adjusting the ilium.

12. a. Children often have asymmetrical growth patterns. Therefore, leg length inequality is unreliable as a standard with pediatric patients. Be sure to check for other indicators of a PI ilium before adjusting.

13. c. The lumbar transverse process is short, sharp, and bladelike in its formation and very susceptible to fracture. It is not used as a segmental contact in any mainstream adjusting procedure.

14. b. The term "posterior" in a subluxation listing generally refers to the side of posteriority. In the right rotational malposition, according to the static Houston Conference listings, the right transverse process has rotated posteriorly, the spinous process has deviated to the left, and the left transverse process has rotated anteriorly. A posterior to anterior thrust on the left transverse would exacerbate the rotational subluxation and is, therefore, contraindicated.

15. b. As a result of immobilization, synovial fluid undergoes fibrofatty consolidation. There is a progression of fibrous tissue and deposition of bone salts, ultimately leading to ankylosis. These degenerative characteristics are descriptive of the connective tissue component of vertebral subluxation complex.

16. a. The trigeminocervical nucleus and the extensive afferent convergence from numerous craniocervical peripheral tissues explain the basis of neck-referred headache.

17. d. Hypoalgesia is incorrect. Patients with reflex sympathetic dystrophy suffer from hyperalgesia, pain to normally innocuous events, and increased sensitivity.

18. d. Collisions occurring at low speeds result in large forces being applied to the lead vehicle. Acceleration causes injuries to the driver and passengers of the lead vehicle.

19. c. Facet jamming is a compressive phenomenon as a result of forced lateral flexion on the ipsilateral side, where the concave curvature of the cervical spine increases.

20. a. Vascular ischemia, embolic complication, and muscle wasting are serious consequences of thoracic outlet syndrome. Severe tissue damage, pulmonary arrest, and neurologic deficit warrant advanced intervention when conservative measures fail.

21. d. An exostosis is a spur or outgrowth from a bone; degeneration, inflammation, and herniation are pathologic changes occurring to intervertebral discs.

22. a. The trigeminocervical nucleus of the fifth cranial nerve descends to about the level of C3 in the cervical cord. Consequently, nociceptive input from muscular and connective tissue structures in the cervical spine can stimulate trigeminothalamic neurons in the trigeminocervical nucleus and lead to head pain.

23. a. *Facilitation* is neurologic term that refers to an increase in the excitability of a neuron. *Facilitated segment* refers to an increase in the excitability of neurons at the segmental vertebral/cord level of spinal subluxation. *Central sensitization* is a more contemporary term used to describe hyperexcitable central neurons. Research suggests that peripheral nociceptive input and peripheral nociceptive sensitization can promote central sensitization.

24. d. While disc herniaton and neurocompression are classically thought of as the cause for pain below the knee, research with injectable nociceptive and analgesic agents has demonstrated that facet joints are also capable of generating this pattern of pain. Trigger points in the gluteus medius can also create a referred pain sensation from the leg and foot.

25. c. Diffuse noxious inhibition, or diffuse noxious inhibitory control, refers to an analgesic mechanism. The adjustment is likely to activate group I through IV afferents, and this is thought to lead to both segmental nociceptive inhibition and a more generalized suprasegmental inhibition. It is posited that chiropractic adjustments can activate the brainstem-derived endogenous analgesic system, which leads to the reduction of nociceptive activity at many cord levels, such that a cervical adjustment may reduce back pain.

26. a. Increased circulating levels of cortisol can occur in response to pain or nociception with pain. With this in mind, it is likely that nociceptive input from a "subluxated" spinal joint can lead to hypercortisolemia.

27. b. While "cord compression" is theorized as a potential outcome of subluxation, it is important to realize that in the clinical setting, spinal cord compression is medical emergency. Canal stenosis due to osteophytes, disc herniation, and hypertrophy of the ligamentum flava are the most common causes.

28. b. The presence of substance P is viewed as an indication that the tissue possesses nociceptive innervation (group III and IV afferents) and is capable of generating the experience of pain. Substance P is released by nociceptive afferents and stimulates resident cells to participate in the inflammatory and nociceptive processes.

29. a. The term *manual therapy* is a generic term encompassing procedures using direct hand contact to treat articulations or soft tissues. The rigor of skill required of the practitioner of manual procedures or manual therapies progresses from that of simple *mobilization*, to that of *manipulation*, to the most controlled clinical application being the *chiropractic adjustment.*

30. b. The term *manual therapy* is a generic term encompassing procedures using direct hand contact to treat articulations or soft tissues. The rigor of skill required of the practitioner of manual procedures or manual therapies progresses from that of simple *mobilization*, to that of *manipulation*, to the most controlled clinical application being the *chiropractic adjustment.*

31. c. Manipulation is a passive manual maneuver during which a joint is quickly brought beyond its restricted physiologic range of movement and beyond its elastic barrier without exceeding the boundaries of anatomic integrity. Some practitioners describe the reference to *manipulation* and *adjustment* as synonyms with both terms having the intended description to include the controlled force, leverage, direction, amplitude, and velocity directed at specific articulations. Other chiropractors make the distinction that *manipulation* is a more general and less specific procedure lacking the skill and the clinical assessment required of the chiropractic adjustive procedure.

32. d. The *adjustment* is a maneuver that is specific in direction, point of contact, amplitude, and velocity, intended to correct a subluxation partly or wholly, improving joint dysfunction and the attending neurologic component of vertebral subluxation. The rigor of skill required of the practitioner of manual procedures or manual therapies progresses from simple *mobilization*, to that of *manipulation*, to the most controlled clinical application being the *chiropractic adjustment*. Some practitioners describe the reference to *manipulation* and to *adjustment* as synonyms with both terms intended to denote the controlled force, leverage, direction, amplitude, and velocity directed at specific articulations. Other chiropractors make the distinction that *manipulation* is a more general and nonspecific procedure, requiring less skill and clinical assessment than that of the chiropractic adjustive procedure.

33. d. *Joint fixation (restriction)* is defined as a temporary immobilization of an articulation. The effects of joint fixation are proposed to include degenerative changes, pain, excitation of alpha-motoneurons (myospasm), excitation of preganglionic sympathetic neurons (vasoconstriction, nociceptive reflexes), and deafferentation of propriospinal tract, dorsal column, and spinocerebellar tracts. Certain authors have referenced the term *joint fixation* as synonymous with the *kinesiopathologic component* or the *hypomobility* associated with vertebral subluxation complex.

34. a. The intervertebral motion segment is richly supplied with mechanoreceptive and nociceptive structures. For this reason, theories suggest that spinal biomechanical dysfunction may result in alternation of normal nociception, mechanoreception, or both. It is proposed that aberrant afferent input, after reaching the spinal cord, may evoke misdirected and/or aberrant neurophysiologic efferent response. *Afferentation* refers to the transmission of afferent nerve impulses. The prefix *dys-* is used to describe activity that is abnormal, difficult, or disordered. In this context, the term *dysafferentation* is used to describe the abnormal afferent input associated with joint complex dysfunction.

35. d. Here, the irritation of the viscera apparently was associated with somatic effects and would thus most closely fit the viscerosomatic reflex hypothesis.

36. b. Spinal movement restriction or somatic joint dysfunction at specific spinal neuromeric levels is hypothesized to evoke sustained afferent activity *(dysafferentation)* that is associated with the sympathetic innervation of the heart. Such sustained afferent impulses from altered joint mechanics are proposed to influence sustained aberrant efferent responses, in this case, proposed to evoke the symptoms of rapid heart rate.

Section Ten Recommended Reading

Bergmann T, Peterson D: *Chiropractic technique,* ed 2, St Louis, 2002, Mosby.

Gatterman M, ed: *Foundations of chiropractic: subluxation,* ed 2, St Louis, 2005, Mosby.

Haldeman S, ed: *Principles and practice of chiropractic,* ed 3, New York, 2005, McGraw-Hill.

Leach R: *The chiropractic theories: a textbook of scientific research,* ed 4, Baltimore, 2004, Williams & Wilkins.

Panjabi M, White A: *Biomechanics in the musculoskeletal system,* New York, 2001, Churchill Livingstone.

Redwood D, Cleveland C, eds: *Fundamentals of chiropractic,* St Louis, 2003, Mosby.

White A, Panjabi M: *Clinical biomechanics of the spine,* ed 2, Philadelphia, 1990, Lippincott.

Chiropractic Practice

Roger Engel, Brian J. Gleberzon, Donald F. Gran,
Jerry Hochman, David M. Sikorski

Spinal Analysis and Evaluation

1. The forces imparted into the pelvic ring from the femur heads in the standing patient tend to cause the pubic symphysis to:
   a. open
   b. close
   c. rotate
   d. laterally translate

2. The correction of foot pronation should cause the femur heads to do what on radiography?
   a. elevate
   b. fall
   c. translate medially
   d. translate laterally

3. Palpatory pain at the origin and insertion of the sartorius muscle may indicate:
   a. posterior rotation of the upper sacroiliac area
   b. anterior rotation of the upper sacroiliac area
   c. internal rotation of the femur head
   d. lateral meniscus tear at the knee

4. Which of these muscles is intrinsically voluntary for sacroiliac joint motion?
   a. piriformis
   b. gluteus maximus
   c. iliopsoas
   d. none of the above

5. A chronic scalene muscle spasm may be found with:
   a. decreased cervical lordosis
   b. increased cervical lordosis
   c. upper cervical subluxation
   d. thoracic subluxation

6. A patient with lumbar pain on extension, a positive McNab's line, and facet arthrosis probably suggests:
   a. spinal stenosis
   b. vertical sacroiliac slippage
   c. facet syndrome
   d. Otto's pelvis

7. Equalization of prone leg lengths on cervical rotation indicates:
   a. rotational fixation of one or more cervical segments
   b. lateral flexion fixation of one or more cervical segments
   c. anterior translation of one or more cervical segments
   d. posterior translation of one or more cervical segments

8. A patient with a right anterior talus subluxation and a right interosseous sacroiliac ligament sprain will show what posture on plumb line analysis?
   a. antalgia
   b. high right shoulder
   c. left head tilt
   d. left pelvic translation

9. A patient with some acetabular degeneration suffers a pelvic trauma by falling on the buttocks during ice-skating. The sacrum is pushed into a frontal plane distortion. Which of these muscles may test weak?
   a. psoas major
   b. piriformis
   c. sartorius
   d. quadratus lumborum

10. An anterior divergence between the atlas plane line and the odontoid perpendicular line would indicate what listing?
    a. AS
    b. AI
    c. PS
    d. PI

11. If the measurement from the base of the spinous process to the lateral margin of the vertebra is greater on the right, what would it indicate?
    a. body rotation on the left
    b. body rotation on the right
    c. convexity to the left
    d. convexity to the right

12. On the lateral cervical view, what do lines that cross closely to the spinous suggest?
    a. flexion malposition
    b. extension malposition
    c. lateral flexion malposition
    d. rotation

13. What would be the preferred method of quantifying the degrees of scoliosis?
    a. Chamberlain's method
    b. McGregor's method
    c. McRae's method
    d. Cobb's method

14. If the pedicle shadows of T8 appear wider on one side than on the other, it would suggest:
    a. posterior body rotation
    b. spinous rotation
    c. laterality
    d. extension

15. Interruption in George's line on a lateral plain film view would suggest:
    a. retrolisthesis
    b. laterolisthesis
    c. lateral flexion
    d. rotation

16. A measurement differing by more than 3 mm from anterior to posterior using Van Akkerveeken's lines suggests:
    a. instability
    b. scoliosis
    c. extension malposition
    d. stenosis

17. Division of the sacral base into four quadrants on the lateral projections to determine the anterior displacement of a spondylolisthesis is called:
    a. Risser-Ferguson method
    b. Harrison method
    c. Meyerding method
    d. Eisenstein method

18. On the weight-bearing A-P pelvic x-ray projection, a measurement from the top of the iliac crest to the inferior margin of the ischial tuberosity that is decreased would suggest:
    a. PI ilium
    b. AS ilium
    c. IN ilium
    d EX ilium

19. With respect to postural landmarks of a person in the prone position, which of the following statements is true?
    a. the inferior borders of the scapula are at the level of T2-T3
    b. the femoral heads are at the level of the L4-L5 interspace
    c. the inferior border of the ribs are at the level of T10-T11
    d. the PSISs are at the level of S2

20. During motion palpation, the two principal movements of the costrovertebral joints are typically described as:
    a. bucket handle and caliper
    b. caliper and flexion
    c. bucket handle and curvilinear
    d. curvilinear and flexion

21. In Bergmann's mnemonic PARTS, proposed as a method to identify a vertebral segment that would respond favorably to spinal manipulation or adjustment, the letter "R" stands for:
    a. restriction
    b. radiculopathy
    c. range of motion
    d. relieving factors

22. In the standing position, a normal plumb line in the lateral view would pass through which of the following group of landmarks?
    a. lateral malleolus, retropatella space, greater trochanter
    b. styloid of the fifth metatarsal, anterior third of the knee, greater trochanter
    c. styloid of the fifth metatarsal, posterior third of the knee, ASIS
    d. lateral malleolus, anterior third of knee, ASIS

23. Which of the following would be considered an ABSOLUTE contraindication to cervical spine manipulation?
    a. if the person were a heavy smoker, moderate drinker and was taking birth control pills
    b. if the person had high cholesterol and was taking corticosteroids
    c. if the person had type 2 diabetes and gout
    d. if the person had a history of acute episodes of rheumatoid arthritis

24. With respect to the associated risk of cervical spine manipulative therapy (cSMT) and stroke, which of the following statements is the MOST accurate statement concerning the current evidence base?
    a. the risk of experiencing a stroke following cSMT is approximately the same as the risk of stroke following the use of non-steroidal anti-inflammatory drugs (NSAIDs)
    b. the risk of experiencing a stroke following cSMT must be considered to be rare, idiosyncratic, and unpredictable
    c. the causal link between cSMT and stroke is well established in the medical and chiropractic literature
    d. there is clear evidence in the literature that delineates those activities or positions that place a patient at greatest risk of sustaining a stroke

25. All of the following tests are used to diagnose joint dysfunction/subluxation of the lumbar spine or sacroiliac joints EXCEPT:
    a. Yeoman's test
    b. Patrick's FABERE figure four test
    c. bowstring test
    d. standing Kemp's test

26. The Waddell tests are used to identify which of the following:
    a. pain of a nonorganic origin
    b. space-occupying lesions
    c. balance and coordination functions
    d. history of alcohol or substance abuse

27. In the upper thoracic and cervical spine, during purportedly normal coupled motion of lateral flexion, the spinous process moves:
    a. toward the concavity of the curve
    b. toward the convexity of the curve
    c. away from the direction of pain
    d. toward the direction of pain

28. The Slump test is suggested for use in:
    a. all spinal disorders
    b. all spinal disorders and most lower limb disorders
    c. all spinal disorders, most lower limb disorders, and some upper limb disorders
    d. all spinal disorders and some upper limb disorders

29. If a patient presents with low back pain that continues into the buttock and leg to below the knee, what is the most likely diagnosis?
    a. lumbar facet syndrome
    b. nerve root irritation due to disc, stenosis, or tumor
    c. cauda equina syndrome
    d. muscle strain

30. In ankylosing spondylitis, which symptom is NOT commonly associated with the condition?
    a. increases in stiffness with activity
    b. onset of back pain before the age of 40
    c. the presence of morning stiffness
    d. men are affected 3 times more often than women

31. If a 25-year-old patient presents with chronic, localized neck pain or stiffness aggravated by specific movements, the most likely diagnosis is:
    a. torticollis
    b. osteoarthritis of the cervical spine
    c. cervical subluxation
    d. cervical disc lesion

32. Sway-back posture is usually associated with:
    a. decreased thoracic kyphosis
    b. shortened hamstring muscles
    c. anterior tilt of the pelvis
    d. flexion of the knees

33. When auscultating for heart sounds, a normal apex beat lies in the:
    a. third left intercostal space (the space below the third rib) within the midclavicular line
    b. fifth left intercostal space (the space below the fifth rib) within the midclavicular line
    c. fifth left intercostal space (the space below the fifth rib) within the midsternal line
    d. third left intercostal space (the space below the third rib) within the midsternal line

34. Movement within the "spinal motion unit" occurs within a three-joint complex. What proportion of the axial compressive load is carried by the intervertebral discs?
    a. 40% to 60%
    b. 50% to 70%
    c. 60% to 80%
    d. 70% to 90%

35. When performing a postural assessment from the lateral view on a "normal" individual, the center of gravity line should fall through:
    a. the line of the sacroiliac joint
    b. the greater trochanter
    c. the anterior aspect of the knee
    d. just posterior to the medial malleolus

36. Postural findings of a high mastoid with level shoulders and no head rotation is suggestive of:
    a. a superior occiput on the high side or an inferior occiput on the low side
    b. a posterior occiput on the high side
    c. a posterior C1 on the low side
    d. a posterior and inferior C2 on the high side

37. Accessory joint motions can best be described as:
    a. involuntary movements necessary for normal joint function
    b. involuntary movements not necessary for normal joint function
    c. voluntary movements necessary for normal joint motion
    d. voluntary movements not necessary for normal joint function

38. The "stance" phase of a normal gait cycle makes up approximately what portion of the complete gait cycle?
    a. one third
    b. one half
    c. two thirds
    d. three fourths

39. At what point is the quality of end-feel or end-play of a joint assessed?
    a. in the joint play (free play) range
    b. at the end of active range of motion
    c. at the end of passive range of motion
    d. at the anatomic barrier

40. Currently, which of the following is a clinician's best tool for evaluating a patient's risk for cerebrovascular accident (CVA)?
    a. personal and familial history
    b. appropriate orthopedic tests
    c. appropriate neurologic tests
    d. cervical radiographic studies

41. Which one of the following tests would likely reproduce the chief complaint in a patient with facet syndrome (capsulitis) at the thoracolumbar junction?
    a. Adam's test
    b. straight leg raising test
    c. Kemp's test
    d. Bechterew's test

42. The referred pain frequently associated with musculoskeletal disorders can typically be described as:
    a. superficial and well defined
    b. superficial and ill defined
    c. deep and well defined
    d. deep and ill defined

43. According to Bergmann and colleagues, a complete loss of end feel (empty end feel) is significant because it may be indicative of joint:
    a. instability
    b. hypomobility
    c. misalignment
    d. restriction

44. The assessment of "joint play" is conducted with the joint:
    a. in loose-packed position
    b. in close-packed position
    c. at mid-passive range of motion
    d. at its physiologic barrier

45. A patient assessed as having a right positive Derefield (R+D) would have the equivalent static and dynamic sacroiliac listings of a right:
    a. posterior-inferior ilium or flexion restriction
    b. posterior-inferior ilium or extension restriction
    c. anterior-superior ilium or flexion restriction
    d. anterior-superior ilium or extension restriction

Answers

1. b. The femur heads provide lateral-to-medial forces into the lower pelvis. The center of the lower pelvis is the pubic symphysis, thereby closing the pubic symphysis.

2. a. Lifting the navicular to reduce pronation and increase the longitudinal arch of the foot will result in the apparent elevation of the other end of the lower extremity, the femur head.

3. a. Posterior rotation of the upper sacroiliac area (as in a PI ilium) will stretch the sartorius muscle, lowering the threshold of sensitivity at the origin and insertion areas where the Golgi tendon organs are located.

4. d. The sacroiliac joints cannot be moved voluntarily; no muscles originate and insert on opposite sides of the sacroiliac joint.

5. a. The scalenes serve to flex the cervical spine. They will cause instability of the first and second ribs, also, if chronically tight.

6. c. Facet syndrome is defined as likely overriding of the lumbar facets associated with hyperextension, accompanied by pain especially during extension. Radiographically, you may see facet arthritic changes.

7. a. Head rotation affects the rotational component of neck motion primarily. Lateral cervical flexion will most directly affect intersegmental lateral bending.

8. d. There will be a muscular effort or compensation to bring the body weight away from the side of injury, thereby reducing shear stresses through the sacroiliac joint and the right foot.

9. b. In this injury, the patient could have physically injured the piriformis muscle in addition to distorting the pelvis. The piriformis also attaches to the greater trochanter of the femur.

10. a. As the atlas tilts anterior and superior, it causes the angle between atlas and axis to increase at the anterior or opens the ADI at the bottom.

11. b. Due to the rounded nature of the vertebral body, as the spinous rotates to one side, it would allow more of the vertebral body to be visible on the opposite side.

12. b. Due to anatomic structures, such as the facets, etc., the vertebrae tend to migrate posterior and inferior when misaligned, causing individual vertebral lines to cross closer to the spinous process.

13. d. Cobb's method is widely accepted as a measurement for the degrees of scoliosis present.

14. a. As a vertebra rotates in the y-axis, the posteriorly rotated side of the body will appear more prominent, therefore allowing more visibility of the pedicle shadow.

15. a. George's line represents the posterior margin of the vertebral bodies, and an interruption would indicate either a posterior or an anterior shifting of the vertebral body.

16. a. Lines that intersect from the inferior vertebral end-plate of the vertebra above with the superior vertebral line of the vertebra below would form a relationship that should be roughly equal. If this relationship is disturbed by more than 3 mm, it may be suggestive of instability.

17. c. Meyerding's method is a widely accepted measurement of translation associated with spondylolisthesis.

18. b. The normal anatomic position of the ilium is angled forward slightly from the superior aspect. Therefore, the shadow projected with x-rays would be decreased if the ilium is misplaced farther anterior.

19. d. Inferior borders of scapula are at the level of T6, inferior borders of the ribs are typically at the level of the midlumbar spine, and the levels the greater trochanters do not intersect the spine. Levels of the PSISs are at the level of S2.

20. a. Vertebrocostal or rib motions are described as caliper and bucket handle.

21. c. Bergmann's PARTS mnemonic, now commonly referenced, stands for the following: P = pain, A = asymmetry/alignment, R = range of motion, T = tone, tonicity, temperature, S = special tests.

22. b. A normal plumb line of a patient in a standing position as seen from the side (lateral view) would fall through the lateral malleolus and anterior third of the knee and intersect the greater trochanter.

23. d. Acute rheumatoid arthritis is associated with destruction of the transverse ligament of the odontoid process. It is considered an absolute contraindication to cervical spine adjusting. The other listed factors (except gout) increase a person's relative risk of stroke, but spinal manipulation is an independent and unrelated factor.

24. b. The risk of stroke or death related to NSAID use is roughly 1:20,000. Best estimates of cSMT and stroke are 1:100,000 (although reported as high as 1:5.6 million). There is not yet a causal link made between cSMT and stroke (the current evidence only supports a temporal link). The evidence does not assist practitioners to identify those activities or positions that place a patient at greater relative risk of stroke. At the current time, the risk of stroke following cSMT must be considered rare, idiosyncratic, and unpredictable.

25. c. Bowstring test is a nerve tension test. The other three tests can elicit or provoke lumbar spine or sacroiliac joint dysfunctions.

26. a. Waddell testing is used to identify patients suffering from pain of a nonorganic origin.

27. b. In the cervical and upper thoracic spine, during normal coupled motion during lateral flexion, the spinous process moves toward the convexity of the curve.

28. c. The Slump test stretches neural and connective tissue components from the pons to the feet.

29. b. Pain below the knee is suggestive of a disc lesion with nerve root irritation.

30. a. In ankylosing spondylitis, some relief of the symptoms is usually achieved with mild to moderate activity.

31. c. The age of the patient makes osteoarthritis less likely. The lack of radiation supports the absence of a disc lesion. Torticollis presents differently and is usually associated with marked restriction of certain cervical movements.

32. b. Sway-back is characterized by flattening of the lumbar curve and an increase in the thoracic curve. The knees are hyperextended and the pelvis is tilted posteriorly. As a result of this, the hamstrings are shortened.

33. b. The apex of the heart lies in the left side of the mediastinum and its sounds are best heard over the prechordium at the left fifth intercostal space at the midclavicular line.

34. c. According to Giles, the disc carries as much as 80% of the compressive load in the lumbar spine.

35. b. The plumb line is supposed to line up with the external auditory meatus, glenohumeral joint, L3 vertebra, greater trochanter, anterior tubercle of the knee, and lateral malleolus.

36. a. Based upon postural analysis, it is sometimes thought that subluxation listings can be a source of spinal asymmetry. In this case, since there is no head rotation or shoulder unleveling, an inferior occiput on the low side, or a superior occiput on the high side, may be present.

37. a. Accessory joint motions are the small amounts of involuntary play allowed by the flexibility of healthy articular soft tissues. These motions are necessary for the joints to properly perform their gross voluntary motions.

38. c. Normal gait involves a "stance" phase, which includes heel strike, midstance, toe off, and contralateral heel strike, plus a "swing" phase, which involves the movement of the ipsilateral leg forward to the next heel strike. These phases normally make up two thirds and one third, respectively, of one complete phase.

39. c. The end feel of a joint is assessed at the limits of its passive range of motion and just prior to reaching the paraphysiologic joint space.

40. a. Currently, no tests or special studies readily available in an outpatient setting exist to accurately determine a patient's risk for CVA. A detailed and focused history and careful observation of the patient during and after assessment and treatment are the best indicators.

41. c. Facet syndrome is characterized by facet imbrication with resultant facet capsulitis and pain. Kemp's test involves rotation, lateral bending, and extension of the patient's trunk, which aggravates the imbrication and the associated pain.

42. d. Referred pain comes from deep somatic tissues that share the same innervations as the responsible site or organ. Because it originates from deep somatic tissues, it characteristically presents as a deep, ill-defined, achy pain.

43. a. A complete lack of end feel may be indicative of a significant compromise to the soft tissue structures that normally limit and protect joint motion. A more detailed examination and assessment of the affected joint are warranted anytime instability is suspected.

44. a. Joint play is assessed at the very beginning of motion when the target joint is in a loose-packed or neutral position, or as close to this position as possible. This is valuable in assessing the soft tissue structures that normally stabilize the joint.

45. b. The finding of right or left positive Derefield (R or L + D) is determined when the apparent short leg, with the patient prone and legs extended, appears to increase in length when the legs are flexed passed 90 degrees. This finding is generally treated by contacting the posterior-superior iliac spine on the involved side and adjusting it with a posterior-to-anterior, inferior-to-superior, and medial-to-lateral vector. The comparable static and dynamic listing would be a posterior-inferior (PI) ilium or extension restriction on the affected side.

Chiropractic Adjustive Technique

1. Regarding side posture pelvic adjusting placing the involved side (contact side) up or down:
    a. it depends on clinical results or patient preference
    b. all children should be adjusted involved side down
    c. all children should be adjusted involved side up
    d. the sacrum is stabilized better with the involved side up

2. There is a functional S1-S2 disc allowing S1 or S2 segmental dysfunction (subluxation) up to the age of:
    a. 1 year
    b. 10 years
    c. 20 years
    d. 40 years

3. The "foundation principle" refers to:
    a. a level pelvis
    b. level knee joints
    c. eyes level with the horizon
    d. hard palate level on the lateral cervical x-ray

4. Most patients presenting with acute severe low back pain usually show signs of subluxation intimately associated with:
    a. bilateral sacroiliac joints
    b. the lumbar disc
    c. contralateral sacroiliac joint
    d. the lumbar facets

5. The P-A thrust used in lumbar side posture adjusting, using a spinous contact, is along which axis?
    a. Z
    b. X
    c. Y
    d. I-S

6. Torque applied to the lumbar segment during a prone lumbar adjustment is applied around which axis?
    a. X
    b. Y
    c. Z
    d. I-S

7. The supine Thompson EX adjustment is easier than the side posture EX adjustment because:
    a. it is done with the involved side down
    b. the patient's involved side leg is placed in a figure four position
    c. the patient's involved side knee is crossed over the other leg
    d. the PSIS is the segmental contact point

8. What type of patient may benefit from use of SOT blocking?
    a. patients with craniosacral dural dysfunction
    b. patients with sacroiliac subluxations
    c. patients with acute low back pain and disc dysfunction
    d. patients with extremity dysfunction

9. A patient presents with inability to laterally flex the lumbar spine to the right or rotate to the left. This restriction may represent a malposition of L5 on sacrum. There is a right convexity of the lumbar spine above L5. The preferred segmental contact point is:
    a. right spinous process
    b. right mammillary process
    c. left spinous process
    d. left mammillary process

10. When considering manipulation of the upper or lower cervical spine, which single head and neck position has been shown to produce the greatest compromise to vertebral artery blood flow?
    a. maximum flexion
    b. maximum extension
    c. maximum lateral flexion
    d. maximum rotation

11. The orientation of the lumbar facets is generally conducive to movement in which plane(s)?
    a. sagittal
    b. coronal
    c. transverse
    d. all planes equally

12. A physician positions a patient in side posture to perform a manipulation intended to induce right rotation at the L1-L2 motor unit. He or she places the patient's left side down, distracts and torsions the trunk into right rotation, then takes a segmental contact point on the L2 vertebra in order to induce left rotation at this segment. This is an example of a(n):
    a. assisted adjustive procedure
    b. resisted adjustive procedure
    c. compressive adjustive procedure
    d. neutral position adjustive procedure

13. The application of a straight posterior-to-anterior (P-A) thrust in the midthoracic spine, in a patient with a normal kyphotic curve, would produce which of the following effects at the target segment relative to the segments above and below?
    a. gapping at the inferior and superior facets
    b. approximation at the inferior and superior facets
    c. gapping at the inferior facets and approximation of the superior facets
    d. approximation of the inferior facets and gapping of the superior facets

14. In the lower cervical spine, rotation is coupled with:
    a. flexion
    b. extension
    c. ipsilateral lateral flexion
    d. contralateral lateral flexion

15. Which one of the following contact points would be most appropriate for correcting a left anterior-superior (AS) ilium, or left sacroiliac flexion restriction, with the patient positioned in side posture and the involved side (left) down?
    a. right sacral ala
    b. left sacral ala
    c. right sacral apex
    d. left sacral apex

16. When performing a rotational manipulation at the occipitoatlantal joints (C0-C1), isolation can be achieved prior to reaching maximum rotation by first inducing slight:
    a. flexion
    b. extension
    c. ipsilateral lateral flexion
    d. contralateral lateral flexion

17. A therapeutic procedure in which the patient voluntarily contracts a particular muscle or muscle group against a specific pressure or force provided by the doctor in order to affect the target joint is characteristic of:
    a. an adjustive procedure
    b. a mobilization procedure
    c. a traction/distraction procedure
    d. an energy procedure

18. In the upper lumbar spine (L1-L3), the motion of rotation is coupled with:
    a. ipsilateral lateral flexion
    b. contralateral lateral flexion
    c. flexion
    d. extension

19. When assessing an elderly patient for chiropractic adjustment, a number of additional concerns need to be considered. They do NOT include:
    a. general decreased flexibility and elasticity of soft tissue
    b. the presence of more degenerative joint disease
    c. functional stability
    d. functional instability

20. Manipulative skills for the lower thoracic spine present a more formidable task to the practitioner for a variety of reasons. One of these reasons is:
    a. the larger number of vertebrae in the thoracic region
    b. the impact of many of the spinal stabilizing muscles crossing the region from the pelvis and lumbar spine regions
    c. the lack of mobility of the region compared to other regions
    d. hypermobility of this area

21. Clinical features of vertebral artery dissection and brainstem ischemia arising from vertebral artery insufficiency include:
    a. pain in the head and neck that is often unilateral and suboccipital
    b. pain that is severe, distinct, and sharp
    c. that the patient reports neck stiffness with no limitation of neck range of motion
    d. a, b, and c

22. In side posture lumbar manipulation, specific segmental localization and intersegmental tension are accomplished by:
    a. flexing the patient's hip beyond 90 degrees
    b. flexing the patient's hip to less than 90 degrees
    c. placing the hip in the anatomic position
    d. extending the patient's hip beyond 20 degrees

23. With diversified technique, examination protocol does NOT include which of the following?
   a. pain
   b. alignment
   c. resistance
   d. temperature

24. You have decided to palpate your patient's SI joint standing. You place your left thumb on the patient left PSIS and your right thumb on the patients left second sacral tubercle. You ask the patient to raise his right lower extremity past 90 degrees. Which of the following are you now palpating?
   a. extension of the left sacroiliac joint
   b. flexion of the right sacroiliac joint
   c. extension of the right sacroiliac joint
   d. flexion of the left sacroiliac joint

25. What are the most common motion findings for choosing a prone thrust approach when treating subluxations in the thoracic spine?
   a. thoracic flexion subluxation
   b. thoracic extension subluxation
   c. cervical extension subluxation
   d. cervical flexion subluxation

26. Contraindications to manipulation are divided into absolute and relative. Which condition would be considered to be an ABSOLUTE contraindication to manipulation in the lumbar spine?
   a. anticoagulant therapy
   b. lateral recess stenosis
   c. abdominal aortic aneurysm
   d. osteoporosis

27. In spondylolisthesis, a grade II represents what percentage of slippage of one bone on another?
   a. 1% to 10%
   b. 1% to 25%
   c. 26% to 35%
   d. 26% to 50%

28. Which of the following technique systems principally addresses subluxation of the sacrum or pelvis, considering all other subluxations compensatory?
   a. Gonstead technique
   b. Logan basic technique
   c. Thompson terminal point technique
   d. Toftness technique

29. Which technique system principally uses changes in posture, often defined mathematically, as its primary outcome measure?
    a. activator methods chiropractic technique
    b. bioenergetic synchronization technique
    c. chiropractic biophysics
    d. Palmer HIO

30. Which of the following technique systems is the only one NOT to eschew the use of rotation either in the setup (preadjustive tension phase) or during the delivery of an adjustment?
    a. applied kinesiology
    b. diversified technique
    c. Gonstead technique
    d. sacro-occipital technique

31. "Pattern analysis," using thermography, would be MOST commonly used by proponents of which of the following technique systems?
    a. chiropractic biophysics
    b. Gonstead technique
    c. Thompson terminal point technique
    d. upper cervical technique

32. Myofascial techniques, such as active release technique or Graston technique, most closely resemble which of the following technique systems?
    a. applied kinesiology
    b. full spine specific (meric) technique
    c. receptor-tonus (Nimmo) technique
    d. spinal biomechanics (Pettibon) technique

33. Craniopathy or cranial technique is a significant component of which of the following pair of technique systems?
    a. applied kinesiology/sacro-occipital techniques
    b. chiropractic biophysics/spinal biomechanics (Pettibon) techniques
    c. Gonstead/Thompson terminal point techniques
    d. network spinal analysis/directional nonforce techniques

34. Palpation for ilium-ishium-sacral motion is accomplished using the:
    a. Kernig and Brudzinski tests
    b. Gillet test
    c. Schober test
    d. Adam's test

35. Which of the following regions of the spine has the strongest evidence of effectiveness for spinal manipulative therapy in terms of number of supportive studies?
    a. cranial region
    b. cervical spine
    c. thoracic spine
    d. lumbar spine

36. Which of the following types of therapies is BEST classified as a low-velocity, low-amplitude oscillating motion?
    a. spinal manipulative therapy
    b. magnetic healing
    c. massage or soft tissue therapies
    d. mobilizations

37. Static palpation findings of edema and tenderness at the posterior superior aspect of the sacroiliac joint would indicate what misalignment?
    a. PI
    b. AS
    c. IN
    d. EX

38. The segmental contact point for the ilium listing of PIEX would be where?
    a. inferolateral PSIS
    b. inferomedial PSIS
    c. superolateral PSIS
    d. superomedial PSIS

39. The line of correction for a side posture AS ilium misalignment would be in what direction?
    a. up the spine
    b. toward the doctor
    c. toward the table
    d. down the femur

40. What is the common pelvis subluxation listing for performing a side posture pull adjustment, involved side down?
    a. PI
    b. AS
    c. IN
    d. EX

41. A posteriorly rotated sacrum may be corrected best by contacting what structure?
    a. lumbosacral junction
    b. S2 tubercle
    c. sacral ala
    d. sacroiliac junction

42. Which adjustive positions lessen the work for the doctor when working with a large or obese patient?
    a. seated
    b. side posture
    c. knee chest
    d. prone

43. What is the MOST appropriate thrust used when adjusting patients on the knee chest table?
    a. thrust and hold
    b. thrust and recoil
    c. thrust and fast release
    d. thrust and slow release

44. The segmental contact point in the imbricated segments of the thoracic spine would include the transverse processes or the:
    a. inferior tip of the spinous process
    b. superior tip of the spinous process
    c. mammillary processes
    d. ribs

45. The appropriate segmental contact point for an anterior superior occiput is the:
    a. mastoid
    b. atlas transverse
    c. glabella
    d. EOP

Answers

1. a. Adjusting the sacrum involved side down allows greater stabilization of the ipsilateral ilium. Due to compounding factors, it may be easier to adjust the pelvis involved side up or down. The same holds true when adjusting children.

2. b. Sacral segments fuse in children at approximately 10 years of age. Until that time, there is some motion, especially between S1 and S2.

3. a. The foundation principle, expounded by Gonstead and Logan, is based on radiographic evidence that the iliac crests, ischial tuberosities, and sacral base are all parallel to the floor. This level foundation serves as a firm base of support for the spine above and also as a reference from which other listings can be compared.

4. b. Most acute low back pain involves the lumbar disc, generally L5-S1. Most chronic pain involves the sacroiliac joints.

5. a. The Z axis is described in texts as the axis passing through the body in a P-A direction. P-A thrust, therefore, is along the Z axis, within the sagittal plane.

6. c. Torque is applied around the axis that passes through the patient's body from posterior to anterior. Torque is applied to reduce lateral bending fixation or wedging of the motor unit. This axis is described by all texts as the z-axis.

7. b. With the supine patient's knee bent and the leg in the figure four position over the other leg, the sacroiliac joint is closed by the patient even before the doctor applied the adjustment.

8. c. Patients with acute low back pain and a bulging disc need immediate pain relief. SOT blocking is unusually effective in providing such "passive antalgia" by reproducing prone antalgia, pulling the nerve root away from the disc.

9. b. Inability to flex to the right indicates an open wedge on the right between L5 and S1. Inability to rotate to the left indicates spinous to the left (body to the right). Right convexity above L5 indicates open wedges above L5 on the right (left scoliosis). In an effort to adjust on the convex side, you must adjust on the right.

10. d. Studies have indicated that rotation, even within normal range, is the head and neck movement or position most likely to induce occlusion of the vertebral artery. This phenomenon may occur in the artery contralateral to the rotation. The addition of extension with the rotation compromises the ipsilateral artery, too, and is thus the most compromising position overall. There is still controversy, however, as to which position may create the most occlusion, because each patient may have a different anatomic variant and response to head positioning.

11. a. The lumbar facets are generally orientated in the sagittal plane, making the lumbar spine most conducive to the motions of flexion and extension.

12. b. Sandoz and Bergmann classified various types of adjustive procedures according to patient position and application of the adjustive force. Positioning the superior segment of the target motor unit into the position of desired correction and then applying a force in the opposite direction to the inferior segment is characteristic of a resisted procedure. Common examples of this type of procedure are short or long lever side posture lumbar pull moves.

13. d. Because of the orientation of the thoracic facets in the coronal plane, with the inferior facets lying posterior to the superior facets of the segment below and anterior to the inferior facets of the segment above, a straight posterior-to-anterior thrust will cause the inferior facet joints to approximate while the superior facets joints separate, or gap.

14. c. Because the lower cervical facets are oriented in a plane that lies somewhere between coronal and transverse, rotation to either side is coupled with ipsilateral lateral flexion. As the head and neck are rotated, the facets on the ipsilateral side glide inferior and posterior, while the contralateral facets tend to glide in a superior and anterior direction, tilting the vertebrae to the side of rotation.

15. b. An anterior-superior (A-S) ilium, or flexion restriction, is generally corrected by moving the ilium of the effected side in a posterior and inferior direction relative to the sacrum, often by applying an posterior-to-anterior and superior-to-inferior force to the ischial tuberosity of the effected side. As an alternative method, the doctor can contact the sacral ala on the effected side and apply a force in a posterior-to-anterior, medial-to-lateral, and inferior-to-superior vector, thus effecting the appropriate correction at the sacroiliac joint.

16. d. Slight lateral flexion towards the side of doctor contact and away from the side of desired rotation correction creates tension at the C0-C1 articulations so that isolation can be achieved prior to reaching maximum rotation of the head and neck.

17. d. Bergmann classified joint manipulative procedures into four basic groups: the adjustment, joint mobilization, manual traction/distraction, and muscle energy techniques (as described by Greenman). The latter are generally described as muscle contractions against controlled resistance to affect a target joint.

18. b. Rotation in the lumbar spine is very limited and coupled with lateral bending. What is unique about this region is that rotation in the upper lumbar segments, L1-L2-L3, couples with contralateral lateral flexion, whereas rotation in the lower segments, L4-L5-S1, couples with ipsilateral lateral flexion. This is an important concept to understand when applying adjustive forces.

19. c. According to Souza, in the elderly patient, early degenerative changes and/or lack of appropriate muscle tone and reaction results in functional instability.

20. b. The number of vertebrae has no bearing on the ability to apply manipulative techniques to a region. Hypermobility and hypomobility are relative states of movement and are not region specific. The presence of differing muscle fiber directions complicates the biomechanical aspects of the lower thoracic spine.

21. d. All of these symptoms may be present in vertebral artery dissection and brainstem ischemia arising from vertebral artery insufficiency.

22. a. Flexion of the hip beyond 90 degrees tensions or stretches the intersegmental tissues and facilitates segmental localization.

23. c. Examination procedures in diversified technique can be summarized by the PART acronym: Pain, Alignment, Range of motion, and Temperature.

24. a. Gillet's test tests SI extension restriction on the contact side when the patient flexes the opposite hip.

25. b. The most common finding for choosing a prone approach to correct subluxations of the thoracic spine is restriction in extension. Flexion restrictions in the thoracic spine would be further flexed with a prone approach. Similarly, cervical extension restrictions would be further extended. Flexion restrictions in the cervical region would be generally unaffected by the prone approach to the thoracic spine except by secondary head movement.

26. c. Anticoagulant therapy is a relative contraindication to manipulation. In many cases, lateral recess stenosis responds well to manipulation, as do osteoporosis patients with musculoskeletal pain syndromes. They are both relative contraindications. Due to the potential serious and sudden consequences of rupture to an abdominal aortic aneurysm and its proximity to the lumbar spine, the presence of this condition is an absolute contraindication to performing lumbar manipulation. It is assumed in this case that the abdominal aortic aneurysm is clinically significant.

27. d. The traditional range for a grade II spondylolisthesis is 26% to 50%, which represents slippage over the second fourth of the bone below by the bone above.

28. a. Logan basic technique principally focuses on the pelvic ("as the goes the sacrum, so goes the spine"). Thompson, Gonstead, and Toftness are full-spine techniques.

29. c. The Harrisons have published their findings of an ideal spine, defined mathematically and determined by postural radiographs, extensively in the literature. Postural assessment is only a relatively small component of AMCT, BEST, and Palmer HIO assessment protocols.

30. b. Only diversified technique permits patient rotation either in the set-up or during the delivery of an adjustment. Virtually all other technique systems advocate against the use of rotation.

31. d. Pattern analysis using thermography is primarily found in the upper cervical milieu.

32. c. Nimmo's receptor tonus technique, developed in the 1950s, focused on muscles and their association with spinal segments.

33. a. Craniopathy constitutes a large component of AK and SOT work. It is not associated with the other technique systems listed.

34. b. Motion palpation of the ilium, ischium, and sacrum complex is accomplished using Gillet's tests.

35. d. The lumbar spine is the most studied region in terms of number of clinical trials investigating the effectiveness of SMT.

36. d. Mobilizations are classified as LVLA oscillating procedures.

37. b. Findings at this part of the joint indicate the joint is opened at the top due to the ilia fixating in a posterior-inferior direction.

38. a. The PIEX indicates a posterior and inferior and lateral rotation misalignment, so correction should be to move it in the opposite direction from inferior to superior and lateral to medial.

39. d. The AS adjustment is performed by the doctor rolling the patient with the thrust made in the direction of the shaft of the femur generally inferior to the doctor's stance.

40. d. To effect the lateral to medial correction needed for an EX misalignment, the most effective means would be a pull maneuver.

41. c. The doctor makes contact with either the pisiform or the thenar on the sacral ala, as far lateral as possible without being on the PSIS.

42. c. The knee chest provides a mechanical advantage to the doctor when adjusting the thoracic or lumbar spines, in particular with large or obese patients.

43. a. Once the joint is brought to maximum preload, a high-velocity, short-amplitude thrust is administered. At the end of the thrust, the segment is held for 1 to 2 seconds.

44. b. Spinous process contacts in the imbricated segments is the uppermost portion of the spinous process to direct the thrust as close to the vertebral body as possible.

45. c. Contact is made with the hypothenar pad of either hand placed over the glabella.

Case Management and Patient Education

1. A 35-year-old man presents with moderate low back pain that developed after moving furniture the previous day. He reports similar episodes following strenuous activity since he was a teenager. After a detailed history is taken, physical examination is conducted, and lumbar radiographs are taken, he is diagnosed with a grade 2 spondylolisthesis with concomitant lumbar sprain/strain. What would be the most appropriate course of action?
   a. send the patient home for bed rest until symptoms subside
   b. proceed with chiropractic care
   c. refer for MRI or CT scanning
   d. refer for surgical consult

2. Which of the following would be the best explanation to offer a new patient regarding the cause of the "cracking" or "popping" sound that accompanies many chiropractic adjustments?
   a. microtears in the joint capsule
   b. the snapping of adjacent ligaments and tendons
   c. sudden changes in intracapsular fluid tension/pressure
   d. the sound of joint surfaces rubbing against each other

3. Which one of the following forms of headache has been shown to be MOST responsive to manipulative care?
   a. temporal arteritis
   b. cervicogenic
   c. tension
   d. cluster

4. A 30-year-old female patient presents with right calf pain and may have a deep vein thrombosis (DVT). What would be the MOST appropriate initial course of action?
   a. prescribe rest and inactivity until symptoms subside
   b. treat with RICE protocols until symptoms subside
   c. treat with massage, muscle stripping, and stretching procedures
   d. refer for medical evaluation

5. When managing a patient with lumbar disc herniation and associated radiculopathy, it is advisable to use caution with lumbar adjustments that involve:
   a. flexion
   b. extension
   c. rotation
   d. lateral flexion

6. After a history, physical examination, and report of findings, an individual declines chiropractic care for the condition and refuses to sign a waiver to that effect. What is the wisest course of action for doctor protection?
   a. try to convince the person that chiropractic is the best hope
   b. try to detain the person until he or she signs the waiver
   c. call them on a daily basis to have them reconsider
   d. send them a certified, return receipt letter detailing the refusal

7. Which one of the following conditions would be considered an absolute contraindication to manipulation?
   a. bone infections
   b. joint hypermobility/instability
   c. inflammatory arthritis
   d. severe pain

8. Which of the following statements is MOST accurate concerning the issue of "informed consent" prior to treatment?
   a. it is only necessary prior to engaging in unusually risky procedures
   b. it is always necessary and may be verbal or implied
   c. it is always necessary and must be in writing
   d. it is only necessary if the patient specifically requests to be informed

9. Vertiginous symptoms elicited during the Dix-Hallpike (or Nylen-Barany) test would be pathognomonic for which of the following clinical conditions?
   a. benign paroxysmal positional vertigo
   b. cervicogenic vertigo
   c. Meniere's disease
   d. Cushing's disease

10. A plan of management used by some chiropractors that theoretically optimizes a person's health, prevents the development of clinical conditions, allows for the identification of emergent conditions, and provides palliative care is best described as:
    a. allopathic care
    b. crisis care
    c. maintenance care
    d. supportive care

11. Which of the following would be considered a secondary preventive strategy of osteoporosis?
    a. provision of external hip protectors
    b. weight-bearing exercise
    c. use of prescription drugs such as bisphosphonates or hormone replacement therapy
    d. dual-energy x-ray absorptiometry (DEXA)

12. Adson's test, Wright's test, and Roos' test (EAST) are used to identify which of the following clinical conditions?
    a. thoracic outlet syndrome
    b. meniscal tears of the knee
    c. disc herniation with neurologic deficits
    d. cervical facet syndrome

13. All of the following are characteristic signs or symptoms of fibromyalgia EXCEPT:
    a. nonrestorative sleep
    b. pain in 11 of 18 characteristic trigger points
    c. diffuse musculoskeletal pain of at least 3 months' duration
    d. abrupt onset of proximal shoulder or pelvic girdle pain

14. Patients should be advised to discontinue or avoid the use of which of the following substances because of its causal link to increased risk of heart disease, lung cancer, diabetes, osteoporosis, and chronic obstructive lung disease?
    a. tobacco
    b. alcohol
    c. ginseng
    d. glucosamine

15. Yerguson's and Speed's tests are used to assess strength and function of which of the following muscles of the shoulder girdle?
    a. biceps
    b. infraspinatus
    c. pectoralis major
    d. supraspinatus

16. In addition to in-office care, all of the following would be appropriate home care, dietary, or lifestyle modifications for patients suffering from gastroesophageal reflux disease (GERD) EXCEPT:
    a. losing of weight if patient weighs at least 20% more than ideal body weight
    b. suggestion to avoid fatty foods, chocolate, mints, caffeine, and alcohol
    c. suggestions to consume larger, rather than several small, meals throughout the day
    d. suggestion to not sleep, lie down, or engage in exercise for 2 or 3 hours immediately following a meal

17. Which of the following is INCORRECT as it pertains to obtaining consent to administer chiropractic treatment to a patient?
    a. the patient must be capable of giving consent (i.e., neither under the influence of drugs or alcohol nor mentally or physically incapable of understanding the nature of the consent)
    b. the individual must be of legal age to give consent
    c. the individual must be informed as to the nature of the consent (i.e., what he or she is consenting to and the likely risks)
    d. informed consent can be provided by a neighbor or relative for minors under the age of 18 as long as there is verbal approval from the legal guardian

18. When prescribing exercise for the osteoporotic patient, what goal should be met?
    a. stimulate bone production and prevent muscle strengthening
    b. stimulate bone production and increase muscle strengthening
    c. increase non–weight-bearing component of exercise routine
    d. resistance exercises should not exceed that provided by daily activities

19. A young male infantryman has facet syndrome in the lumbar spine. Which management strategy will likely make the patient WORSE?
    a. placing gel inserts into his running shoes
    b. maintaining aerobic conditioning by running on level surfaces, preferably dirt or grass
    c. mobilizing his lumbar spine into flexion on a mechanized table
    d. maintaining aerobic conditioning by swimming 500 meters of the breast stroke

20. How does sciatic pain resulting from diabetic neuropathy differ from sciatic pain resulting from spinal disease?
    a. symptoms are relatively chronic in onset and develop over several months
    b. there is usually no back pain associated with sciatica of diabetic neuropathy
    c. sciatic pain is relieved by forward bending
    d. the sciatic pain is usually unilateral

21. Ankle clonus is a sign of:
    a. upper motor neuron lesion
    b. lower motor neuron lesion
    c. injured ankle tendon
    d. torn plantarflexor muscle of the foot

22. When testing a patient with cervical distraction in the neutral position, an increase in neck pain usually indicates:
    a. pressure on a cervical nerve root
    b. rotator cuff tear
    c. vertebral artery ischemia
    d. cervical joint capsule sprain

23. If a patient presents with repeated substernal pressure that lasts 2 to 3 minutes and is relieved by rest, the MOST likely diagnosis is:
    a. pericarditis
    b. mitral valve prolapse
    c. angina pectoris
    d. subluxation of the sternum

24. Unilateral pneumothorax is characterized by:
    a. decreased or absent chest movement over involved side
    b. tracheal deviation toward the side of involvement
    c. increased breath sounds over side of involvement
    d. hyporesonant percussion note

25. A patient with a chronically tight psoas muscle should do which of the following stretches?
    a. extend the involved (tight psoas) side leg off the bed supine
    b. forced foot dorsiflexion
    c. flex forward and toward the involved (tight psoas) side
    d. flex the hip on the involved side and laterally flex away

26. Stretching of tight pectoralis muscles for posturally induced dorsal pain can be performed by:
    a. approximating the elbows anterior to the rib cage
    b. rolling the bent elbows clockwise and counterclockwise while the hands are placed firmly on the lateral rib cage
    c. leaning into a corner with the arms elevated to shoulder level or higher and contracting the pectoralis muscles
    d. clasping the hands behind the neck, bringing the elbows together and lifting the elbows as high as possible

27. For a patient with a right convexity scoliotic lumbar curve, it makes sense to:
    a. strengthen the right-sided lumbar muscles
    b. strengthen the left-sided lumbar muscles
    c. stretch the right-sided lumbar muscles
    d. stretch the muscles on the convex side of the curvature

28. A runner presents with radiographic evidence of heel spurs and reports pain when the large toe or the entire foot is brought into dorsiflexion. Besides foot manipulation, what other modality may play an important role in proper management of this patient?
    a. foot orthotics for pronation or supination
    b. taping of the posterior aspect of the ankle
    c. manipulation of the knee
    d. forced dorsiflexion applied to the ankle joint daily

29. A 12-year-old overweight female patient presents with a right limp and right hip pain that began after a fall on an icy sidewalk. Radiographs show asymmetry of the positioning of the femur heads within the acetabuli. Correct patient management would be:
    a. sacroiliac joint manipulation
    b. referral for orthopedic consultation
    c. hip joint manipulation
    d. SOT blocking

30. Pelvic tilts strengthen the:
    a. hamstrings and upper abdominals
    b. upper abdominals and gluteals
    c. hamstrings and gluteals
    d. lower abdominals and psoas

31. For the best protection of lumbar mechanics, the driver's car seat should be positioned:
    a. as far from the steering wheel as possible
    b. with the front of the seat lower than the back of the seat
    c. with the entire seat bottom level with the floor of the car
    d. as close to the steering wheel as practical

32. The sacroiliac belt (trochanter belt) is recommended for which of these situations?
    a. lumbar disc bulge
    b. facet syndrome
    c. sacroiliac instability
    d. canal stenosis

33. Which of the following is MOST appropriate for rehabilitation management of the middle-aged female patient with hip joint osteoarthritis?
    a. Pilates
    b. impact-style aerobics
    c. long walks
    d. pool exercises and weight reduction

34. The patient has the right under an "informed consent" to:
    a. have the doctor of his or her choice
    b. accept or reject treatment
    c. choose the technique used
    d. request specific therapeutic procedures

35. A patient would have a claim of abandonment when:
    a. the doctor gives a one month opportunity to secure another care provider
    b. the patient no longer has a need for continued care
    c. the doctor owed a duty to the patient
    d. the physician refused to see the patient over a weekend

36. Patients with back and leg pain suggestive of a disc herniation are absolute contraindications for chiropractic manipulative intervention when what additional sign is present?
    a. bowel and bladder disturbances
    b. positive MRI for disc bulge
    c. positive Valsalva maneuver
    d. difficulty standing erect

37. What is the preferred method of measurement for analysis of scoliosis?
    a. Cobb's method
    b. Meyerding's method
    c. Risser's method
    d. Jackson's method

38. Signs of brainstem ischemia, such as vertigo or dizziness, following a spinal manipulation would warrant what actions by the doctor?
    a. remanipulate the segment in the opposite direction
    b. observe the patient
    c. send patient home with icing instructions
    d. refer immediately to emergency department

39. Migraine headaches classically demonstrate what symptoms?
    a. throbbing pain
    b. focal pain in the suboccipital region
    c. visual aura of scintillating scotoma
    d. pain behind one eye

40. Ilium misalignments occur in infants or toddlers due most often to:
    a. trauma
    b. birth process
    c. sleep positioning
    d. sitting up

41. Risk factors for low back pain during pregnancy include previous low back pain, multiparity, and:
    a. middle age
    b. young age
    c. bone density
    d. structural malformation

Answers

1. b. Grade 2 spondylolisthesis in an adult without recent history of trauma is generally considered stable, even if symptomatic, and may respond favorably to chiropractic manipulative care. Referral for further studies and medical consultation should generally be considered with grades 3 and 4 in adults and grades 1 and 2 in children.

2. c. As indicated by Sandoz, the characteristic cavitation associated with a chiropractic adjustment occurs when the fluid tension or pressure barrier that exists between synovial joint surfaces in an encapsulated environment is overcome by the manipulative force.

3. b. Souza lists manipulation as a primary treatment for cervicogenic headache based on a study published by Nilsson. The other headaches listed have had less favorable results from manipulation or may require medical intervention, as with temporal arteritis.

4. d. Deep vein thrombosis (DVT) is a potentially serious condition that requires special studies to properly identify and possible anticoagulant therapy for treatment. Medical referral is indicated as soon as DVT is suspected.

5. c. The rotary component of lumbar adjusting, especially in the side posture position, is believed to place the disc annulus under the greatest amount of stress and to increase the likelihood of complications associated with manual manipulation in patients with lumbar radiculopathy. Manipulation can be used given special care to minimize or eliminate rotation and with careful monitoring of patient signs and symptoms during and after the procedure.

6. d. Any time a patient refuses recommended procedures or treatment and refuses to authenticate an indication of their decision, special caution should be taken. Risk management experts recommend that a certified letter be sent with return receipt outlining the individual's informed decision to forgo the recommended procedure(s) against the doctor's advice. A copy of the letter and the returned receipt should be kept in the patient's file.

7. a. Of the conditions listed, all are relative contraindications to manipulative therapy with the exception of bone infections e.g., tuberculosis), which carry a high risk of pathologic fracture with adjustive therapy and are thus categorized as an absolute contraindication by Bergmann et al. Patients having relative contraindications may be manipulated with caution and with special consideration given to the type of manipulation methods used.

8. b. Informed consent from the patient is always required prior to undertaking any procedure or treatment. Because of the relatively low risk of serious complications associated with manual therapies, it is generally agreed upon by risk management experts that this consent can be either verbal or implied. More specific information and consent are required in writing for particularly risky procedures or for patients who are at particular risk from a procedure. It is, however, a wise precaution to have the patient sign an informed consent form prior to any diagnostic or therapeutic procedure.

9. a. A positive response elicited to the Dix-Hallpike test confirms a diagnosis of benign paroxysmal positional vertigo.

10. c. Maintenance care is a type of management that is delivered to theoretically optimize a person's health, prevent the development or reoccurrence of a clinical condition, or allow for the detection of a clinical condition early in its development. Crisis care is care provided only when symptoms are present. Supportive care is a type of care that, when not provided, results in the reemergence of a patient's symptoms.

11. d. Secondary preventive strategies are those that seek to identify a problem or clinical condition before it presents clinically. DEXA is the most sensitive method to identify the presence and degree of osteoporosis.

12. a. The Adson's, Wright's, and Roos' (Elevated Arm Stress Test) tests are used to identify a patient with thoracic outlet syndrome.

13. d. Fibromyalgia is diagnosed by pain in 11 of 18 characteristic trigger points, nonrestorative sleep, and diffuse musculoskeletal pain of at least 3 months' duration. Abrupt onset of proximal shoulder or pelvic girdle pain is characteristic of polymyalgia rheumatica.

14. a. The use of tobacco has been causally linked to increased in heart disease, lung cancer, diabetes, osteoporosis, and chronic obstructive lung disease.

15. a. Yerguson's and Speed's tests are used to assess the strength of the biceps muscle.

16. c. Patients should be advised to consume small meals throughout the day if they have symptoms of GERD.

17. d. Choices "a," "b," and "c" are correct, and all of these elements need to be considered when obtaining consent. Informed consent for a minor can be given only by the parent or legal guardian and must include the person's signature.

18. b. According to Souza, to induce a bone mass response, exercise must provide mechanical loading through either pull of muscle on bone or weight bearing.

19. d. Repetitive activities that induce extension and axial loading will generally aggravate a symptomatic lumbar facet syndrome. The breast stroke is an extension activity. Conditioned athletes will often not find running to be problematic on softer surfaces as long as they avoid running downhill. Gel inserts may help reduce ground-body impact forces and loading to the lumbar spine.

20. b. Symptoms are usually acute in onset and develop over several days. Forward bending does not relieve the symptoms, and the sciatica is usually bilateral due to the systemic nature of diabetes. Back pain is usually absent in diabetic sciatic pain.

21. a. Ankle clonus, rapid multiple beat clonus on rapid passive dorsiflexion of the foot, strongly suggests upper motor neuron lesion of the spinal cord or brain.

22. d. Cervical distraction decreases the pressure on nerve roots, has no effect on rotator cuff tears, and does not compromise the vertebral artery when done in the neutral position.

23. c. Pericarditis lasts for seconds and radiates to arm and/or neck. Mitral valve prolapse is not related to exertion. Substernal pain is not typical of subluxation of the sternum and would return on commencement of movement following rest.

24. a. Usually, with a unilateral pneumothorax, the trachea is deviated away from the side of involvement and there is a decrease in breath sounds on the affected side. Percussion may be hyperresonant.

25. a. The psoas runs from the anterior lumbar spine and discs to the lesser trochanter. Extending the involved side leg off the table will increase the separation of the trochanter and the lumbar spine, thereby stretching the psoas muscle.

26. c. Isometric contractions after a muscle is stretched help induce relaxation of extrafusal muscle fibers. Having the corner of the room to stretch the arms posteriorly stretches the pectoralis muscles. Contracting the stretched pectoralis muscles reflexly relaxes dorsal spinal muscles.

27. a. Scoliotic curves, secondary to imbalance of paraspinal muscles, exhibit signs of convex side weaknesses and concave side spasms. Muscle procedures for scoliosis should include strengthening of the convex spinal muscles and stretching of the concave spinal muscles.

28. a. Pronation or supination is the most common cause of heel spurs. The use of orthotics restores normal positioning of the plantar fascia and removes tendon stress associated with loss of the longitudinal arch.

29. b. This case should remind the examining doctor of the most likely presentation of a slipped femoral epiphysis. Manipulation of this patient's hip joint may speed up avascular necrosis, while sacroiliac manipulation is ignoring the cause of the problem. Immediate referral is advised.

30. c. Pelvic tilts involve bringing the posterior lower pelvis inferiorly and the pubic region superiorly, while the entire pelvis is brought anteriorly. The hamstrings will pull the posterior pelvis inferiorly and the gluteals flex the pelvis.

31. d. With the seat close to the pedals, the lumbopelvic region is flexed, separating the posterior facets and disc space at L5-S1. Adding a lumbar pillow supports the lumbar curve at the same time.

32. c. The trochanter belt holds the sacroiliac joints together long enough for gelation to occur within the interosseous ligaments between visits. Instability is reduced as ligamentous stability is restored. The belt helps hold the joint surfaces together long enough for muscle splinting to decrease.

33. d. Pool exercises and weight reduction reduce load on the hip joints while allowing the patient to gain muscle strength and flexibility. Pilates would be too strenuous for most women with hip joint osteoarthritis, while long walks and impact exercises would further irritate the inflamed joint.

34. b. Informed consent is the prerequisite for treatment. The starting point for an informed consent analysis is recognizing that, except in rare situations, the patient has the right to accept or reject treatment.

35. c. Abandonment occurs when the doctor, without proper notice, unilaterally severs his professional relationship with a patient who is in need of ongoing health care services.

36. a. Cases of bowel and bladder disturbance, leg weakness, and rectal and genital changes after a manipulation should alert the chiropractor that immediate surgical decompression for cauda equine syndrome was indicated.

37. a. A report by Goldberg indicated an average intraobserver disagreement 1.9 degrees using Cobb's method.

38. b. When signs of brainstem ischemia occur, the doctor should cease manipulation, observe the patient, and refer if symptoms do not subside.

39. c. Throbbing pain or pain behind one eye most often is associated with vascular headaches. Focal pain in the suboccipital region is known more for suboccipital headaches.

40. a. The simple or compound ilium misalignment does not occur in the newborn, infant, or toddler unless it is trauma induced.

41. b. Low back pain risk factors during pregnancy include previous back pain or injury, a young age, or multiparity.

Section Eleven Recommended Reading

Anrig C, Plaugher G: *Pediatric chiropractic,* Baltimore, 1998, Lippincott Williams & Wilkins.

Bergmann T, Peterson D, Lawrence D: *Chiropractic technique,* ed 2, New York, 2002, Churchill Livingstone.

Byfield D, Kinsinger S: *A manual therapist's guide to surface anatomy and palpation skills,* Oxford, 2002, Butterworth Heinemann.

Campbell L, Ladenheim C, Sherman R, Sportelli L: *Risk management in chiropractic,* Fincastle, Va, 1990, Health Services Publications.

Chaitow L: *Palpation and assessment skills,* ed 2, New York, 2003, Churchill Livingstone.

Cooperstein R, Gleberzon BJ: *Technique systems in chiropractic,* Oxford, 2004, Churchill Livingstone.

Cox J: *Low back pain: mechanism, diagnosis and treatment,* ed 6, Baltimore, 1999, Lippincott Williams & Wilkins.

Gatterman M: *Chiropractic management of spine related disorders,* ed 2, Baltimore, 2003, Lippincott Williams & Wilkins.

Gleberzon BJ: *Chiropractic care of the older patient,* Oxford, 2001, Butterworth Heinemann.

Haldeman S, ed: *Principles and practice of chiropractic,* ed 3, Norwalk, Conn, 2005, Appleton & Lange.

Herkowitz H, Rothman R, eds: *Rothman-Simeone: the spine,* ed 4, Philadelphia, 1999, WB Saunders.

Kendall F, McCreary E: *Muscles: testing and function with posture and pain,* ed 5, Philadelphia, 2005, Lippincott Williams & Wilkins.

Kirkaldy-Willis W, Bernard T: *Managing low back pain,* ed 4, New York, 1999, Churchill Livingstone.

Landenheim C: *Professional chiropractic practice: ethics, business, jurisprudence and risk management,* Norwalk, Ia, 2001, Practice Makers Products.

Liebensen C, ed: *Rehabilitation of the spine: a practitioner's manual,* ed 2, Philadelphia, 2005, Lippincott Williams & Wilkins.

Magee D: *Orthopedic physical assessment,* revised ed 4, Philadelphia, 2005, WB Saunders.

Marchiori D: *Clinical imaging: with skeletal, chest, and abdomen pattern differentials,* ed 2, St Louis, 2005, Mosby.

Plaugher G, ed: *Textbook of clinical chiropractic: a specific biomechanical approach,* Baltimore, 1993, Williams & Wilkins.

Simons D, Simons S, Travell J: *Myofascial pain and dysfunction: the trigger point manual (volumes 1&2): the upper half of the body,* ed 2, Philadelphia, 1999, Lippincott Williams & Wilkins.

Souza T: *Differential diagnosis and management for the chiropractor: protocols and algorithms,* ed 3, Sudbury, Mass, 2005, Jones and Bartlett.

Yochum T, Rowe L: *Essentials of skeletal radiology: volumes 1-2,* ed 3, Baltimore, 2004, Lippincott Williams & Wilkins.

SECTION TWELVE

Associated Clinical Sciences

Gynecology and Obstetrics

Robyn Beirman

1. A vaginal discharge that is frothy, malodorous, and green-yellow in color is most likely due to infection with:
   a. *Chlamydia trachomatis*
   b. *Trichomonas vaginalis*
   c. *Candida albicans*
   d. *Gardnerella vaginalis*

2. Which of the following statements about genital herpes is INACCURATE?
   a. it may be caused by herpes simplex 1 or herpes simplex 2
   b. it may be transmitted even in the absence of genital lesions
   c. it is often accompanied by dysuria and a vaginal discharge
   d. incubation period is usually 7 to 10 days

3. Excessive uterine blood loss, which is either intermenstrual or acyclic, is called:
   a. menorrhagia
   b. metrorrhagia
   c. polymenorrhea
   d. metrostaxis

4. The LEAST likely cause of left iliac fossa pain in a 30-year-old is:
   a. acute salpingitis
   b. ectopic pregnancy
   c. acute cervicitis
   d. torsion of an ovarian cyst

5. Which of the following is NOT a major risk factor for carcinoma of the breast?
   a. diet rich in animal protein and saturated fats
   b. family history of ovarian cancer
   c. late menarche and early pregnancy
   d. presence of *BRCA1* or *BRCA2* gene

6. The LEAST likely cause of infertility is:
   a. polycystic ovarian syndrome
   b. uterine fibroids
   c. hyperprolactinemia
   d. endometriosis

7. A 48-year-old woman presents with a 6-day history of heavy vaginal bleeding. Her last menstrual period was 2 weeks earlier. There have been no similar episodes in the past. The LEAST likely cause of her problem is that:
   a. she has endometriosis
   b. she is perimenopausal
   c. she has a physiologic ovarian cyst
   d. she is having a miscarriage

8. A 27-year-old nulliparous woman presents with dysmenorrhea. Pain occurs prior to bleeding and is relieved soon after the onset of bleeding. Low-grade chronic pelvic pain also occurs intermittently. She is unaware of any prior sexually transmitted diseases. She complains of irritability and an intermittent chronic white, odorless vaginal discharge. Symptoms have been present for approximately 2 years. The most likely cause is:
   a. primary dysmenorrhea
   b. endometriosis
   c. pelvic inflammatory disease (PID)
   d. adenomyosis

9. Spontaneous abortions in the first trimester are most commonly due to:
   a. insufficient hormone production for the maintenance of pregnancy
   b. abnormalities of the embryo
   c. maternal disease
   d. uterine abnormalities

10. To make the diagnosis of endometriosis, the MOST appropriate investigative technique would be:
    a. ultrasonography
    b. computed tomography
    c. hysterosalpingography
    d. laparoscopy

11. Which of the following is NOT usually elevated in the blood of a patient with polycystic ovarian syndrome?
    a. sex hormone–binding globulin (SHBG)
    b. insulin
    c. luteinizing hormone (LH)
    d. androgens

12. Which of the following is NOT characteristic of preeclampsia?
    a. hypertension
    b. convulsions
    c. proteinuria
    d. edema

13. Primary dysmenorrhea is associated with:
    a. anovulatory cycles
    b. multiparity
    c. decreased endometrial prostaglandin synthesis
    d. pain mainly on days of heaviest flow

14. Risk factors that predispose a woman to endometrial carcinoma include all of the following EXCEPT:
    a. endometrial hyperplasia
    b. early menopause
    c. obesity
    d. excessive unopposed estrogen

15. Which one of the following statements about pelvic inflammatory disease is INACCURATE?
    a. it is commonly caused by *Neisseria* species
    b. it can involve any part of the reproductive tract from vagina to ovary
    c. it may result in chronic pelvic pain, infertility, or ectopic pregnancies
    d. it may be sexually transmitted or occur postpartum

16. Bilateral breast lumps, associated with tenderness, are MOST likely to be due to:
    a. fibroadenoma
    b. fibroadenosis
    c. Paget's disease of the nipple
    d. fat necrosis

Answers

1. b. *Trichomonas vaginalis* is the only infective agent to cause this type of discharge. The discharge associated with *Chlamydia trachomatis* is mucopurulent, that of *Candida albicans* is thick and white, and *Gardnerella vaginalis* is characterized by a white-gray discharge with a fishy odor.

2. d. Incubation period for herpes simplex infections is more commonly 2 to 7 days. Although the majority of genital herpes infections is caused by herpes simplex 2, some (approximately 10% to 30% in United States) are due to herpes simplex 1.

3. c. Menorrhagia refers to excess menstrual blood loss; polymenorrhea refers to menstrual cycles that are less than 21 days in duration (often with a heavy flow); and metrostaxis describes a situation in which there is continuous bleeding from the uterus.

4. c. Acute cervicitis usually presents with a vaginal discharge, bleeding, and possibly dyspareunia but not iliac fossa pain. The other three disorders would have iliac fossa pain as a major clinical manifestation.

5. c. The greater the number of ovulatory cycles a woman has prior to her first pregnancy, the greater is the risk of breast cancer. Thus, late menarche and early pregnancy are not risk factors.

6. b. Polycystic ovarian syndrome and hyperprolactinemia can cause infertility due to the inhibition of ovulation. Endometriosis can cause infertility via a number of mechanisms, including the interference of ovum pickup and transport through the uterine tube. Fibroids may cause complications during pregnancy but rarely cause infertility.

7. a. Endometriosis is unlikely to present for the first time in a 48-year-old woman. Although menstrual irregularities can occur in this disorder, it would be an unusual primary presentation. The symptoms described are more typical of the other three scenarios.

8. c. Dysmenorrhea that is relieved with the onset of menstruation suggests an etiology associated with pelvic congestion. Although some congestion will occur with endometriosis and adenomyosis, the presence of a chronic vaginal discharge and chronic pelvic pain increases the likelihood that this woman has PID. A history of STDs is not always found, as many of these infections are asymptomatic.

9. b. It has been estimated that 80% to 90% of miscarriages occur in the first trimester, the vast majority as a result of abnormalities of the product of conception. Insufficient hormone production is an important, but not as common, cause of miscarriage between 8 and 12 weeks. Maternal disease is a cause of miscarriage, most commonly in the second trimester. Uterine abnormalities can cause miscarriage, but this is not a common cause.

10. d. Direct visualization and biopsy of endometrial deposits are required to make a positive diagnosis. Ultrasonography and computed tomography may be useful in assessing extent but are not usually sufficient for the initial diagnosis.

11. a. Insulin resistance in this disorder results in hyperinsulinemia. This, plus the elevated levels of LH and altered LH–to–follicle-stimulating hormone ratio, stimulates androgen secretion from the ovaries, as well as reducing the level of SHBG.

12. b. Convulsions (and/or coma) may occur in eclampsia, not preeclampsia. Hypertension after the 20th week of gestation, plus proteinuria and/or edema, is known as preeclampsia.

13. d. Primary dysmenorrhea is usually associated with ovulatory cycles, an increase in prostaglandin production in the secretory endometrium, and is more common in nulliparous women.

14. b. Obesity is thought to be the most significant of the risk factors for endometrial carcinoma. This cancer is often preceded by endometrial hyperplasia, as well as unopposed estrogen levels. Late onset of menopause also increases the risk.

15. b. Pelvic inflammatory disease is defined as an infection of the upper female genital tract in that it involves one or more of the following structures: cervix, uterus, uterine tubes, or ovaries.

16. b. Fibroadenoma, Paget's disease of the nipple, and fat necrosis are usually unilateral, not bilateral. Fibroadenoma and Paget's disease are usually nontender. Fibroadenosis (i.e., chronic mastitis) most commonly presents with multiple, bilateral tender breast lumps.

CHAPTER 72

Geriatrics

Lisa Zaynab Killinger

CONTENT AREAS

- Anatomic and physiologic process of aging
- Geriatric disorders and case management

1. According to the Centers for Disease Control and Prevention, which group of elderly Americans suffers from the highest incidences of hypertension, heart disease, and diabetes?
   a. Caucasian
   b. Native American
   c. African American
   d. Asian American

2. What assessment tool might be used to aid in differentiation between delirium and dementia in an aging patient?
   a. Barthel Index
   b. Rand 36
   c. Mini-Mental State Examination
   d. Fall Hazard Checklist

3. Evidence-based health promotion recommendations for the patient at risk for heart disease would include:
   a. a diet high in meat-based proteins and complex carbohydrates
   b. losing weight, limiting alcohol intake, and exercising regularly
   c. increasing the amount of dietary fiber and calories from unsaturated fat
   d. losing weight, increasing dietary sodium and potassium, and exercising regularly

4. According to the United States Bureau of the Census statistics, which portion of the geriatric population is the fastest growing?
   a. Caucasian
   b. ethnic minorities
   c. males
   d. poor

5. What is the number one cause of death in both male and female elderly persons?
   a. cancer
   b. stroke
   c. diabetes
   d. heart disease

6. The "Get Up and Go" test, a common geriatric assessment tool, is a measure of:
   a. cognitive status
   b. bladder function
   c. functional status
   d. socioeconomic status

7. According to *Healthy People 2010*, which group of elderly persons has nearly twice the incidence of disability due to chronic low back pain compared with Caucasians:
   a. Native Americans
   b. African Americans
   c. Hispanics
   d. Asian Americans

8. Which of the following is NOT a contributing factor to the greater potential for drug toxicity in the older patient?
   a. lower lean body mass
   b. higher fat stores
   c. decreased water content of body
   d. increased gastric acidity

9. The rate of poverty in this population is roughly three times that of Caucasian elderly.
   a. Asian Americans
   b. Hispanic Americans
   c. African Americans
   d. mixed ethnicity

10. Which of the following statements is TRUE related to persons over age 65?
    a. they fear crime more and have the highest rate of criminal victimization compared with all other age groups
    b. they have more acute illnesses and more chronic illnesses as a group
    c. there are significant disparities between the poverty levels and health statuses of persons of various ethnicities and their Caucasian counterparts
    d. they make up less than 10% of the population

11. Which of the following is NOT a risk factor for osteoporosis?
    a. smoking
    b. European descent
    c. heavy alcohol or caffeine use
    d. diet high in soy-based products

12. Which is NOT a sign of stroke?
    a. difficulty speaking
    b. loss of strength or coordination in a limb
    c. dizziness or unsteadiness
    d. decreased blood pressure

13. Which of the following is NOT a recommendation made in the "Food Pyramid for Persons Over Age 65"?
    a. calcium and vitamin D supplements
    b. vitamin B12 supplements
    c. at least 6 glasses of water per day
    d. vitamin A supplements

14. The most common form of this type of confusion has a slow, insidious onset.
    a. dysphagia
    b. depression
    c. delirium
    d. dementia

15. What is the single most important lifestyle recommendation you can offer a patient with osteoporosis to delay or prevent disability due to this disease?
    a. increase in physical activity levels
    b. multimineral supplement
    c. decrease in the dietary intake of fat
    d. decreased caffeine consumption

16. Which of the following is NOT an appropriate recommendation to help prevent falls in the home of an aged patient?
    a. proper and adequate nutrition
    b. a regular, carefully designed exercise program
    c. installation of rails near steps and in tub area
    d. use of dim lighting in hallways to prevent glare

17. Two "normal" musculoskeletal changes seen in the aging patient are:
    a. decreased muscle mass and increased bone density
    b. decreased bone density and decreased ligament elasticity
    c. decreased lung capacity and increased lean body mass
    d. increased ligament elasticity and decreased lean body mass

18. Asking the elderly patient about which of the following abilities might be a part of a functional status assessment?
    a. ability to remember name, date, year, and season
    b. ability to do laundry, get dressed, and prepare meals
    c. ability to name an object placed in their hand
    d. ability to recall the name of objects placed in the patient's hand

19. Which of the following is NOT considered a consequence of "normal aging"?
    a. decreased muscle mass
    b. decreased production of stomach acids
    c. decreased sense of hearing, vision, smell, and taste
    d. increased ligament elasticity

20. Which of the following lists includes the three stages of degeneration according to the Kirkaldy-Willis model of spinal degeneration?
    a. dysfunction, instability, and stabilization
    b. instability, subluxation, and stabilization
    c. stabilization, misalignment, and subluxation
    d. dysfunction, instability, and degeneration

21. Appropriate recommendations for a chiropractor to offer an elderly patient with stress incontinence might include:
    a. decreasing fluid intake
    b. Kegel exercises to strengthen the muscles of the pelvic floor
    c. pharmaceutical intervention
    d. increasing calcium intake

22. Which of the following lists contain three preventable risk factors for osteoporosis?
    a. family history of osteoporosis, diet high in protein, fair skin
    b. fair skin, small frame, early menopause
    c. sedentary lifestyle, avoidance of dairy products, smoking
    d. alcohol consumption, smoking, diet high in soy-based proteins

23. The American Cancer Society recommends that persons over the age 50 consume ___ grams of fiber per day to help prevent colon cancer.
    a. 10
    b. 20
    c. 30
    d. 40

Answers

1.   c.   The Centers for Disease Control and Prevention, or CDC, tracks statistics on health in various populations. In this case, disparities in health status are identified to help focus future health promotion/ prevention efforts to those with the greatest need.

2.   c.   The chiropractic textbook *The Aging Body, Conservative Management of Common Neuromusculoskeletal Conditions* offers an excellent discussion of comprehensive geriatric assessment. The Mini-Mental State Examination (MMSE) has long been considered by many health professionals as the gold standard in assessing cognitive concerns related to aging.

3.   b.   The *Clinician's Handbook of Preventive Services* offers a guide to health professionals on sound, evidence-based prevention recommendations related to leading health concerns. Health disease, the leading cause of death in both men and women over 65, may be prevented or controlled through the listed lifestyle changes. Sodium intake should also be restricted.

4.   b.   The U.S. Bureau of the Census and other government organizations track the growth of various subsets in our population. Our nation is aging and becoming increasingly diverse, with Caucasian elderly soon to be in the minority.

5.   d.   According to the CDC, heart disease is the leading cause of death in the elderly. Cancer and stroke are the second and third leading causes of death, respectively.

6.   c.   The chiropractic textbook *The Aging Body, Conservative Management of Common Neuromusculoskeletal Conditions* offers an excellent discussion of comprehensive geriatric assessment. An important part of geriatric assessment is the functional assessment (how well a patient performs regular activities of daily living). Functional assessment can be assessed using a "Get Up and Go" or "Up and Go" test and other assessments such as the Functional Status Index test.

7.   a.   *Healthy People 2010* is the major "State of the Union in Health" document in the United States. It compiles health information and research and sets goals for improving the health of the nation. In this case, disparities in health status are identified to help focus future health promotion/prevention efforts on those with the greatest need.

8. d. In numerous physiology textbooks, including *The Science of Geriatrics* by J. E. Morley and colleagues, age-related changes are discussed in the context of drug metabolism. As the patient ages, gastric acidity, or secretion of acid from the stomach, decreases. This factor is not as significant as the other listed changes related to an increased potential for drug toxicity in aging patients.

9. c. *Healthy People 2010* identifies poverty as a key barrier to good health and disparities in poverty among various population subgroups. This question is also seen on the Palmore Facts on Aging quiz, considered the gold standard for assessing student's baseline knowledge about the geriatric patient population.

10. c. This question is also seen on the Palmore Facts on Aging quiz, considered the gold standard for assessing student's baseline knowledge about the geriatric patient population. Older patients do fear crime more but are not the victims of as much crime as are young inner city males. The elderly make up over 13% of the U.S. population as of 2005.

11. d. Chiropractors should become familiar with the risk factors related to osteoporosis: smoking, fair skin, European or Asian descent, alcohol use, smoking, sedentary lifestyle, early menopause, etc. Diets high in soy products, and their related isoflavones, may be protective against osteoporosis.

12. d. Stroke is the third leading cause of death in aging patients. Chiropractors should be intimately familiar with the signs and symptoms of strokes, particularly because stroke patients may present to a chiropractor with the all too common complaint of headache. The National Chiropractic Mutual Insurance Company is a good source of information on this topic.

13. d. The nutritional recommendations for aging persons differ from those in younger persons. The aging need fewer calories, must be encouraged to consume six glasses of water per day to combat the ubiquitous problems of dehydration and constipation, and are also encouraged to take calcium and vitamin D and B12 supplements to combat the poor absorption of these nutrients in aging persons and osteoporosis.

14. d. Differential diagnoses for delirium, dementia, and depression are part of a comprehensive geriatric assessment. Dementia is known for its gradual, insidious onset, whereas delirium is often a rapid onset triggered by infection, trauma, or drug toxicity.

15. a. The body of scientific literature on osteoporosis indicates that the most important intervention is the addition of physical activity, particularly weight-bearing exercise, to prevent bone loss and build bone in even the oldest, most frail patients. Concurrent use of calcium and vitamin D supplementation is also recommended. Caffeine may aggravate osteoporosis but not to the extent of sedentary habits. See *Chiropractic Care of the Aging Patient* by Gleberzon (editor).

16. d. Low light vision is compromised with aging, so increased lighting is required in the homes of aging persons. Choices a through d are actually sound recommendations. Any standard fall hazard checklist or home safety checklist to assess the environmental safety of an older adult will include the listed items.

17. b. Most geriatrics texts will list common age-related changes. Muscle mass, bone density, ligament elasticity, and lean body mass all commonly decline with aging, but most of these changes can be reversed with increases in physical activity.

18. b. The chiropractic textbook *The Aging Body, Conservative Management of Common Neuromusculoskeletal Conditions* offers an excellent discussion of comprehensive geriatric assessment. An important part of geriatric assessment is the functional assessment (how well a patient performs regular activities of daily living).

19. d. Most geriatrics texts will list common age-related changes. Muscle mass, bone density, ligament elasticity, all five senses, stomach acid production, and lean body mass all commonly decline with aging.

20. a. The Kirkaldy-Willis model is discussed in both chiropractic and other health professional texts and research articles. This topic is discussed in a chiropractic context in the chapter on aging in the textbook *Fundamentals of Chiropractic* by Redwood and Cleveland (editors).

21. b. Common to many geriatrics texts is a discussion of incontinence, a leading cause of institutionalization in the elderly. While many interventions are pharmaceutical or surgical in nature, evidence points to favorable outcomes in patients who simply strengthen pelvic floor musculature through focused exercises.

22. c. Chiropractors should become familiar with the preventable risk factors related to osteoporosis: smoking, alcohol use, sedentary lifestyle, etc.

23. c. Because colorectal cancer is the third leading cause of cancer death in the aging population, good evidence-based prevention recommendations should be understood by chiropractors or any health professional caring for older patients. The American Cancer Society makes a recommendation of 30 grams/day, based on the best available scientific evidence.

Clinical Psychology

Rodger Tepe

1. Which of the following defense mechanisms BEST represents the process of attributing one's own unacceptable characteristics to others?
    a. displacement
    b. projection
    c. repression
    d. reaction formation

2. Depressive syndrome symptoms (a dysphoric mood) present for more than 2 years, separated by occasional periods of normal mood, is most typical of:
    a. major depressive episode
    b. bipolar disorder
    c. cyclothymic disorder
    d. dysthymic disorder

3. A binge-purge eating cycle is most typical of:
    a. bulimia nervosa
    b. anorexia nervosa
    c. obesity
    d. rumination disorder

4. Intense fear of gaining weight or becoming fat, even though being already underweight, is most typical of:
    a. bulimia nervosa
    b. anorexia nervosa
    c. obesity
    d. rumination disorder

5. Circadian rhythm sleep disorder may be diagnosed if which of the following is present?
    a. the sleep disturbance occurs during the course of a comorbid mental disorder
    b. the sleep disturbance mismatches the sleep-wake schedule required by the person's environment and/or her or her circadian sleep-wake pattern
    c. the sleep disturbance is comorbid with the physiologic effects of a general medical condition
    d. the sleep disturbance is due to a sleep-related breathing condition

6. Disregard for the rights of others; repeatedly performing acts that are grounds for arrest; reckless disregard for the safety of self or others; and lack of remorse are most typical of:
    a. borderline personality disorder
    b. histrionic personality disorder
    c. paranoid schizophrenia
    d. antisocial personality disorder

7. The BEST diagnosis for a child showing marked impairment in the use of multiple nonverbal behaviors, failure to develop appropriate peer relationships, lack of spontaneous seeking to share enjoyment, and lack of social or emotional reciprocity would be which of the following?
    a. autistic disorder
    b. mental retardation
    c. attention-deficit/hyperactivity disorder
    d. oppositional defiant disorder

8. An individual who deals with emotional conflict by attributing exaggerated positive qualities to others is most likely to be using which of the following defense mechanisms?
    a. omnipotence
    b. rationalization
    c. idealization
    d. sublimation

9. In *DSM-VI*, major depressive episode belongs in which of the following classifications of mental disorders?
    a. anxiety disorders
    b. psychotic disorders
    c. mood disorders
    d. adjustment disorders

10. In *DSM-VI*, posttraumatic stress disorder belongs in which of the following classifications of mental disorders?
    a. anxiety disorders
    b. psychotic disorders
    c. mood disorders
    d. adjustment disorders

11. Anxiety about or avoidance of places or situations from which escape might be difficult is most typical of which of the following disorders?
    a. acute stress disorder
    b. social phobia
    c. generalized anxiety disorder
    d. agoraphobia

12. Which of the following is the MOST typical symptom of schizophrenia?
    a. peculiarities of voluntary movement
    b. blunted or flat affect
    c. disturbance consisting of 1 month of delusions, hallucinations, and grossly disorganized behavior
    d. disturbance of at least 6 months that includes at least 1 month of delusions, hallucinations, and grossly disorganized behavior

13. A preoccupation with fears of having, or the idea that one has, a serious disease based on the person's misinterpretation of bodily symptoms is MOST consistent with a diagnosis of:
    a. hypochondriasis
    b. conversion disorder
    c. somatization disorder
    d. body dysmorphic disorder

14. A history of many physical complaints beginning before the age of 30 that occur over a period of years and result in treatment being sought or significant impairment in social, occupational, or other important areas of functioning is MOST consistent with a diagnosis of:
    a. hypochondriasis
    b. conversion disorder
    c. somatization disorder
    d. body dysmorphic disorder

15. A clinical presentation in which pain in one or more anatomic
     sites is the predominant focus and is accompanied by (1) significant
     distress, (2) impairment in social, occupational, or other functioning,
     (3) psychological factors that are judged to be involved, and
     (4) symptom(s) that are not intentionally feigned is most consistent
     with a diagnosis of:
     a. hypochondriasis
     b. conversion disorder
     c. pain disorder
     d. body dysmorphic disorder

Answers

1. b. By definition, projection consists of attributing one's unacceptable characteristics to others as an anxiety-reducing mechanism. The ability to recognize basic defense mechanisms is important to physicians as part of general communication skill and because pain and illness often escalate the use of defense strategies.

2. d. A dsythymic disorder consists precisely of a 2 (or more)-year course of dysphoric mood with exacerbations, remissions separated by occasional periods of "normal" mood lasting not longer than 2 months.

3. a. Although some persons with anorexia nervosa may occasionally binge and purge, binging and purging is most typical of bulimia nervosa.

4. b. Along with body weight less than 85% of normal, disturbance of body image and (in females) amenorrhea, intense fear of gaining weight is a distinguishing characteristic of anorexia nervosa.

5. b. The mismatched sleep-wake cycle referred to in this question is, again, the definition of circadian rhythm sleep disorder, which distinguishes it from other dyssomnias.

6. d. Considered the quintessential "criminal" personality, antisocial personality disorder is easily distinguished from other ego-syntonic personality disorders as per the characteristics in the stem of the question.

7. a. Autistic disorder is defined in the question. It does happen that uninformed doctors may misdiagnose autism as Asperger's or ADHD. Considering the extent of improper diagnosis and treatment of this group of disorders, referral for diagnostic consultation/ second opinion should be considered.

8. a. Omnipotence is a less familiar defense mechanism than projection, rationalization, etc., but is worth knowing about in today's world where the word "codependence" has become a part of America's working vocabulary (albeit misunderstood). Like other mechanisms that externalize, omnipotence can become dysfunctional if overused.

9. c. Considering the high rate of comorbidity between chronic pain and depression, chiropractors should be knowledgeable about and able to differentially diagnose the commonly occurring mood disorders and understand how they fit into the categories of mental illness diagnoses. The over prescription of analgesics and antidepressant drugs adds to the importance of referral for second opinions and comanagement with conservative caregivers.

10. a. PTSD will be seen in chiropractic practices particularly related to vehicle accidents and perhaps other severe physical trauma–related injuries. This must be understood as an anxiety disorder to result in proper treatment and/or referral/comanagement.

11. d. It is reasonable to expect a primary care physician to know the difference between agoraphobia and social or other phobias. The definition is in the question.

12. d. Although not commonly seen in outpatient settings, chiropractors should be able to identify schizophrenia as a potentially self or other harmful condition and be able to make appropriate case note entries and referrals.

13. a. Differentiating hypochondriasis from other somatoform disorders is important for chiropractors in the sense that the unfortunate term "it is all in your head" is often misused in relationship to hypochondriacs, who present their bewildering, inconsistent array of symptoms with effusive language and strong emotion. Although these patients can be difficult to manage, they need help and may also have other illnesses mixed in among the hypochondriacal symptoms.

14. c. Somatization disorder can be confused with hypochondriasis because both present with a mixed/inconsistent variety of symptoms that cannot be substantiated with orthopedic or lab tests etc., and are presented in a dramatic or effusive manner. The key distinction here is that hypochondriasis involves the exaggeration of a true sensation while somatization disorder involves no necessarily true sensation and is more multisymptomatic across systems than hypochondriasis.

15. c. There are several questions from the somatoform disorders due to their prevalence in outpatient settings and the confusion they can cause to sincere physicians who want to believe what their patients tell them. There is also greater litigation exposure with this group in addition to more "wear and tear" on the doctor. Symptoms typically will not resolve or will be substituted, which is upsetting to doctor and patient alike. Headache and back pain can be difficult to substantiate other than by patient report and are the most frequently occurring examples of pain disorder. Previous editions of DSM referred to this as psychogenic pain disorder, which may have been easier to understand by non-mental health professionals.

Dermatology

Antonio E. Bifero

1. A 17-year-old student with a history of herpetic gingivostomatitis develops a generalized and symmetric patchy rash 1 to 2 mm in diameter, which is painful and itchy. The lesions have two concentric rings with a central core. There is some erosion in the oral mucosa. Choose the correct diagnosis.
    a. urticaria
    b. pemphigus vulgaris
    c. erythema multiforme
    d. secondary syphilis

2. An 18-year-old man is plowing a field on a hillside. The tractor strikes a large rock and tips over, pinning him underneath. The ground is muddy, and he is able to work his way free. He discovers a deep, penetrating puncture wound to his calf. He walks home and washes the soil off the wound site and puts a bandage over it. A week later, the wound is healing, and the leg is not swollen, but he begins to experience generalized muscle spasms, with stiffness and pain in his shoulders and back. He has difficulty with eating and swallowing, with painful and stiff jaw and facial muscles. What is the diagnosis?
    a. tetanus
    b. toxic shock syndrome
    c. gas gangrene
    d. none of the above

3. A 19-year-old woman presents to your office following femoral hernia reduction surgery with fever, vomiting, mild diarrhea, and myalgias. Symptoms began suddenly with onset of a pruritic maculopapular rash. Physical examination reveals a temperature of 39°C and hypotension. The erythroderma is distributed on the palms and soles of feet and has begun to desquamate. Choose the correct diagnosis.
    a. cellulitis
    b. tinea corporus
    c. scarlet fever
    d. toxic shock syndrome

4. A 23-year-old man complains of severe pruritic vesicular lesions on the webs of the fingers and wrists. His younger sister complains of the same condition. What is the MOST likely diagnosis?
   a. bullous impetigo
   b. Norwegian itch (scabies)
   c. atopic dermatitis
   d. tinea versicolor

5. In mid summer, a 3-year-old was taken to the emergency department with a 3-day history of fever, malaise, abdominal pain, nausea, and vomiting. Physical exam revealed a temperature of 103°F. Food poisoning was the diagnosis and he was released. Three days later, the patient reported to another emergency department with persistent fever, anorexia, diffuse myalgias, irritability, photophobia, cough, nausea, and vomiting. A second physical exam showed hepatosplenomegaly and a diffuse erythematous maculopapular rash with petechiae on the trunk, arms, legs, palms, and soles. Lab results included an elevated white blood cell (WBC) count of 12.5×10^9 cells/L (normal range: 3.0 to 9.1×10^9 cells/L), thrombocytopenia, elevated AST of 279 U/L (normal: ≤43 U/L), and elevated ALT of 77 U/L (normal: ≤47 U/L). The patient was transferred to a pediatric intensive care unit, where she had declining mental status, metabolic acidosis, and respiratory failure; the patient died 6 days after treatment was initially sought. What is the diagnosis?
   a. Rocky Mountain spotted fever
   b. scrub typhus
   c. varicella zoster
   d. fifth disease

6. Which of the following produces a primary lesion characterized as an ulcer and a secondary lesion characterized as a rash?
   a. *Rickettsia prowazekii*
   b. *Rickettsia typhi*
   c. rickettsia pox
   d. *Coxiella burnetii*

7. An ill-looking 58-year-old man with a 20-year history of diabetes mellitus presents with severe pain and swelling of his right arm that started days after minor trauma. His temperature is 103.6°F. Examination of the arm reveals a 13-cm area of dark red epidermal induration. Large bullae filled with purple fluid are seen in the center of the wound. Some parts are black in color. Crepitus is felt with palpation of the arm. Labs show leukocytosis and elevated serum CPK. Which of the following is the most likely diagnosis?
   a. erysipelas
   b. folliculitis
   c. cellulitis
   d. necrotizing fasciitis

8. A 68-year-old homeless man presents to the emergency department with a history of dull vision, night blindness, xerophthalmia, neuritis, muscular weakness, and muscle atrophy. Numerous pleomorphic follicular keratotic papules are noted over the posterolateral aspect of the arms, chest, neck, and face. He states he first noticed the skin lesions 3 months ago on his arms. The hands and feet are spared. What is the diagnosis?
    a. pellagra
    b. phrynoderma
    c. hypervitaminosis A
    d. comedos

9. A 9-year-old boy presents with patchy baldness of 2 weeks' duration. He states that a few of his classmates have the same condition. Upon inspection, you notice multiple scaly lesions on the scalp. What is the diagnosis?
    a. tinea capitis
    b. tinea corporus
    c. androgenetic alopecia
    d. none of the above

10. A 64-year-old man presented with a generalized, blistering rash of 3 weeks' duration. The lesions appeared first in the mouth and nail folds with gradual involvement of the groin, face, and trunk. On examination, there was extensive blistering and large areas of denuded skin. Laboratory investigations showed a normal CBC and biochemical profile. His serum contained anti-keratinocyte antibodies. What is the diagnosis?
    a. Senear-Usher syndrome
    b. pemphigus vulgaris
    c. dermatitis herpetiformis
    d. erythema multiforme

11. A 25-year-old woman presents with a 2-year history of spots on her face, trunk, and back. She is extremely self-conscious of it, and it seems to be worse when tanning. Physical exam is unremarkable. What is the diagnosis?
    a. leprosy
    b. vitiligo
    c. tinea versicolor
    d. piebaldism

12. Which of the following would be the correct term for a dermatophyte fingernail infection?
    a. tinea corporus
    b. tinea manuum
    c. onychomycosis
    d. tinea captious

13. A 7-year-old child presents to your office for evaluation of a peculiar growth on her hand that does not itch. On examination, you find numerous flesh-colored papules roughly 3 mm in diameter with umbilication. What is the diagnosis?
    a. herpetic Whitlow
    b. verruca vulgaris
    c. molluscum contagiosum
    d. atopic dermatitis

14. A 20-year-old man camping in the Ohio River valley develops pruritic erythematous plaques and vesicles over the face, neck, and arms 5 days into the hike. Some appear to have sharp edges and others have begun to crust. No history of fever or chills is noted. What is the diagnosis?
    a. atopic dermatitis
    b. impetigo
    c. erythema infectiosum
    d. acute contact dermatitis

Answers

1. c. Erythema multiforme is the most likely diagnosis in this patient. The lesions are generalized and can occur in the oral mucosa. Classically, they look like a target and are both pruritic and burning. Pemphigus vulgaris is a chronic bullous autoimmune disease manifesting in the fourth and fifth decades of life. Secondary syphilis appears 2 to 6 months after the primary infection and usually consists of a maculopapular rash on the hands and feet. Urticaria is characterized by itchy wheals lasting several hours.

2. a. Tetanus is caused by the exotoxin of the anaerobic bacterium *Clostridium tetani*. Spores are ubiquitous in soil and germinate in deeper tissues where the partial pressure of oxygen is lower. Toxic shock is an acute febrile illness with a fulminant course, it does not produce tetanospasm.

3. c. Toxic shock syndrome is a toxin-mediated systemwide disease caused by the bacteria *Staphylococcus aureus*. It is characterized by high fever, vomiting, and a diffuse macular rash that may involve the mucous membranes. Desquamation of the involved area usually ensues. High-risk factors include surgical wounds, nasal packs, burns, and vaginal tampons, to name a few. Cellulitis is an acute infection of the dermis and hypodermis with erythema, heat, and tenderness at point of entry of bacteria. Tinea corporus is a chronic fungal infection of the skin that has a benign course and does not fit the clinic picture described. Scarlet fever is an exotoxin-induced complication of group A streptococcal infections usually seen in children. It produces a scarlatinform rash that spreads centrifugally.

4. b. Scabies is a skin infection caused by the mite that is spread via skin contact. There is intense itching. Impetigo is an infectious skin disease caused by *S. aureus* or *S. pyogenes* that presents with vesicular lesions on the face circumscribing the nostrils or the lips that crust. Atopic dermatitis or eczema is a skin hypersensitivity. Tinea versicolor is an asymptomatic dermatophytosis characterized by scaling macules with sharp margins on the trunk.

5. a. Rocky Mountain spotted fever (RMSF) is the most common fatal tick-borne illness reported in children in the United States. The early stage is characterized by macular rash and fever, even though most patients are not reported as having the triad of fever, rash, and tick-related tissue trauma. More often, the rash appears several days after onset of fever and can become petechial. RMSF can result in severe systemic manifestations, like pneumonitis, myocarditis, hepatitis, acute renal failure, encephalitis, gangrene, and death. Scrub typhus is not endemic in the United States and is transmitted by the bite of an infected mite. The rash is papular at first and then necrotic but ultimately evolves into an eschar. Varicella zoster (chickenpox) presents with a diffuse pruritic vesicular rash and is not described as fatal. The fifth disease (human parvovirus B19) presents as a "slapped-cheek" rash on the face with a diffuse red rash on the trunk and limbs with low-grade fever. The condition abates without treatment within 1 week.

6. c. Rickettsial pox is transmitted by the mouse mite and presents with fever; unlike other rickettsial diseases, it has a rash that starts on the extremities and moves to the hands and feet. Approximately 1 week before the fever, a red papule appears at the bite site that develops into an eschar. *Rickettsia typhi* and *Rickettsia prowazekii* cause endemic and epidemic typhus, respectively. They present as a severe illness with fever and rash only; no ulcers or eschars are identified. Q fever, caused by *C. burnetii,* presents only with flulike illness and no skin lesions.

7. d. Necrotizing faciitis due to group A streptococci starts with a painful induration of the underlying soft tissue and develops rapidly into an eschar and necrotic mass leading to sepsis. Cellulitis is a deep local invasion without necrosis.

8. b. Phrynoderma (hypovitaminosis A) is deficiency disease that involves the integument and usually begins as hyperkeratotic follicular eruptions on the anterolateral thighs or posterolateral arms, moving centrally to include the thorax, neck, and face. Diminution of dark adaptation is a tell-tale sign of vitamin A deficiency. Comedos are usually found on the face in association with normally functioning glandular tissue. Pellagra is a niacin deficiency characterized by scaly skin sores that initially are red and pruritic and have a burning sensation.

9. a. Tinea capitis (scalp ringworm) is a fungal skin infection chiefly occurring in young schoolboys more than in girls. Most are noninflammatory, producing scaly lesions or "gray patching." Tinea corporus is ringworm of the body. Alopecia is a genetically determined disorder usually affecting man in their fourth and fifth decades.

10. b. Pemphigus is a chronic autoimmune blistering disease of the skin and mucous membranes seen in older patients and characterized by intradermal blistering. The buccal mucosa is usually the first site of involvement. Senear-Usher syndrome is an overlap syndrome with features of lupus erythematosus. Dermatitis herpetiformis represents extremely itchy grouped vesicles most frequently located on extensor surfaces and associated with gluten sensitivity. Erythema multiforme lesions are generalized target lesions that are burning and pruritic.

11. b. Vitiligo (leukoderma) is an autoimmunity-induced destruction of melanocytes resulting in blotching of the skin. Tanning enhances the contrast between normal skin and affected skin. It has been implicated in people with autoimmune disorders or adrenal insufficiency. Leprosy is a destructive chronic bacterial infection of skin and nervous system. Tinea versicolor is an asymptomatic dermatosis characterized by hypopigmented or hyperpigmented scaly macules on the trunk. Piebaldism is a rare autosomal dominant disorder of melanocyte development characterized by congenital white forelock and multiple symmetrical hypopigmented or depigmented macules.

12. c. Onychomycosis (tinea unguium) is a chronic fungal infection that affects the toenails and fingernails and can involve any component of the nail unit, including the nail matrix, the nail bed, or the nail plate. Tinea corporus (ringworm) affects the body, and tinea manuum affects the hand.

13. c. Molluscum contagiosum is a self-limiting viral disease due to the pox virus and is frequently seen in kids, sexually active adults, and the immunocompromised. There is a central keratotic plug (umbilication) and it resolves spontaneously. Verrucae vulgaris are due to human papilloma virus and have no umbilication. Keratocanthoma is found on the face typically.

14. d. Contact dermatitis can be due to a chemical irritant or allergen causing a type IV hypersensitivity reaction. The most likely cause in this case would be poison ivy resin, which tends to be pruritic, localized, and linear in distribution correlating with contact to exposed skin. Impetigo is a bacterial infection of the epidermis seen around the nose and lips characterized by weeping vesicles that crust. Erythema infectiosum (fifth disease) is primarily a childhood viral disease characterized by a "slapped-check" appearance. Atopic dermatitis is an autosomal dominant inflammatory reaction involving the hands, wrists, neck, feet, and face usually associated with a family history of asthma.

CHAPTER 75

Sexually Transmitted Diseases

Antonio E. Bifero

1. A 25-year-old enlisted man presents with a painless sore on his penis that progressed over a period of 3 weeks. He has a past history of drug abuse and prior sexually transmitted disease. On inspection you noticed a 2-cm ulcer on the shaft of the penis. The margins are raised with some induration. The right inguinal lymph node is palpable. His temperature is 37°C, and pulse, blood pressure, and respirations are all normal. What is the diagnosis?
    a. chancroid
    b. genital herpes
    c. primary syphilis
    d. none of the above

2. What is the MOST likely cause of primary syphilis?
    a. *Treponema pallidum*
    b. herpes simplex virus type II
    c. *Haemophilus ducreyi*
    d. none of the above

3. A 25-year-old homosexual man presents to a free clinic with abrupt onset of dysuria and purulent meatal discharge of 2 days' duration. He admits to having three new partners in the past 8 days. Examination reveals adnexal tenderness bilaterally and right lateral knee pain on palpation. The urethra is stripped, and a gram stain of the material was positive. Based on the information provided, what is the diagnosis?
    a. Reiter's syndrome
    b. Steven-Johnson syndrome
    c. nongonococcal urethritis
    d. gonococcal urethritis

4. A 27-year-old man presents with a complaint of red, raised, soft growths on the shaft and prepuce of the penis. A biopsy was taken to look for potential malignancy. Choose the most likely diagnosis.
   a. condylomata lata
   b. genital herpes
   c. condyloma acuminatum
   d. Peyronie's disease

5. A 27-year-old Caucasian woman presents to the emergency department with a 3-day history of fever, chills, severe headache, stiff neck, and myalgia. Two days prior to this, she noticed genital lesions that were very painful. Loud noises and bright lights disturb her. She admits to having had a sexual relationship with a new boyfriend. No prior history of sexually transmitted diseases is noted. What is the MOST likely diagnosis?
   a. primary syphilis
   b. secondary syphilis
   c. first episode of HSV2 genital herpes
   d. bacterial meningitis caused by *Neisseria gonorrhoeae*

6. What ulcerative genital infections are MOST often associated with lymphadenopathy and therefore NOT likely a cause of the patient's symptoms in the preceding question?
   a. chancroid
   b. granuloma inguinale
   c. lymphogranuloma venereum
   d. a, b, and c

7. A 21-year-old woman presents to the clinic with a foul-smelling yellow vaginal discharge of 5 days' duration and lower quadrant pain. She has reported having casual sex with two partners in the past month. A bimanual pelvic exam revealed adnexal tenderness on the left. What is the diagnosis?
   a. gonococcal urethritis
   b. pelvic inflammatory disease
   c. bacterial vaginosis
   d. vulvovaginitis

8. A 34-year-old African American man presents with unilateral inguinal
    pain of 6 days' duration. He admits that 10 days earlier he noticed
    a small herpetiform ulcer on the prepuce. He has had one new sexual
    partner. On examination, the right inguinal nodes are firm and slightly
    painful, and you observe a positive grove sign. He has some
    constitutional signs and symptoms. What is the diagnosis?
    a. genital herpes
    b. incarcerated inguinal hernia
    c. lymphogranuloma venereum
    d. granuloma inguinale

9. A 40-year-old homosexual man presents to the clinic with a 1-year
    history of nights sweats and flulike symptoms. He lost over 25 pounds
    in the past 5 months. On examination, he is pale and thin with a
    temperature of 38.5°C. He has extensive psoriasis and generalized
    lymphadenopathy. A chest film shows pulmonary infiltrates in the left
    lower lobe. What is the diagnosis?
    a. HIV syndrome
    b. chronic fatigue syndrome
    c. hepatitis A infection
    d. fever of unknown origin

1.　c.　Primary syphilis has an incubation of 3 weeks and presents with a mildly tender papule that ulcerates over a few weeks. Genital herpes is a viral infection that has an incubation period of no more than 1 week. The lesions are markedly painful and can sometimes ulcerate. It is usually accompanied by that includes fever, malaise, and headaches. Chancroid presents with a painful ulcer after a short incubation period of 3 to 5 days.

2.　a.　*Treponema pallidum* is a fragile spirochete that causes syphilis. Pathogenic isoforms have never been cultured continuously on artificial media in vitro. HSV2 is a virus that causes location eruptions in genital herpes. *Haemophilus ducreyi* is a gram-negative bacillus that causes chancroid.

3.　d.　Mucopurulent discharge, dysuria, rapid onset, inguinal tenderness, and positive gram stain are diagnostic of gonococcal infection (NGU). NGU follows a gradual onset characterized by a viscid clear discharge in only 35% of cases. Steven-Johnson syndrome is a serious systemic disorder with vesicobullous lesions involving the skin and mucous membranes. Reiter's syndrome includes NGU, uveitis, arthritis, and skin lesions.

4.　c.　Condyloma acuminatum, also known as venereal warts, are usually described as being red or flesh-colored growths caused by the human papilloma virus through sexual contact. Genital herpes presents with painful vesicles on an erythematous base. Condyloma lata is a sequela of secondary syphilis and are described as being flat, pale warty erosions that develop in warm, moist areas such as the perineum and genital areas. Peyronie's disease is a unilateral bending of the penis caused by fibrotic scaring that forms on the tunica of the corpus cavernosum.

5.　c.　Primary syphilis does not usually have constitutional symptoms, and many people do not know they have been infected. Secondary syphilis presents with a disseminated rash. *Neisseria gonorrhoeae* does not cause meningitis.

6.　d.　Chancroid is caused by *H. ducreyi*; lymphogranuloma venereum is most commonly caused by *C. trachomatis*. Granuloma inguinale caused by *Calymmatobacterium granulomatis* produces a hard, indurated granulomatous lesion. All are associated with inguinal lymph node invasion.

7. b. Yellow purulent cervical discharge, lower abdominal pain elicited by movement of the cervix, or palpation of adnexal areas is characteristic of pelvic inflammatory disease. Approximately 50% of cases are caused by *N. gonorrhoeae*. Vaginitis and bacterial vaginosis are characterized by a foul-smelling vaginal discharge without adnexal tenderness or abdominal complaints.

8. c. Lymphogranuloma venereum is caused by *Chlamydia trachomatis* and presents in three stages. The transient primary lesion could be a papule, a shallow ulcer or erosion, or a small herpetiform lesion (usually found in the coronal sulcus, prepuce, or glans) and is easily missed. The secondary stage involves unilateral inguinal lymphadenitis as opposed to granuloma inguinale.

9. a. History of fulminant spiking fevers, weight loss, and generalized lymphadenopathy in individuals with opportunistic infections are characteristic of HIV syndrome. Chronic fatigue syndrome is associated with extreme debilitating fatigue that worsens of over months and may include myalgias, lymphadenopathy, and brain fog. Hepatitis A is an acute infection with flulike illness and jaundice. Fever of unknown origin is defined as a temperature of greater than 101°F for at least 3 weeks that remains undiagnosed after 1 week of investigation.

Toxicology

Jesse Thomas Coats

1. Constriction of the pupils (miosis) may be due to exposure to which one of the following agents?
   a. organophosphates
   b. lysergic acid diethylamide (LSD)
   c. cocaine
   d. amphetamines

2. Respiration rate and depth may be depressed by exposure to which one of the following toxic compounds?
   a. cyanide
   b. carbon monoxide
   c. alcohol
   d. strychnine

3. Which one of the following antidotes may be used for ingestion of toxic levels of warfarin?
   a. atropine
   b. dimercaprol
   c. Fab' fragments
   d. phytonadione

4. "Sudden sniffers death syndrome" is used to describe the preferred route of administration of which of the following toxic agents?
   a. organophosphates
   b. ammoniates
   c. glycols
   d. halogenated hydrocarbons

5. Which one of the following naturally occurring methylxanthines is responsible for most fatalities in this class of compounds due to poisoning?
    a. caffeine
    b. theophylline
    c. theobromine
    d. guarna

6. Convulsions caused by drug poisoning are most commonly associated with:
    a. phenobarbital
    b. diazepam
    c. strychnine
    d. chlorpromazine

7. Alkalinization of the urine with sodium bicarbonate is useful in the treatment of poisoning with:
    a. aspirin
    b. amphetamine
    c. morphine
    d. phencyclidine

8. Which one of the following statements is FALSE about arsenic poisoning?
    a. acute poisoning causes severe diarrhea and difficulty swallowing
    b. signs of chronic poisoning include peripheral neuritis, hypotension, and anemia
    c. death following acute intoxication may be due to hypovolemic shock
    d. gingivitis, stomatitis, and salivation can occur

9. Which of the following is an agent useful in the treatment of severe poisoning by organophosphate insecticides, such as parathion?
    a. ethylenediaminetetraacetic acid (EDTA)
    b. pralidoxime (2-PAM)
    c. N-acetylcysteine
    d. diethyldithiocarbamic acid

10. Use of activated charcoal may be contraindicated in treatment of poisoning by which one of the following drugs?
    a. phenobarbital
    b. carbamazepine (Tegretol)
    c. proxyphene (Darvon)
    d. methanol

11. Regarding methanol intoxication, which one of the following statements is INCONSISTENT with the toxic state?
   a. blurred vision and hyperemia of the optic disc may develop
   b. it may produce bradycardia, coma, and seizures
   c. treatment includes administration of ethanol
   d. ascorbic acid corrects the metabolic alkalosis

Answers

1. a. Organophosphates cause cholinergic toxic effects, whereas all of the other choices produce adrenergic toxic effects.

2. a. Alcohol causes respiratory depression, whereas all of the other choices stimulate respiration.

3. d. Warfarin ties up vitamin K, making vitamin K replenishment a prudent health care measure.

4. d. Halogenated hydrocarbons such as freon and various aerosol propellants are the choice for inhaled intoxicants.

5. b. There are about 100 deaths reported a year from toxicity by theophylline, whereas the numbers of deaths from caffeine, theobromine, and guarna deaths are negligible.

6. c. Strychnine is known to cause convulsions, whereas all of the other choices are often used as anticonvulsants.

7. a. Aspirin intoxication is treated by alkalinization of the urine to increase urinary excretion of aspirin and its metabolites. Acidification of the urine is the treatment of choice for toxicity from the remaining choices.

8. d. These signs and symptoms are commonly associated with acute mercury poisoning, not arsenic.

9. b. 2-PAM is the agent of choice for treatment of organophosphate poisoning. The reader should be aware of classic antidote/toxin pairs such as use of *N*-acetylcysteine to counteract poisoning with acetaminophen.

10. d. Methanol or wood alcohol is not absorbed by activated charcoal, because neither has an attraction for each other.

11. d. Methanol causes metabolic acidosis, not alkalosis; thus ascorbic acid is not useful to reverse acidosis.

Pediatrics

Jesse Thomas Coats

1. Which one of the following childhood conditions has clinical features of nondescriptive maculopapular rash of short duration of 2 to 3 days, 14- to 20-day incubation period, fever, malaise, and cervical and occipital lymphadenopathy?
   a. polio
   b. mumps
   c. rubella
   d. measles

2. Which one of the following conditions most commonly demonstrates café-au-lait spots on lower lumbar region, buttocks, and chest?
   a. diaper dermatitis
   b. spina bifida occulta
   c. neurofibromatosis
   d. pyronephritis

3. Which one of the following is used to assess for any presence of a spinal cord lesion?
   a. rooting
   b. sucking
   c. Moro response
   d. Galant's test

4. When triaging for child abuse, which of the following pairs correctly corresponds with dating bruises?
   a. 1 to 2 days—red or blue
   b. 2 to 4 weeks—yellow
   c. 5 to 7 days—green
   d. 10 to 14 days—red and swollen

5. Which one of the following tests is an excellent test of upper extremity pyramidal function?
    a. asymmetrical tonic neck reflex
    b. Landau maneuver
    c. parachute reflex
    d. palmar grasp

6. Which one of the following conditions is occasionally observed with Klippel-Feil syndrome?
    a. Sprengel's deformity
    b. Klumpke's deformity
    c. Erb's deformity
    d. radial head dislocation

7. Which one of the following infant neurologic reflex tests is BEST for assessment of central nervous system function?
    a. acoustic blink
    b. sucking
    c. Moro response
    d. Galant's test

8. Which one of the following statements about Reye's syndrome is FALSE?
    a. it is an encephalopathy with fatty degeneration of the viscera
    b. it is suspected when an upper respiratory tract infection is followed by excessive vomiting and convulsions
    c. it is usually complicated by liver dysfunction and hypoglycemia
    d. children should be given aspirin during an influenza infection

9. Which one of the following is considered to be the MOST critical neonatal neurologic test to perform?
    a. rooting
    b. sucking
    c. Moro response
    d. Galant's test

10. Os odontoideum is most commonly associated with which one of the following conditions?
    a. Hodgkin's lymphoma
    b. Klippel-Feil syndrome
    c. Down syndrome
    d. Turner's syndrome

11. Which one of the following physical assessments of a child is INCORRECT?
    a. oral thrush is most commonly caused by streptococcal infection
    b. more than 90% of cases of sore throat and fever in children are due to vial infection
    c. average heart rate can be as high as 140 at birth
    d. average respiratory rate can be 30 to 75 in newborns

12. Which one of the following time periods corresponds best with closure of the skull landmark known as the bregma, or the "baby's soft spot"?
    a. 6 to 12 months
    b. 12 to 18 months
    c. 18 to 24 months
    d. 24 to 36 months

13. Which one of the following tests might support the diagnosis of cerebral palsy?
    a. asymmetrical tonic neck reflex
    b. Landau maneuver
    c. parachute reflex
    d. palmar grasp

14. Which one of the following tests may be performed to identify a hemiparesis or brachial plexus injury?
    a. rooting
    b. sucking
    c. Moro response
    d. Galant's test

15. Which one of the following is a common finding for both slipped capital femoral epiphysis and Legg-Calve-Perthés disease?
    a. complication includes avascular necrosis and ankylosis
    b. more common in boys and who are short
    c. may complain of pain in the groin or knee
    d. the child should be weight bearing

16. Which one of the following bones is the first bone to calcify in utero and is also the most common bone to be fractured during the birth process?
    a. clavicle
    b. patella
    c. rib
    d. skull

17. Which one of the following conditions is LEAST likely to be associated with activity-related injuries?
    a. Osgood-Schlatter disease
    b. nursemaid's elbow
    c. slipped capital femoral epiphysis
    d. spondylolysis

18. Which one of the following statements concerning neonatal findings is INCORRECT?
    a. inconsolable crying is one of the pathognomonic signs of colic
    b. generalized or central cyanosis including the tongue and lips may be associated with congenital heart disease or lung disease
    c. Apgar score of 7 to 10 is normal at 1 minute of birth
    d. Mongolian spots should be referred to perform a biopsy

19. Which one of the following statements about asthma in children is INCORRECT?
    a. asthma is the most common chronic lung disorder in children
    b. cold, dry air is often the stimulus for exercise-induced asthma
    c. children with allergic asthma will often suffer from eczema as well
    d. chiropractic techniques do not work on "wet" asthma but are quite effective on "dry" asthma

Answers

1. c. This is a classic natural history for rubella. None of the other diseases or conditions are close to matching this presentation. The reader should, however, become familiar with the other conditions for they make good testing material in similar format.

2. c. Be careful not to get used to matching buzzwords. None of the others match.

3. d. Galant's test is for spinal lesion detection, whereas the other choices are more often used to detect central or brainstem lesions.

4. c. The natural progression for contusions/bruises is as follows: 1 to 2 days, red and swollen; 2 to 4 days, red or black to blue; 5 to 7 days, green; 10 to 14 days, yellow.

5. c. Parachute test is used to test pyramidal function, whereas the remaining choices more often are used to test extrapyramidal function.

6. a. Sprengel's deformity is commonly associated with Klippel-Feil syndrome.

7. a. Of the available answers, acoustic blink is best for assessment of central nervous system function.

8. d. Children under 13 years of age should not be given aspirin for this is the most well known mechanism by which Reye's syndrome develops.

9. c. The Moro response occurs when there is a quick change in the infant's position. This will cause the infant to throw the arms outward, open the hands, and throw back the head. The other reflexes/tests are less important. It is a critical neonatal neurologic test especially adapted to identify hemiparesis or brachial plexus injury.

10. c. Os odontoideum is associated with Down syndrome and represents a congenital disorder of the dens of C2.

11. a. Oral thrush is caused most commonly by the *Candida* organism with some variation in the species.

12.   b.   The anterior fontanel known as bregma, or the "baby's soft spot," closes or ossifies at about 12 to 18 months old.

13.   d.   Palmar grasp test is a fast, efficient, and classic test for cerebral palsy.

14.   c.   Moro response is a critical neonatal neurologic test especially adapted to identify hemiparesis or brachial plexus injury.

15.   c.   Hip pathology may also refer pain to the knee.

16.   a.   The clavicle is the first bone to ossify in utero.

17.   c.   This injury can be very insidious and often one cannot identify an injury that precipitated it.

18.   d.   Mongolian spots are benign and should never necessitate biopsy.

19.   d.   Recent past has generated more research referencing the positive clinical outcomes regarding treatment and management of asthma with chiropractic manual manipulation, regardless of the etiology.

Emergency Procedures

Bart N. Green

1. You see chest movement in an unconscious patient after opening the airway. Next you should:
   a. listen and feel for air exchange
   b. assume the patient is breathing
   c. perform chest compressions
   d. none of the above

2. The most important step to take upon involvement in an emergency is to:
   a. let the patient know that you have arrived
   b. assess the scene and environment
   c. make sure that you have plenty of gloves
   d. immediately care for the patient

3. Small bubbles of air trapped under the skin of the neck and chest region and usually caused by pneumothorax are called:
   a. pneumothorax
   b. myocardial infarction
   c. le petit bubels
   d. subcutaneous emphysema

4. The rate of compression for adult CPR is:
   a. 120 per minute
   b. 100 per minute
   c. 80 per minute
   d. 90 per minute

5. When performing rescue breathing on adults, give _____ ventilations every __ seconds.
   a. 2 and 10
   b. 1 and 5
   c. 1 and 3
   d. 1 and 2

6. While performing CPR, the patient begins to vomit. You should:
   a. roll the patient on his side and clean out his mouth
   b. continue doing CPR
   c. stop performing CPR and wait for the paramedics
   d. roll the patient on his side, clean out his mouth, and reassess airway, breathing, and circulation

7. What is the BEST method for controlling bleeding and should be attempted first?
   a. elevation
   b. direct pressure
   c. trauma dressing
   d. tourniquet

8. You have applied a pressure dressing and bandage to a hemorrhage and the dressing becomes blood soaked. What should you do next?
   a. apply a tourniquet above the injury site
   b. remove the dressing and apply a new, clean one
   c. apply additional dressings on top of it and hold firmly in place
   d. apply an ice pack to the site

9. When caring for a fractured, dislocated, or sprained extremity, when is it important to check for pulses, sensation, and motor function?
   a. after the splint has been removed at the hospital
   b. before applying a splint
   c. before and after applying a splint
   d. during the detailed physical exam of the patient, usually en route to the hospital

10. What type of splint is used for a clavicle or scapula fracture?
    a. air splint
    b. fixation splint
    c. sling and swathe
    d. traction splint

11. The most frequent poisoning occurs in what age group?
    a. children
    b. parents
    c. senior citizens
    d. teenagers

12. A child ingests an unknown amount of aspirin. If the child is conscious, the poison control center is likely to tell you to do which of the following?
    a. induce vomiting
    b. have him drink milk
    c. have him drink soda pop
    d. administer activated charcoal

13. While working in the biochemistry lab, someone spills dry acid on his arm. You should:
    a. flush the arm with a base solution
    b. pour water on his arm
    c. brush off the dry acid, then wash the arm with water
    d. brush off the dry acid and wrap the arm in gauze; transport to the emergency department

14. What is the FIRST thing that you should do when caring for a burn patient?
    a. remove the patient from the source of burn
    b. cool the patient with sterile water
    c. place dry dressings over the burn
    d. call the local burn center

15. Which of the following is the MOST likely serious complication of electrical shock injury?
    a. hypoperfusion
    b. cardiac arrest
    c. full-thickness burn at the exit point
    d. stroke

Answers

1. a. After positioning the airway for an unconscious victim, the rescuer should place his or her cheek near the victim's mouth and listen for breathing and feel for breaths against his or her cheek to indicate that the patient is voluntarily able to move air in and out of the lungs.

2. b. It is imperative for a rescuer to ensure that the scene is safe to enter prior to providing emergency rescue. This ensures that the rescuer does not become an additional victim.

3. d. When a patient has a punctured lung, resulting in pneumothorax or hemopnumothorax, air can leak into the subcutaneous tissues, thus creating subcutaneous emphysema. This may be detectable by the rescuer pinching a small amount of the patient's skin, located inferior to the clavicle, and rolling it between the fingers. It will feel like the crunching of small air bubbles or Rice Crispies.

4. b. According to the 2000 American Heart Association CPR guidelines, CPR compression is standardized as 100 compressions per minute for all ages of victims.

5. b. Artificial respiration, also known as rescue breathing, is delivered at a rate of 1 breath every 5 seconds.

6. d. When a patient vomits during CPR, it may a sign of successful resuscitation or from gastric reflexes. To ensure that the patient's airway is clear and to prevent aspiration pneumonia, it is important to clear the airway and then reassess the patient's vital functions of breathing and circulation before continuing with any further rescue care. Reassessing vital functions makes no assumption about the patient's cardiovascular status.

7. b. Direct pressure is the first line of defense for external hemorrhage. If it is unsuccessful, then elevation and pressure applied to pulse pressure points are added sequentially. Tourniquets are used as a last resort.

8. c. When a bandage becomes soaked, additional dressings should be placed over the soaked one. Removing a bandage may result in further bleeding by tearing away the clot.

9. c. Pulse, sensation, and motor function are assessed before splinting to assess the integrity of extremity neurovascular function. They are checked again after splinting to ensure that the splint is not applied too tightly.

10. c. A sling and swathe is used for proximal upper extremity musculoskeletal injuries to secure the injured limb. There is no other splint available for clavicle and shoulder injuries.

11. a. Unfortunately, children are the most common casualties resulting from poisoning. Children are more likely to ingest toxic substances due to their inability to read labels and because poisons are often not kept in protected areas around the home.

12. d. Activated charcoal is a substance used to counteract the toxicity of certain toxins. It helps prevent the poison from being absorbed from the stomach into the body.

13. c. Dry acid may become more corrosive if immediately mixed with water. Therefore, the best approach to emergency care is to brush the dry acid off of the skin with a dry brush, cloth, or gauze and then flush the area with copious amounts of water.

14. a. To avoid more potential burns from explosives or corrosive material, the patient should be moved to a safe area before burn care is rendered.

15. b. Electrical shock may interfere with the electrical conductivity of the nerve fibers in and around the heart. Therefore, cardiac arrest is a likely complication.

CHAPTER 79

Jurisprudence, Ethics, and Basic Economics

Bart N. Green

1. Which law covers you for malpractice suits if you are providing care in good faith to a victim at the scene of an auto accident and you have no preexisting obligation to care for this person?
   a. Pratt and Whitney law
   b. Hawthorne law
   c. health care compliance law
   d. Good Samaritan law

2. You happen across a person on the sidewalk who appears to be unconscious and bleeding. You immediately begin to care for the patient. You acted with:
   a. implied consent
   b. expressed consent
   c. informed consent
   d. minor consent

3. A branch of philosophy investigating how human actions can be judged as right or wrong is called:
   a. epistemology
   b. epidemiology
   c. ethics
   d. deontology

4. In 1993, the Health Insurance Portability and Accountability Act (HIPAA) was enacted for what purpose?
   a. to protect clinicians from lawsuits arising out of malpractice
   b. to protect patients' privacy pertaining to personal and private medical information
   c. to protect researchers from sanctions by funding agencies
   d. to protect insurance companies from lawsuits when moving health records

5. Which of the following describes the principle of beneficence?
    a. an individual's ability to make the distinction between right or wrong conduct
    b. an act of creating a positive balance in a practice yearly budget
    c. an act of kindness that results in a positive outcome or removal of harm
    d. acting in the patient's best interest without first retaining patient consent

6. "Professional misconduct, improper discharge of professional duties, or failure to meet the standards of care of a professional resulting in harm to another" defines:
    a. consent
    b. malpractice
    c. nonmaleficence
    d. battery

7. Which of the following represents ACCEPTABLE professional behavior for a chiropractor?
    a. providing care to a dentist in exchange for dental work
    b. dating a new and attractive patient while he or she is still under the chiropractor's care
    c. owning a diagnostic imaging service and referring patients from one's clinical practice to the imaging service
    d. conducting a research study on patients without the patients knowing about it

Answers

1. d. Good Samaritan laws were enacted in the 1960s to protect health care providers from malpractice lawsuits when they provide care to patients in emergency situations. Providers should have no preexisting obligation to provide that care and should provide it in good faith and for no remuneration.

2. a. Implied consent is obtained when the victim cannot provide expressed or informed consent, such as in the case of an unconscious victim needing emergency care.

3. c. Ethics involves the study of human decisions and behavior surrounding the issues of right and wrong. Ethics are based upon various societal norms.

4. b. HIPAA is federal legislation that protects personal health record information when it is transferred between health care providers and between health care providers and third party payers. Patients have the right to view all disclosures of their information to various parties and to restrict the dissemination of this information.

5. c. Beneficence is an ethical principle pertaining to doing what is good, kind, helpful, or generous. Choice "a" describes personal morals and ethics. Choice "b" is a distracter. Choice "d" represents the process of implied consent (if the patient is unable to give informed consent).

6. b. The question is one definition of malpractice. Choice c means that one does no harm to others, and choice d is the unlawful and unwanted touching or striking of one person by another, with the intention of bringing about a harmful or offensive contact.

7. a. It is acceptable for a doctor to render services for no financial payment but to swap services. This is an act known as bartering and is probably the oldest form of payment known to man. However, in our modern society, it is expected that such bartering is appropriately accounted for in personal financial records.

Section Twelve Recommended Reading

Abrams W, Beers M, Berkow R, eds: *The Merck manual of geriatrics,* ed 3, Whitehouse Station, NJ, 2000, Merck Research Laboratories.

American Academy of Orthopaedic Surgeons: *Emergency care and transportation for the sick and injured,* ed 9, Sudbury, Mass, 2005, Jones and Bartlett.

American National Red Cross: *First aid: responding to emergencies,* ed 3, St Louis, 2001, Mosby.

Beers M, Berkow R, *The Merck manual of diagnosis and therapy,* ed 17, Whitehouse Station, NJ, 2004, Merck Research Laboratories.

Bougie J, Morgenthal P: *The aging body: conservative management of common neuromusculoskeletal conditions,* New York, 2001, McGraw-Hill.

Campbell L, Ladenheim C, Sherman R, Sportelli L: *Risk management in chiropractic,* Fincastle, Va, 1990, Health Services Publications.

DeCherney A, Nathan L, eds: *Current obstetric & gynecologic diagnosis & treatment,* ed 10, Norwalk, Conn, 2006, Appleton & Lange.

Goldman H: *Review of general psychiatry,* ed 5, Norwalk, Conn, 2000, Appleton & Lange.

Habif T: *Clinical dermatology: A color guide to diagnosis and therapy,* ed 4, St Louis, 2004, Mosby.

Hay W, Levin M, Sondheimer J, Deterding R: *Current pediatric diagnosis & treatment,* ed 17, Stamford, Conn, 2005, Appleton & Lange.

Hazzard W, Blass J, Halter J, Ouslander J, Tinetti M: *Principles of geriatric medicine and gerontology,* ed 5, New York, 2003, McGraw-Hill.

Olson K: *Poisoning & drug overdose,* ed 4, East Norwalk, Conn, 2004, Appleton & Lange.

Redwood D, Cleveland C: *Fundamentals of chiropractic,* St Louis, 2003, Mosby.

Scott R: *Legal aspects of documenting patient care for rehabilitation professionals,* ed 3, Gaithersburg, Md, 2006, Aspen Publishers.

Task Force on DSM-IV: *Diagnostic and statistical manual of mental disorders DSM-IV-TR,* ed 4, Washington, DC, 2000, American Psychiatric Press.

US Department of Health and Human Services: *Healthy people 2010,* Washington, DC, 2000, Department of Health and Human Services.

US Department of Health and Human Services: *Clinician's handbook of preventive services,* ed 2, Washington, DC, 1998, US Government Printing Office.

Index

Discogenic pain, 424, 436

Discrete enlarged lymph nodes, 367, 377

Discs. *See* Intervertebral discs

Disease simulation model, 510, 518

Diseases. *See also Specific disease*
   animals and, 302, 304
   calcium ions and, 474, 481
   communicable, 301, 304
   elderly and, 602, 605
   endemic, 302, 303, 304, 305
   handwashing and, 303, 305
   kidneys and, 380, 383, 479
   liver and, 367, 377
   osteoclasts and, 244, 248
   prevalence rates of, 302, 305
   spinal cord and, 470, 479, 583, 589
   vertical transmission and, 301, 304

Distal convoluted tubules, 46, 48, 147, 149

Distal ileum, 153

Distal tubules, 146, 148

Diuretics, 147, 149

Diversified adjustments
   components of, 569, 575
   description of, 535, 542
   rotation and, 570, 576

Dix-Hallpike test, 580, 588

DNA
   prokaryotic cells and, 277, 280
   radiography and, 453, 457
   thymine and, 201, 204
   uracil and, 202, 205

DNA polymerase, 202, 204

Docosahexenoic acid (DHA), 178, 182

Dopamine, 187, 190

Dorsal columns, 527, 533

Dorsal respiratory group, 141, 143

Dorsolateral tract of Lissauer, 85, 89

Double emulsion film, 452, 456

Down syndrome, 636, 639

Drug toxicity, 602, 606

DSM-VI, 610, 611, 614

Dual innervation, 98, 102

Dual-energy x-ray absorptiometry (DEXA), 581, 588

Duchenne muscular dystrophy, 241, 246

Ductus arteriosus, 30, 33

Duodenum, 35, 36, 38

Dura mater, 74, 79

Dysafferentiation, 540, 546

Dysmenorrhea, 597, 599

Dysplasia, 224, 226

Dysplastic spondylolysis, 476, 483

Dysthymic disorders, 609, 613

Dystrophin, 241, 246

Dystrophy, 472, 480

E

Ears, temperature measurement and, 335, 337

Eaton agent, 258, 267

Eaton-Lambert syndrome, 361, 373

Edema, 263, 271, 597, 599

Edema in kwashiorkor, 189, 191

Eicosanoids, 180, 185

Eicosapentanoic acid (EPA), 178, 182

Elastic recoil, 141, 143

Elbows, 19, 22, 26

Elderly
   dementia in, 251, 254
   diet recommendations for, 603, 606
   forms of abuse of, 237, 239
   heart disease and, 602, 605
   musculoskeletal changes and, 603, 607
   poverty and, 602, 606
   urinary tract infections in, 264, 272

Electrical shock injury, 643, 645

Electromagnetic radiation, 450, 454

Electromyograms, 125, 128

Electron acceleration, 452, 456

Electron transport systems, 216, 217

Elevated Arm Stress Test, 588

Embryonic midgut, 35, 38

EMG studies, 379, 382

Emphysema
   alpha-1 antitrypsin and, 260, 269
   examination findings of, 368, 378
   lung bullae and, 356, 370
   presentation of, 343, 345

Encephalitis, 290, 299

Encephalopathy, 252, 255

Endemic diseases, 302, 303, 304, 305

End-feel, 557, 558, 562, 563

Endocarditis, 258, 267, 292, 300

Endochondral ossification, 13, 15

Endocrine secretions, 50, 51

Endometrial carcinomas, 597, 599

Endometrial hyperplasia, 259, 268, 597, 599

Endometriosis, 596, 598, 599

Endotoxins, 277, 280

End-play, 557, 562

Energy, 181, 185

Energy procedures, 568, 575

Enteric disease, 286, 295

Enterocytes, 152, 154

Enterohemorrhagic *E. coli*, 287, 296

Entheses, 462, 466

Enthesopathy, 466

Environmental Protection Agency, 310

Enzymes, 213, 216, 217

Epicondylar fractures, 427, 440

Epicondylitis, 242, 246

Epidemiology, 301, 302, 304, 305

Epidermis, 5, 8

Epilepsy, 325, 328

Epinephrine, 101, 160, 161, 197, 199

Epiphyseal cartilage, 13, 15

Epiphyseal discs, 11, 14

Epithelial cells, 45, 47

Erb-Duchenne paralysis, 100, 415, 420

Erector spinae muscle group, 60, 66, 69

Erythema infectiosum, 287, 296, 624

Erythema multiforme, 617, 621

Erythropoietin, 159, 161, 259, 268

Escherichia coli, 283, 287, 293, 296

Esophageal bleeding, 379, 382

Esophageal dysmotility, 235

Esophagus, 326, 328

Estrogen, 259, 268, 597, 599

Ethics, 647, 649

Ethmoid bone, 57, 62

Ethnic minorities, 601, 602, 605, 606

Eversion, 415, 421

Ewing's sarcoma, 243, 248

EX adjustments, 566, 573

Excitable membranes, 113, 118

Excitation-contraction coupling, 126, 129

Exocytosis, 113, 118, 154

Exostosis, 544

Expiration, 141, 143

Extension, 512, 520

Extension malposition, 553, 560

Extensor hallicus longus, 404, 408

Extrafusal fibers, 124, 127

F

Facet arthrosis, 475, 482

Facet jamming, 538, 544

Facet joints
   classification of, 76, 81
   foramen and, 55, 60
   injuries to, 432, 443
   innervation of, 74, 78

Facet syndrome, 507, 515
   Kemp's test and, 557, 562
   management of, 582, 589
   symptoms of, 513, 521, 552, 559

Facilitated lesions, 511, 519

Facilitated segmens, 538, 544

Facilitation, 510, 517

Facilitative lesions, 508, 516

FAD, 202, 204

Fajersztajn's sign, 401, 406

Falciform ligaments, 31, 33

Falls, 603, 607

Familial hypercholesterolemia, 229, 231

Family histories, 327, 329

Fascial plane lines, 461, 465

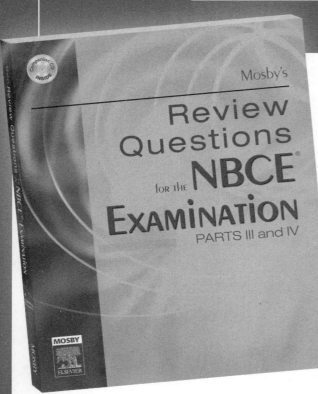
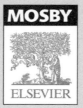